an integrative approach to language disorders in children

an integrative approach to language disorders in children

Elizabeth Carrow-Woolfolk, Ph.D.

Consultant in Language/Learning Disorders
Houston, Texas

Joan I. Lynch, Ed.D.

Associate Professor of Language Science
The University of Texas
Health Science Center
Houston, Texas

Grune & Stratton
A Subsidiary of Harcourt Brace Jovanovich, Publishers
New York   London
Paris   San Diego   San Francisco   São Paulo
Sydney   Tokyo   Toronto

Library of Congress Cataloging in Publication Data

Carrow-Woolfolk, Elizabeth.
  Integrative approach to language disorders in children.

  Bibliography: p. 451
  Includes index.
  1. Language disorders in children.   2. Children—
Language.   I. Lynch, Joan.   II. Title.
RJ496.L35C37   618.92'855   81-7180
ISBN 0-8089-1406-5   AACR2

  Grune & Stratton, Inc.
  111 Fifth Avenue
  New York, New York 10003

  Distributed in the United Kingdom by
  Academic Press Inc. (London) Ltd.
  24/28 Oval Road, London NW 1

Library of Congress Catalog Number 81-7180
International Standard Book Number 0-8089-1406-5

Printed in the United States of America

to our families:
Bob and Robin,
and John and Carrie

also to Pat,
and to the other children
who have taught us about
language disorders

contents

preface

This book is about language disorders. We wrote it for individuals who are concerned with children who have such disorders, professionals whose responsibility it is to assist language-disordered children in the school or clinic, and students whose responsibility it is to learn about these children. Although our focus is on the practical aspects of language disorders, we believe that practice must be strongly undergirded by theory and research, and thus we have attempted to present a balance of all three.

The book is both integrative and multidimensional. As is suggested by the title, the primary purpose of the text is to present an integrative approach to language, its acquisition, and its disorders in children. Consequently we have integrated material on four levels. Theory is integrated with research and clinical observation, because we believe that this combination provides the best understanding of language disorders. At a second level of integration, we relate viewpoints from the fields of psychology, linguistics, and speech pathology to demonstrate how positions from different disciplines are compatible with and even necessary to a valid and complete understanding of the nature of language and its disorders. The third level of integration relates the literature on normal language acquisition to the clinical needs of professionals who deal with language disorders. Lastly, and probably most importantly, we attempt to integrate the various components of the language system and to explore how they are related within the child.

Just as the book is integrative in several aspects, it is multidimensional in many ways. Our central theme, in fact, is the multidimensional aspect of language: we view language as being composed of four major dimensions, the cognitive, the linguistic, the performance, and the environmental/communicative dimensions. Although we consider the description of linguistic behavior to be an important task of the language specialist, the significance of understanding the child who has the linguistic problem is stressed. Language disorders do not exist in the language but in the child. This emphasis on the child requires a description of the variations of linguistic problems associated with different disorders. Consideration of the variety of manifestations of language disorders may increase the readers' appreciation of their diversity as well as their commonality, particularly the similarity of the effect of divergent pathologies on the linguistic code.

The book is organized into four major sections. Part One provides the foundation for understanding language disorders by describing in detail the four dimensions of language used in the integrative approach. Part Two describes the child's acquisition of the linguistic code, a necessary prerequisite to understanding language disorders and the children who have them. Part Three applies the integrative theory to language disorders and reviews procedures and positions in assessment and intervention. Part Four discusses the manifestations of language disorders in children with mental retardation, hearing impairment, autism, clinical language disorders, and traumatic aphasia. Unique to this section on language disorders is the consideration of the problems displayed by bilingual children and those with disorders of reading and writing.

A special feature of the book is the use of asides to the text. These items were chosen to contribute an added dimension of current interest, personal insight, or clinical experience to the topic under discussion. Several topics peripheral to the approach to language used in this text have been excluded, however. A discussion of the relationship between impairment of specific areas of the brain and specific types of language disorders has been omitted, for example. Also language disorders associated with cleft palate, cerebral palsy, and multiple handicaps are not specifically reviewed.

Throughout the text we have attempted to provide a historical perspective. A surprising number of innovations are historically grounded. An understanding of historical positions and their modifications provides appreciation of the cycles of change that ideas undergo and leaves the reader with a healthy mistrust of any single solution, explanation, or theory. To enrich this historical context, short biographical sketches of individuals who have made important contributions to the fields of language and language disorders are included. Our criteria for selection of these individuals were as follows: (1) Some of their publications appeared in press prior to 1971. (2) Their theories have had a continuing impact on work with the language disordered. (3) Their publications have covered more than a single specialized area of language. (4) Their contributions include books and/or tests in addition to articles. (5) Their work has been referenced in one or more chapters of this volume, *or* their philosophy has had significant impact on a large number of researchers or language specialists. As these sketches are read, the web of professional colleagueship may become apparent, suggesting the debt that all of us owe to those who taught us.

In a book about language, some statement about the special terms we have used is in order. It cannot be denied that the choice of words, including pronouns, can reinforce discriminatory attitudes. Yet total avoidance of sex-identified words may result in awkward and stilted writing. Since a majority of language-disordered children are male, all *children* in this book are referred to as "he," except when a particular person is being discussed. All *adults* are referred to as "she"—again, unless there is obvious reference to a particular individual. The term "language specialist" is used to refer to those individuals who are interested in language and language research from a theoretical standpoint as well as to those whose primary interest is the educational management and/or clinical remediation of children with language disorders.

There are many people we would like to thank for their suggestions and contributions to the preparation of this book. We thank our colleagues, Gerald

Siegal and Laurence Leonard, for reading portions of the manuscript. We thank our research assistants and typists, Fachon Walker, Pat Reed, and Susan White. The editorial and production staff of Grune and Stratton also deserve our special thanks for their extraordinary concern and care as they supervised the transition of all of our words and ideas into print. We also thank the children with language disorders, whose struggles to learn language provided continued incentive for us to understand their problems. And finally we thank our families and friends for their patience and support.

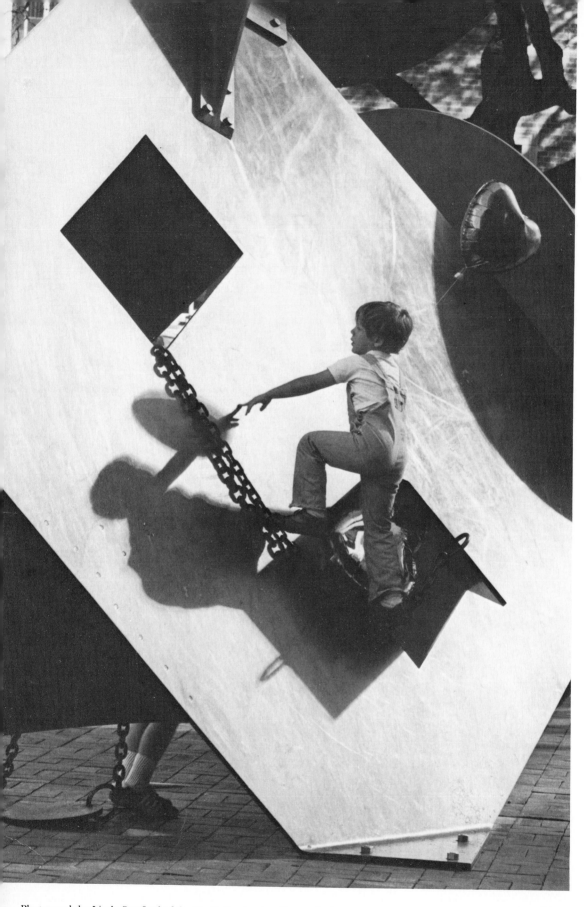

Photograph by Linda Stanford of the Media Production Center, University of Texas Health Science Center at Houston.

part one
foundations
of language

language

IT IS IMPOSSIBLE to attempt a description of disordered language without first defining language itself. That, however, is a difficult task. There are many disciplines that have language as a major interest for theoretical speculation, research examination, or clinical application. But because each discipline has its own concerns, each respective definition involves only one or another aspect of language. The study of the management of language disorders, however, cannot limit its concern to a single aspect of language; a theoretical description that is comprehensive enough to encompass the clinical manifestations of language disorders and yet specific enough to provide a basis for clinical assessment and intervention is needed.

This chapter introduces a model that will be used as a basis for the discussion of language disorders in this book. The description includes (1) a general discussion of the perspectives through which language will be viewed; (2) a definition of the scope and nature of language, which establishes the limits of the presentation; and (3) an introduction to the four dimensions of language, which will be used as bases for subsequent chapters.

The Historical Perspective

PERSPECTIVES FOR THE STUDY OF LANGUAGE

For centuries, language has been a focus of concern for scientists and philosophers, and many efforts have been made to discover its nature and characteristics and to propose theories regarding its origin and development. Scholars have continually projected new or rediscovered interpretations of language as well as new terminologies for describing it. Each attempt at analysis and description, at synthesis and theory, in which novel theories and descriptions have been integrated with historic views of language, has expanded the existing knowledge of language and its parameters. When new theories are not integrated with the evolutionary history of language, the theories represent a narrow and specific point of view and contribute little to the language paradigm.

The point of view held by the authors of this book is that the wealth of past knowledge is essential to the preservation of a stable framework for understanding language and interpreting its disorders. New ideas are not seen as replacements for the old but as supplements, clarifications, and expansions of theories that may stimulate new ideas and insights. Thus, the basic definition of language does not change with new ideas; it is rather modified by them.

The necessity of holding the old while examining the new is of particular importance to the individual concerned with language disorders. Unless a broad historic base is used, there is a danger of following changes in the focus of language theory with changes in the assessment and intervention of language-disordered children. If this happens, children are taught according to the current views on language regardless of needs and abilities and regardless of the validity of the current theory. This can result in confusion on the part of the clinicians and failure to effect language change in the children. Throughout this book, therefore, current theory and practice are presented within an historical framework wherever possible. The evolution of thought about language and its disorders is used as a basis for the presentation of current ideas. Brief summaries of the lives and contributions of scholars important in the field of language or language disorders are also presented.

The Disorders Perspective

In literature on disordered language, the emphasis is often on the theories and description of normal language and its development. The linguistic, the psychological, or the social method of describing normal language is used to describe disordered language as well as to identify and clinically manage the language-disordered child. Although any one of these descriptions alone may not be broad enough to describe the disorder, the concept of language disorder is forced into the description and made to "fit." The developmental stages, sequences, and descriptions of normal language are assumed to be the same for disordered language, and consequently, plans for intervention are often exclusively based on such normative data.

There seems to be validity, however, in choosing disordered language as the center of emphasis in both the theoretical and practical aspects of language. Definitions and descriptions should be chosen for their ability to account for observed disorders in language. Each theory, however imperfect, must reflect the actual language behavior of children, particularly those with disorders. A language-disorder theory should reflect the complexity of language. It is impossible to ignore aspects of language because they are difficult to understand or explain or cannot be measured or observed accurately.

The center of emphasis in this book is *disordered* language. The authors believe that an intellectual venture into language theory may provide an enlightening exercise for the scholar; however, the language specialist, faced with a person who is deficient in communication skills, cannot afford to be purely intellectual about language, unless the theory provides a means of understanding and helping to change the problem. In other words, a valid and useful theory of language must take abnormalities into account.

The Integrative Perspective

Uncritical acceptance of any single point of view about language as a basis for making decisions about disordered language forces an emphasis on one aspect only of disordered language. Individuals who are "developmentalists" will reject any view of language that includes the behavioral processes. Individuals who focus on semantics tend to ignore syntax. When the pragmatic aspect of language gained renewed interest, other aspects of language were neglected or rejected. There seems to be a propensity in the specialty of disordered language to consider the various views of language mutually exclusive. Specialists seem to forget that theories are theories and that the real world of disordered language does not change with each different theory. When there is a focus on one aspect of language, such as pragmatics, a language-disordered child may still have syntactic, cognitive, or semantic problems.

The integrative perspective of this book, then, focuses on the child instead of the theory. The child is not divided into a syntactic part, a pragmatic part, etc. It is the specialists who fragment the language-disordered child. It may seem simpler to choose one aspect or theory of language than to attempt to integrate all viewpoints and theories; however, the only valid way to begin to understand language disorders and the language-disordered child is to study and understand *all* aspects and dimensions of language.

This text, then, will not support one view over another, but will attempt to integrate theories and approaches so that language specialists may assist language-disordered children in a comprehensive and realistic way.

Language and Communication

Early scholars distinguished between the terms *language* and *communication,* usually considering language to be a human method of communication (Sapir, 1921). The distinction became more pronounced as the terms were applied more broadly to very different kinds of functions and events. Communication came to include all methods of exchange of information. In human interpersonal exchanges, for example, vocal tone, gestures, and instinctive cries were considered as part of the total communication system, whereas language referred to the linguistic code only. With advances in mass media, telecommunications, and information theory, mathematicians, physicists, and engineers adopted the term communication to refer to all systems that included a sender, a receiver, and message transmission, and could be quantified and modified (Cherry, 1957). The comparison of the human model of communication with the engineering model was called *cybernetics* (Mysak, 1966; N. Weiner, 1948).

As communication began to be used to describe any type of message transmission, language became reserved for those types of communication that were *coded,* that is, organized into a systematic, arbitrary set of symbols. Although language was (and still is) used to describe other codes—the manual coded signs used by the deaf, the codes used by computers—it was primarily applied to the *vocal* code of humans. Language came to be defined, then, in terms of the auditory-vocal linguistic code and its structural and semantic rules. (Although this definition is memorized by students learning about language, the coded feature is considered by the authors of this book to be only one dimension of language.)

It is possible to consider communication without language, but not vice versa. Communication is the purpose of language—the "what, when, where, why and how something is said . . ." (Muma, 1978, p. 118). Phylogenetically, the concept of communication predates that of language. The primitive instinctive exchanges, looks, and gestures of humans transmitted information prior to the use of a formal code to represent ideas and feelings. Ontogenetically, the act of communication takes place between a child and a caretaker through cries, looks, and touch prior to the child's understanding and use of the human vocal code. On the other hand, communication is the *main* function of language. Language cannot be defined or described without considering its purpose and function.

Language and Speech

The language-disorders specialist needs to distinguish between concepts of *speech* and language. In clinical practice, there is evidence of two separate but related activities; (1) speaking and (2) using a linguistic code involving rules of grammar, semantics, and pragmatics. The literature has not clearly distinguished between the terms speech and language. J. W. Black and Moore (1955) described speech as behavior in which words serve both as a substitute stimuli to evoke responses and also as substitute responses. J. W. Black and Moore's definition does not distinguish speech from language, for both spoken and written words can serve as substitute stimuli; they were defining human language exchange. On the other hand, Eisenson, Auer, and Irwin (1963, p. 6) do make this distinction; they described speech as a means of expressing language: "Speech is a medium that employs an oral linguistic code that enables one human being to express feelings and to communicate thoughts to another human being.... Man produces linguistic forms for speech through his oral (articulatory), vocal and pantomimic mechanisms." This same distinction was provided by de Saussure (1959), who stated that language (langue) exists collectively in a group, whereas speech (parole) exists in the individual.

It is possible to speak or to utter sounds in certain sequences and yet not have language. Sapir (1921, p. 10) wrote that a speech-sound, even when spoken, "is very far from being an element of language." Some persons who have sustained brain damage and are aphasic are able to produce "English" with good intonation and inflection, but with no meaningful words. Many of these patients also lack the ability to understand what is said to them, although their hearing is normal. Such persons display speech without language. It is also possible to have language without the ability to speak. This is vividly exemplified by the deaf who do not speak, yet who have a perfectly adequate language expressed in signs.

Speech is not necessarily language and language is not always speech, although there is a close relationship between them (Cutting & Kavanagh, 1975). As Cazden (1971) pointed out, language is knowledge in our heads, and speech is the realization of that knowledge in behavior; it is language, primarily, that makes meaningful speech possible. De Saussure (1959, p. 14) also made some interesting observations regarding language and speech: "In separating language from speaking we are at the same time separating (1) what is social from what is individual; and (2) what is essential from what is accessory and more or less accidental. . . ." He continued his distinction by saying that

Edward Sapir

Edward Sapir was born in Germany in 1884 and moved with his parents to the United States as a child. He obtained his degrees at Columbia University and subsequently gained a reputation as an anthropologist. Sapir has been recognized as an expert on American Indian languages and was one of the first to explore the relationship between the study of language and anthropology. Although Sapir was the author of many scholarly articles, he produced only a single book, *Language: An Introduction to the Study of Speech,* in which he emphasized the theme of the relationship between thought, language, and culture. He did not consider language to be instinctive; he described language emergence as having social prerequisites. Although he described language as but the "outward" facet of thought, he did not conceive of thought or reason without it. Sapir's book remains in active circulation and is considered a classic in the field.

Ferdinand de Saussaure

Ferdinand de Saussaure was born into a distinguished and educated Swiss family. He entered Geneva University in 1875 at the age of 17 and became interested in linguistics, concentrating on Indo-Europe-an languages. In graduate studies at Leipzig University, instead of concentrating on historical linguistics (the usual focus at that time), he became interested in investigating phonology. He later became a member of the Linguistic Society of Paris, and because of his work with synchronic linguistics, he is now regarded as the founder of modern structural linguistics. Actually, his work was so advanced for his time that it was little understood until some time after his death. His best known publication, *Course in General Linguistics,* was published posthumously in 1915.

De Saussaure's main contribution to the understanding of language was his attempts to clarify terminology. He differentiated between language (langue) and speech (parole), describing language as knowledge that can be studied even when not spoken. He also drew attention to the role of language as a system of classification. Later linguists considered his ideas a theoretical foundation to the newer trends in linguistic study.

language is not a function of the speaker but a product that is passively assimilated by the individual. Speaking, according to de Saussure (1959) is a willful and intellectual individual act. Within the act he distinguishes between the speaker who uses the language code for expressing his own thoughts; and the psychological mechanism by which the speaker exteriorizes the code.

Definitions of Language

The linguist Sapir (1921, p. 8) defined language as "... a purely human and non-instinctive method of communicating ideas, emotions, and desires by means of a system of voluntarily produced symbols which are auditory and produced by the organs of speech." The important elements in Sapir's definition are that (1) language is a function exclusive to humans; (2) it is learned; (3) it is one method of communicating; (4) it is systematic; (5) it is symbolic; and (6) the symbols are vocal (heard and spoken). The arbitrariness of the symbols is pointed out by Hughes (1962), who defined language as a system of arbitrary vocal symbols by which thought is conveyed from one human being to another. Hill's (1958, p. 9) definition brought out the concept of *meaning* in language. He said, "The entities of language are symbols, that is, they have meaning, but the connection between symbols and things is arbitrary and socially controlled."

Bloomfield, Langer, and Lenneberg used definitions that are limited to one aspect of language. Bloomfield's concern (1933) was with language as an object to be known; he proposed that the study of language was the study of the coordination of sounds with meaning. Langer (1942, p. 96) stressed the intellectual function of language, writing that "the essence of language is the formulation and expression of conceptions rather than the communication of natural wants." She believed that the tendency to see reality symbolically is the real keynote of language. The communicative and behavioral functions of language were considered by the neuropsychologist, Lenneberg (1973, p. 6) to be its most important characteristics— not the labels or "names." He said that "language is relational . . . to teach someone to speak is essentially to invite him to relate aspects of the environment."

Historic ideas about language, particularly those by C. W. Morris (1938), who described the three aspects of language as syntactic, semantic, and pragmatic, have been placed within the framework of contemporary terminology by linguists, particularly Bloom and Lahey (1978). They discussed language within the framework of its content, its form, and its function and the integration among these aspects. Their definition attempts to integrate the classic philosophical concern with meaning (content) with that of the psycholinguistic insights into phonological, lexical, and syntactic development (form) as well as the currently revived interest in pragmatics (function). It omits, however, the aspect of human language that describes the behavioral processes of understanding and producing language. The primary subject of a purely linguistic description of language is linguistic knowledge rather than linguistic behavior. The linguistic definition considers the cognitive system, which forms the content of the linguistic code, and the communicative environment, in which the linguistic code is used, to be nonlinguistic aspects of language.

Taken together, the definitions of Sapir, Hill, Lenneberg, Bloom, et al., characterize human language as (1) symbolic; (2) representative of categories of reality events; (3) arbitrary; (4) systematic; (5) coded; (6) vocal—the most usual form of the symbols is auditory-vocal, even when not spoken; (7) used to communicate ideas; (8) a means of relationship with others; and (9) a behavioral process.

The definitions differ from each other in that some specialists view language primarily as an object to be studied. The ele-

Susanne K. Langer

Language scholars feel that Langer has made an important contribution to the understanding of the nature of language by providing philosophical insights into symbolization and its use by humans. Upon finishing her studies at Radcliffe, she taught philosophy at several major universities. She authored several books on philosophy, but it is *Philosophy in a New Key* that language specialists consider her major work.

Langer's work examines the logic and meaning of symbols; her resulting interpretation forms the basis of her elaboration and integration of the significance of language, ritual, myth, and music in human mentality. For Langer, verbal symbols *are*, in fact, "the new key." Her work illustrates the importance of the study of language in philosophy, as well as the influence of philosophy on the study of language.

ments of language are identified and classified, and the rules by which those elements may be combined are analyzed (for instance Bloomfield's definition states that the study of the coordination of sounds with meanings is the study of language). Other specialists consider language to be a behavioral process; as, for example, Sapir, who considers language as a means of communicating ideas by means of symbols that are auditory and produced by the organs of speech. Still others see language as communication that involves the interaction of a speaker and a listener and an environment where each has the potential to modify the behavior of others. A description of language as a means of relationship is provided by Lenneberg, who states that to teach someone to speak is essentially to invite the speaker to relate aspects of the environment.

Each of these views of language represents in a valid manner *some aspect* of language. Language, however, is none of these because it is all of these.

FOUR DIMENSIONS OF LANGUAGE: AN INTEGRATIVE VIEW

The basic interest of the psychologist is the *system* by which children learn: the manner in which they learn to perceive, remember, understand, formulate, and produce a meaningful linguistic code. The focus of the linguist is on the *knowledge* of the syntactic, semantic, and pragmatic rules of the linguistic code and the manner in which these rules are used in expressive language. These two approaches, together with the understanding of the social forces that regulate the emergence and performance of language, should be part of an integrative approach to language—one that considers *all* viewpoints important to the understanding of the language-disordered child.

The major thesis of this text, therefore, is that in order to understand the complex human behavioral system of language, it is important to study and integrate its characteristics in terms of four major components or dimensions. The four dimensions are as follows:

1. *The dimension of linguistic knowledge.* This is the dimension of the linguistic code viewed as an object for study. Linguistics is concerned with the lexicon and with the phonological, grammatic, semantic, and pragmatic rules that comprise the system by which a message is transmitted. The code and these rules make up the task the child must learn in order to use language.
2. *The cognitive dimension.* This is the dimension of the cognitive system by which language is learned, i.e., the sensory, perceptual, memory, conceptual, and representational abilities humans must possess in order to acquire the rules that govern the code and its meaning.

3. *The dimension of language performance.* This is the dimension of the behavioral processes humans learn and use in order to handle the code internally, in transmission from external to internal states, and vice versa. These behavioral processes include comprehension and production of language.
4. *The dimension of communicative environment.* This is the dimension of the communication relationship that supports the exchange between two persons. This includes the internal motivations, desires, and needs to communicate on the part of the speaker, as well as the environmental factors that stimulate, support, and maintain the language as it emerges.

This text will use these four dimensions of language, instead of the traditional definition of language, as the model from which to describe normal and disordered language. (The complexity of this method of defining language reflects the complexity of language.) In this way, it will be possible to integrate the various approaches to language with one another as well as with the historic views.

the dimension of linguistic knowledge

2

A LINGUISTIC CODE can exist in the abstract, that is, it can be described without anyone speaking or understanding it. The description of a code may include the vocabulary, the grammar, the meanings associated with the lexicon (as in a dictionary) and with the grammar, and the rules governing the appropriateness of structure in specified contexts. This type of description of language focuses on the linguistic code itself; it can be studied without the intention of understanding or speaking the language. The linguistic code, in this sense, is invariant; if someone wants to learn the language described in the book, he must master the rules described—the same rules that others have had to master to speak the language.

Although hundreds of linguistic codes are used by humans, they have common characteristics and similar structures. The characteristics make them functional codes—codes that are symbolic, systematic, arbitrary, and usually vocal. Each code has a grammatical, semantic, and a pragmatic structure. The rules governing the structure are different for each language, however, resulting in the great diversity among languages.

This chapter describes the characteristics common to all language as well as the nature of the structure of language codes. An introductory presentation of three types of structure—the grammatical, the semantic, and the pragmatic—is provided. A more detailed discussion of syntax, semantics, and pragmatics from a developmental point of view will be presented in Chapters 7, 8, and 9.

CHARACTERISTICS OF THE LINGUISTIC CODE

Symbolic Aspects of the Code

One of the most important characteristics of human language is its symbolic nature. A *symbol* is something that stands for or in the place of something else. A symbol *refers* to things, that is, it represents them. Symbols have no basic, necessary, or inherent relationship to those things they represent. They differ from *signals* in that they do not announce the object—they refer to it. Saying the word *war* does not necessarily mean that a war is taking place or is even imminent; a picture of a dove may symbolize peace although the dove itself has no power to bring about peace.

A symbol differs in important ways from a *sign* or *signal*. A sign leads to or indicates a thing, and a *natural sign* has a direct relation to its object. Examples of *natural signs* (physical, chemical, or biological) include smoke signaling fire or dark clouds signaling rain. In this type of sign, the sign reveals its meaning in a nonarbitrary way. In *learned signals*, the sign announces the object it has come to be associated with, as a whistle may signal food to a specific group of people, or a specific flag may signal that the ship on which it flies is from a particular country. The learned sign has no direct relation to its object. In distinguishing between signs and symbols, Cassirer (1953–1957) described signs as having a sort of physical or substantial being and symbols as having only functional value. He believed that a sign or signal is related to the thing to which it refers in a fixed and unique way; a symbol is extremely variable.

The inconstancy of symbols is evident in many ways. The *referents* for symbols (that to which the symbol refers) may change with time; words change in meaning as society changes. A refer-

The drawings function as abstract signs since they all indicate that what they signify is nearby. All of them are learned signs except the last, which has not yet become associated with the thing it indicates. (From Sam and Sib, *reprinted courtesy of King Features.)*

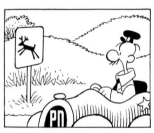
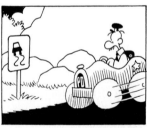
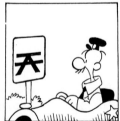

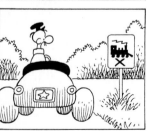
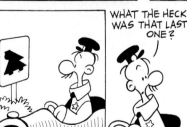
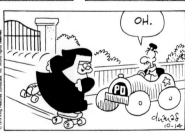

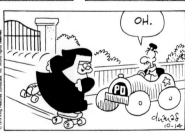WHAT THE HECK WAS THAT LAST ONE?

OH.

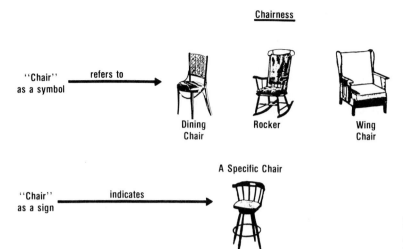

Chairness

"Chair" as a symbol — refers to → Dining Chair, Rocker, Wing Chair

A Specific Chair

"Chair" as a sign — indicates →

Figure 2-1
An example of the difference between a symbol and a sign.

ent can be symbolized by more than one symbol (*big, huge,* and *large* mean essentially the same thing). A single symbol can have more than one referent (*pen* can refer to a writing instrument as well as an enclosure for pigs). Furthermore, the meaning of a symbol is not always the same as the referent. The referent of *burn you* may not be what the teenager has in mind when he says it. Thus, the meaning and the referent of the word can be different.

Language can be and is used by humans in both a signifying and in a symbolizing manner. When words are used as signifiers, they indicate concrete, specific objects or situations, e.g., a mother who looks at her child, points, and says *"chair"* is signaling a specific chair. In their symbolic use, words refer to classes of things. Sapir (1921, p.12) wrote "The elements of language, the symbols that ticket off experience, must therefore be associated with whole groups, delimited classes, of experience ..." The word *chair,* for example, does not mean a specific bedroom or office chair, but refers to "chairness." When the word *chair* is used to indicate a specific piece of furniture, it means that the specific object is a member of the class *chair* (Fig. 2-1).

Not all words represent classes of things; if they did, the communication of our thoughts and ideas would be severely restricted. Words may also represent events, relations, and ideas. Words that do represent classes of things are usually easily understood. Words such as *truth, love* and *honesty,* however, do not have such specific meanings; the meaning one brings to the symbol is related to the experiences one has relative to its referent.

The symbolic function of language includes not only the meanings of words, but also the meanings of word endings and word order and word combinations. The meanings derived from symbols combined in particular and unique ways, as in words that have specialized endings or that are combined in sentences, are even more complicated to comprehend.

Language must have at least two components to be considered language: symbols and their meaning. A sequence of sounds or words is symbolic *only* when it is associated with meaning. Symbols do not need to be sound symbols, however. They can be, and sometimes are, manual symbols. It would seem appropriate, therefore, to consider the term *linguistic* as refering to both the structure (form) of the language *and* the meanings that are associated with the structure (content). However, the term *linguistics* is frequently used to refer to the structure only (Bloom & Lahey, 1978), implying that the structure or form is the language, and that the meaning or content is a related "nonlinguistic" component. Neither the structural or conceptual system alone is language—language is the relationship between the two.

Systematic Aspects of the Code

A second important aspect of language is its systematic nature. In language, symbols are structured into a code in which the arrangements within and between the elements are governed by rules. Carroll (1964, p. 14) stated that the central concept in linguistics is structure, which is, "the ordered or patterned set of contrasts or oppositions which are presumed to be discoverable in a language, whether in the units of sound, the grammatical inflections, the syntactical arrangements or even the meaning of linguistic forms."

The structure of each language is governed by its own set of rules. In most of the grammatical systems, however, there are three levels of structure: the phonological, the morphological, and the syntactic, which in turn are built upon the basic element of the language, the *lexicon*. The structure of these levels forms the code by which humans communicate.

At the phonemic level, the system's structure dictates the particular sequence or combination of sounds that are acceptable by the rules of a specific language. In English, for example, the sequence "spr" is acceptable, and it would be possible to invent a new word, "sprill," to meet the requirements of the rules of the language. However, it would be difficult to convince speakers of English that "ftz" is an acceptable combination. The phonemic system also dictates that the past tense is pronounced /t/ after jump and /d/ after wag. The rules state that the pronunciation in this case depends on the preceding sound, whether it is voiced or voiceless.

At the morphological level, combinations of sounds, called words, signal meanings. Single sounds or combinations of sounds that are not referred to as words, but as morphemes, also signal meaning, such as /s/, which signals plurality when used at the end of certain nouns, or /t/ and /d/, which signal past tense when used at the ends of verbs. The morphological rules explain the system of expressing a particular grammatical meaning, such as "plural" or "past," in that language.

At the syntactic level, each particular language system demands that certain classes of words be placed in certain sequential relationships to other classes in order for meaning to emerge. The utterance "cat milk drinking the is" contains acceptable English words, but for the native speaker of English the utterance is meaningless. This utterance does not follow the rules of the language, which require, for example, that the class of words of which *the* is a member should precede the class of words of which *cat* is a member. Word order conveys specific meaning. This is illustrated by transposing the words *man* and *boy* in the utterance, "The man pushes the boy," thereby changing the direction of the action from boy to man.

The structure of the language makes it possible to convey considerable information within a limited number of units of utterance. By compressing both the sound units and the meaningful units, more information can be communicated in less time. Sounds are compressed by temporally overlapping one sound with another in speaking. Meaningful units are compressed by using coded endings to words, as well as word order, to convey meaning. Consider the way in which language permits large chunks of information to be handled by a limited memory. The following ideas

There is more than one boy.
They play baseball.
They belong to a team.
They play on a field.
The team owns the field.
The event of playing occurred in the past.

can all be uttered in one sentence:

The boys played baseball on their team's field.

The rules of language are not only syntactic; the semantic (meaning) and pragmatic (function) systems are also governed by rules. The rules governing the meaning and use of a particular language are less well known than those governing the syntax. These rules describe how specific grammatic structures are related to meaning and the contexts in which specific grammar and usage are appropriate.

Although the typical speaker is constantly using the rules of his language to formulate linguistic utterances, he more than likely is not able to formally state the rules that he uses, unless he is a linguistic scientist or a student of language.

Arbitrary Characteristics of the Code

The symbols of language are arbitrary. There is no inherent relationship between the particular spoken, written, or signed word and the object, idea, or class of objects it symbolizes. In the English vocal system, there is no logical explanation for the assignment of the sound sequence /καυ/ *(cow)* to the domesticated four-legged animal that gives milk. The same animal is referred to as *vaca* in Spanish and *vache* in French, indicating that a particular sound sequence is based upon preference or accident within a specific linguistic culture.

Although the original choice of a particular symbol is arbitrary, the use of the symbol by the speaker of a language is no longer arbitrary. The speaker of a particular language must use the symbol already agreed upon if he wishes to communicate with others in his linguistic society.

Writing also expresses the arbitrary nature of language. Letters and written characters differ from language to language. Some languages, such as Arabic and Hebrew, are read from right to left on the page, whereas certain oriental languages are read from bottom to top. Chinese writing is unique in an even greater respect; this graphic system assigns a separate symbol to each word—not each sound. Consequently, Chinese can be read by persons who cannot understand each other's spoken dialect of Chinese.

Vocal Characteristics of the Code

Primacy of Vocal Symbols

Although, as previously stated, there are many ways in which the term language can be used, this book considers vocal language as the primary communication medium used by humans. Humans have in the past and present used other means (pictograph, idiograph, manual signs, etc.) to exchange ideas. Howev-

---

Humpty Dumpty had a clear understanding of the arbitrariness of words and the loose connection between words and meaning.

"I don't know what you mean by 'glory,' " Alice said.

Humpty Dumpty smiled contemptuously. "Of course you don't—till I tell you. I meant 'there's a nice knock-down argument for you!' "

"But 'glory' doesn't mean 'a nice knock-down argument,' " Alice objected.

"When I use a word," Humpty Dumpty said, in rather a scornful tone, "it means just what I choose it to mean—nothing more or less."

"The question is," said Alice, "whether you *can* make words mean so many different things."

"The question is," said Humpty Dumpty, "which is to be master—that's all."*

*From Lewis Carroll: *Through the Looking Glass.* New York: Random House, 1946, p. 94. Reprinted with permission.

---

er, the method that is used most frequently, is most economical in use of time, and is most simple in terms of coding is the vocal system. In this system, sounds that occur either alone or in a specific sequence are associated with classes of objects. These vocalizations are grouped into specific sequences called *words*. The word meanings may be modified by adding sounds to the sequence, either at the beginning or at the end of the word. For example, /s/ may be added to the word *cake*, thereby changing the meaning from singular to plural. Words are sequenced into *sentences;* this word order also influences meaning. Although the code is a vocal code, it does not necessarily have to be spoken; a mute person can understand the code, and a deaf person may be taught to produce the sounds of the code. The sound code may be expressed or received through writing even if it cannot be heard or spoken—the written or graphic system is a visual–motor expression of the auditory–vocal system.

Relation of Vocal to Graphic and Manual Symbols

Although the language code was originally a sound code only, humans developed, at a later period, a graphic system to represent the individual sounds. In a language such as English, the graphic system represents the vocal sound system on an almost one-to-one basis—there is a connection between the graphic sign or letter and the sound it represents. The linear sequences of sounds that occur in time when spoken are transferred to a spatial sequence of graphic signs that represent these sounds. The sequence of the first to the last sound in a word is translated to a sequence of letters.

Speech refers to the oral expression of the linguistic codes, i.e., the articulation of the specific sounds of language in their specific order by the peripheral organs of the vocal mechanism. *Writing* refers to the graphic expression of language by use of characters representing the vocal sounds of which the code is composed. In English, these characters are ordered from left to right.

The manual expression of language sometimes follows the vocal code, as in finger spelling, and other times uses a separate code, as in sign language. Sign language is a visual–motor language. All dialects of sign language taught in the United States are included in the label American Sign Language (Ameslan). Ameslan has no spoken or written vocabulary and is often supplemented by finger spelling, which consists of hand signs representing each letter of the alphabet. Sign language maximizes the use of visual imagery and space. Whereas oral language occurs in a linear auditory–vocal sequence, the components of a sign must be articulated simultaneously.

The Grammar of Language: Syntactics

The early study of linguistics was descriptive in nature. The current approach is to describe language in terms of abstract rules. The scientific study of the syntactic and morphophonemic structure of language has provided a theoretical basis for studies of how children acquire language as well as for studies of disordered language.

Descriptive Model of Grammar

The early study of language in the United States was stimulated by the need of a method to record the languages of the Indians of North America. The linguists of the early twentieth century developed systematic methods of recording and analysizing languages. These methods were the basis for the training of most linguists of that time. Standard field methods were developed to assist in the accumulation of data from individuals who spoke Indian languages, languages that had never been written or read (Boas, 1911).

The earliest methods of language analysis were purely descriptive. Initially, attempts were made to utilize traditional European grammatical categories for studying the structures of the Indian languages, but the linguists found that these languages did not fit into their traditional grammatic systems. Boas and his contemporaries Bloomfield and Sapir then developed an approach called *structuralism,* which stated that "every language has its own unique grammatical structure and that the task of the linguist is to discover for each language the categories of description appropriate to it" (Lyons, 1970, p. 27).

During this period, linguists attempted to mold the study of language into a scientific discipline. Bloomfield (1933) excluded from study those aspects of language that could not be rigorously observed and examined. He based his theory of linguistic description on behaviorism, which was prominent at that time in psychology. According to the behaviorists, the only significant factors in human behavior were those that could be described in terms of a stimulus and a response. Any behavior that could not be described in such terms was not of concern to them.

Leonard Bloomfield

A great figure in American linguistics, Leonard Bloomfield began his professional career after receiving his Ph.D. from the University of Chicago in 1909 and doing postgraduate work at the University of Leipzig in 1913 and 1914. His scholarly interest was initially directed toward the study of Germanic philology. However, his first book, *Introduction to the Study of Language,* was a prelude to what was to be his lifelong concern—to make linguistics a science. Bloomfield's interest in linguistic science did not prevent his involvement in the pragmatic aspects of linguistics, however. The teaching of reading and of foreign languages were of great concern to him. Bloomfield is also well-known for his work with other languages, especially those of Algonquian and Cree groups of American Indians.

Avram Noam Chomsky

Scholars and students in the field of linguistics consider Avram Noam Chomsky's widely acclaimed theories of grammar among the most dynamic and influential ideas about language of the last quarter century. Chomsky received his Ph.D. at Pennsylvania State University, having studied linguistics, mathematics, and philosophy. Since 1955, he has been on the faculty at the Massachusetts Institute of Technology, where he is presently Professor of Linguistics.

Chomsky's early interest in linguistics was influenced by his father, a Hebrew scholar of considerable repute. The system of transformational generative grammar, for which Chomsky became famous, developed from his studies in modern logic and mathematics. In the area of political debate, Chomsky is known for his criticism of American foreign policy.

Early publications include *Synatatic Structures; Aspects of the Theory of Syntax; Current Issues in Linguistic Theory;* and *Language and Mind.* More recent publications are concerned with both politics and linguistics: *Reflections on Language; The Logical Structure of Linguistic Theory;* and *Human Rights and American Foreign Policy.* Chomsky's publications and teaching have influenced not only linguistics but also the study of psycholinguistics, child language, and language disorders.

Generative Model of Grammar

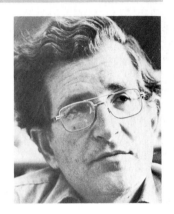

The philosophy and methods of descriptive linguists were rejected in 1957, when, in his book entitled *Syntactic Structures,* Noam Chomsky heralded a new era in linguistic study. Chomsky postulated that grammar is a theory or hypothesis of language that accounts for the utterances produced by the native speaker. This was a new definition of grammar; until Chomsky, the word grammar had implied the grade-school struggle with sentence diagramming and rules regarding the use of *I* versus *me* and *can* versus *may.* These dictums constituted a *prescriptive* grammar and were very different from Chomsky's *generative* idea of grammar.

The ultimate goal of a grammar, as described by Chomsky, is to specify rules that can generate only well-formed utterances. Everyone who speaks a language knows these rules intuitively without ever having formally studied them. By means of these rules, a speaker can generate an infinite number of structures.

As viewed by Chomsky, linguistic theory is concerned primarily with an ideal speaker-listener in a homogenous speech community. Chomsky calls speaker-listener's intuitive knowledge of the rules of his language *linguistic competence,* and the actual use of language in concrete situations, *linguistic performance.* The linguist's task, according to Chomsky, is to define the underlying system of rules that has been mastered and used by the speaker-listener. The linguist deduces this system by utilizing the data of performance, i.e., what the speakers say. Thus, Chomsky's grammar provides a structural description of a specific sentence and how it is used and understood by the ideal speaker-listener. In addition to this, the grammar provides the formulation of generative rules and attempts to specify what the speaker actually knows about language and how it can be used.

The grammar has three major components: (1) phonological; (2) syntactic; and (3) morphological. The *phonological* system is made up of speech sounds called *phonemes.* The phonemes of a language are the sounds that distinguish meaning in that language. For example, /b/ and /v/ are phonemes in English; if they are interchanged in words, there is a corresponding change in meaning, e.g., *base/vase*. In Spanish, /b/ and /v/ are members of the same phoneme and can be interchanged *without* changing or distinguishing meaning. In each language, phonemes are combined according to rules that originally were purely arbitrary. English is transcribed phonetically by using 24 consonants and 15 simple vowel sounds.

The term *morpheme* refers to the smallest meaningful unit in a language, whether it is a word or part of a word. Words are *free* morphemes. Meaningful prefixes and suffixes are *bound* morphemes; for example, the morpheme *un* carries the meaning of negation, as in the words unfashionable, unsinkable, and unforgivable.

Syntax is used to describe the manner in which the order of words can have grammatic significance. Compare these two sentences:

> The boy ate the fish.
> The fish ate the boy.

Both sentences contain exactly the same words, but the order of words makes the difference between a mundane comment on what a child had for lunch and a sensational news item. The rules that permit the speaker to modify words (by adding morphemes) and sentences (by the arrangement of words) constitute the *morphosyntactic* system of langauge.

According to Chomsky's theory, the syntactic component of a grammar specifies for each sentence (1) a *deep structure* that determines its *semantic* interpretation and (2) a *surface structure* that determines its *phonetic* interpretation. A deep structure that carries the meaning of a dog chasing a cat may have any of the following surface structures: (1) The cat is chased by the dog; (2) The dog chases the cat; or (3) The dog is chasing the cat.

The syntactic component has a *base,* or system of rules, which generates a restricted set of *basic strings,* each with an associated structural description called a base *phrase-marker.* A phrase-marker is a graphic representation of how a speaker of English understands a sentence. The surface structure is generated from the basic strings by application of *transformations.* A transformation is stated in the form of a rule, which is applied to one member of a pair of constructions and alters that member to produce the second member of the pair. For example, the construction, "The dog bit the cat" is altered by transformation to "When was the cat bitten by the dog?" The first construction above is termed the *input string,* and the second is termed the *output string.*

A transformational grammar is organized in three sections. The first is the *phrase structure segment,* which describes strings of comparatively simple structure. The second section—the transformational segment—describes all the transformations by which the output strings of the first section are carried into the *terminal strings*. The third section is the *morphophonemic section,* which describes all the processes by which the terminal strings are given shapes identifiable as utterances, i.e., by which the terminal strings undergo phonetic interpretation (Fig. 2-2).

Phrase structure rules divide a sentence initially into two parts (called *constitutents*), but instead of dividing the surface structure, the rules are abstract notations that are applicable to the deep structure. For example, it may be desirable to divide the sentence, "The dog bit the cat" into two constitutents. A logical division would be:

The dog + bit the cat

Using phrase structure rules, instead, the sentence would be written in an abstract notation:

Noun Phrase (NP) + Verb Phrase (VP)

The two phrase structures can be divided again. The noun phrase in the sentence above is made up of the article or determiner, *the,* and the noun, *dog.* The verb phrase is composed of the verb, *bit* and the noun phrase, *the cat,* which in turn is made up of the determiner, *the,* and the noun, *cat.* This same phrase structure rule can be applied to any sentence. The tree diagram (Fig. 2-3) illustrates the use of phrase structure rules.

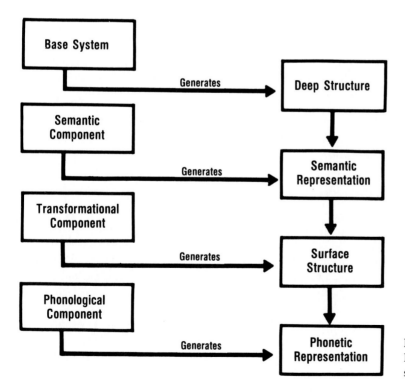

Figure 2-2
Illustration of the general structure of grammar.

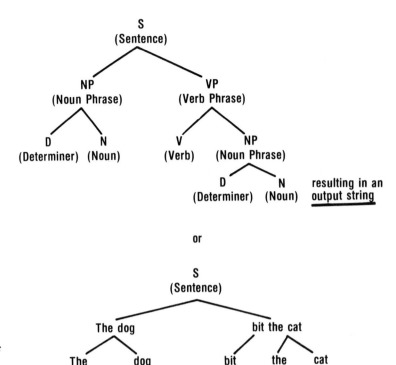

Figure 2-3
A tree diagram of the phrase structure of a sentence.

The analysis of sentences into small units, which in turn can be analyzed into their respective constitutents, illustrates the *hierarchical structure* of language.

Linguists' description of language has moved beyond the analysis of the basic structures to analysis of semantics. Not only do linguists today state that every grammar must have a linguistic component, but they also attempt to relate meaning to structure.

The Meaning of the Linguistic Code: Semantics

Definition of Semantics

For language to be language, there must be a correspondence between the reality of the concrete world of objects existing in space, changing in time, and bound together by physical, psychological, and logical relationships, and the reality of language structure (Church, 1961). The term for this relationship is *semantics,* which describes the way in which meanings are *marked* into the phonological, lexical, and morphosyntactic systems in a particular language. In this interpretation, the content, when viewed separately from the linguistic structure, does not constitute semantic elements or relations. In semantics, there must be a relation between content and structure.

From the discussion of symbols in the early part of this chapter, it may seem that the referent of the symbol is the same as its "meaning." In theory, this is true; symbols do refer to concepts or ideas of reality. In actuality, however, that to which a symbol, or group of symbols, refers may not be the meaning it has for an individual (e.g., words used in slang expressions). Individuals structure reality uniquely both because their biological make-up receives different information about reality, and because they have had particular experiences with reality. Individuals, therefore, bring "meaning" to symbols; they do not get meaning from them. Regarding this, Church (1961, p. 124) has stated ". . . we can make meaningful statements which are factually untrue, which are nonsensical (but still meaningful), which deal with hypothetical rather than actual situations, or which may even postulate the absence or nonexistence of something."

Although many linguists and psychologists have considered the study of meaning in language outside of their concern, those who study child language and its development, and, even more importantly, those who are concerned with language disorders, cannot omit this aspect of language.

Psychological and Linguistic Views of Meaning

When discussing "meaning," the psychologist and the linguist often refer to two different aspects of the topic. The psychologists who have addressed themselves to the study of the meaning of language have been concerned with the psychological process by which a linguistic stimulus can evoke meaning in the listener. The linguist's interest, on the other hand, has been the manner in which the language structure represents the content of language. Psychologists have begun with the external language stimulus and its language response and theorized to an internal process, usually referred to as a *mediation process.* Linguists have started with surface structure and interpolated to deep structure and semantic intentions.

Psychological Theories of Meaning. Within the field of psychology itself, there have been divergent positions taken relative to the study of meaning. These positions represent two schools of psychology: the behavioristic and the cognitive. Representing the former approach is Bousfield (Cofer, 1961, p. 81), who stated "It seems to me that meaning is not only an unnecessary concept for verbal learning but a concept bound to lead to confusion. Like the concept of emotion, it is ambiguous, and it is tied up with philosophical considerations going beyond the domain of psychology." Skinner (1967, pp 322–324) took a similar point of view: "A complimentary practice has been to assign an independent existence to meanings. . . . But can we identify the meaning of an utterance in an objective way? . . . The only solution is to reject the traditional formulation of verbal behavior in terms of meanings."

Sometimes the referent and the meaning of the word are confused! (From The Family Circus, *by Bil Keane, reprinted courtesy of The Register and Tribune Syndicate, Inc.)*

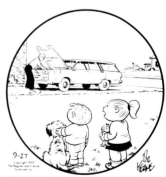

"Cinderella's coach turned into a pumpkin, but daddy says our car's turning into a lemon."

In general, the behaviorists described meaning in terms of observable phenomena, particularly the responses of the organism to stimuli and the effects of variation one had on the other. Other psychological theories accepted the existence of nonmaterial events (thoughts, or ideas) and sought to correlate these with material ones. Ogden and Richards (1953, p. 99), for example, illustrated the relationship of thoughts, words, and things by a diagram called the triangle of reference (Fig. 2-4). In the triangle of reference, the three factors (thought or reference, symbol, and referent) involved when any statement is made or comprehended are at the corners of the triangle; the relationship of these three factors are represented by the sides. As can be seen, the relation between the symbol and the referent is different from the other two relations, implying an indirect connection between them. (In other words, the symbol or word spoken causes a thought and the thought relates to the referent. There is no real connection, however, between the symbol or word, e.g., *dog*, and the actual animal. This approach to meaning introduced cognitive elements into the description of language even though it limited the consideration of meaning to that of reference.

The mediation theory of Osgood (1967, 1968) is a modification of the behavioristic view of language. He based his theory, which explains what he called "sign behavior," upon a general theory of learning. The question he posed about sign (symbol) behavior was, Under what conditions does a stimulus (word) that is not the significate (referent or object) become a sign of the significate? He used *significate* to mean the referent or that to which a sign refers. He did not believe that the relation of signs to their significates could be explained on the basis of simple conditioning because people do not interpret the same words in the same manner.

In his theory, Osgood described meaning in terms of a representational mediation process. He believed that a pattern of

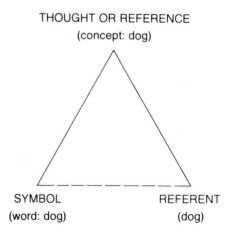

THOUGHT OR REFERENCE
(concept: dog)

SYMBOL
(word: dog)

REFERENT
(dog)

Figure 2-4
The triangle of reference. (Adapted with permission from Ogden and Richards, 1953, p. 9.)

George Armitage Miller

Miller is one of a number of American psychologists who, early in their academic and scholarly careers, developed an interest in the study of language. He received his education in psychology at Harvard University and soon after published his first book, entitled *Language and Communication*. In 1976, he published *Language and Perception* (with Philip N. Johnson-Laird).

Although Miller is probably best known for his theory of memory, in which he described the limits of memory in terms of the number of chunks of information that can be stored by the human brain, his major contribution to the understanding of language is his attempt to integrate psychology and linguistics. His theoretical preferences are on the side of the cognitive theorist; he believes that human behavior (e.g., language) cannot be interpreted or understood according to classical conditioning.

stimulation that is not the significate (object or referent) is a sign of that significate, if it evokes in the organism a mediating process. A word that is not the referent or object (*dog*) is a sign of that referent (the animal itself) if it evokes in a person's thought a process that relates the word to the dog. Osgood made no attempt in his definition to resolve the question of the underlying nature of the representational mediators. He did, however, separate the stimulus-response paradigm of the behaviorists into two stages: decoding and encoding. This was of particular importance to the area of language disorders because it gave comprehension a distinct role.

G. A. Miller (1965, 1967) also disagreed with the behavioristic interpretation of meaning. He believed that meaning is too complicated a phenomenon to be explained wholly in terms of conditioning, chaining responses, etc. He argued for a cognitive approach.

> If we accept a realistic statement of the problem, I believe we will also be forced to accept a more cognitive approach to it; to talk about hypothesis testing instead of discrimination learning, about the evaluation of hypotheses instead of the reinforcement of responses, about rules instead of habits, about productivity instead of generalization, about innate and universal human capacities instead of special methods of teaching vocal responses, about symbols instead of conditioned stimuli, about sentences instead of words or vocal noises, about linguistic structure instead of chains of responses—in short, about language instead of learning theory (Miller, 1965, p. 20).

Miller suggested that psychologists forgo the study of language if they found the hypothetical constructs needed for understanding meaning to be too complex, arbitrary, improbable, and mentalistic.

Linguistic Approaches to Meaning. As was true of the psychologists, early linguists preferred that other sciences define the meaning of the linguistic form because of the difficulty in defining most meaning and of demonstrating its consistency. One of these early linguists, Bloomfield (1933, p. 139), defined meaning in behavioristic terms: "We have defined the *meaning* of a linguistic form as the situation in which the speaker utters it and the response which it calls forth in the hearer."

Other linguists (N. Chomsky, 1957; Katz & Foder, 1967) supported the view that a linguistic description of a language should include the study of its semantic features. The use of grammatical explanations only seemed to ignore the fact that some sentences may differ in grammatical structure while being identical in meaning and vice versa.

Linguists who have provided theories of meaning have attempted to describe "how" language means and not how the individual learns the meaning of language. Approaches to the study of meaning by linguists are of three major types: (1) study of the relationship between the complexity of meaning and the complexity of transformations; (2) analysis of the features of words that contribute to meaning; and (3) study of verb cases that reflect meanings of word relations. These procedures have been adapted for use in teaching the language-disordered child.

• *Transformation Complexity Hypothesis.* One attempt to understand the relation between meaning and the linguistic code has been by investigating the relationship of the complexity of meaning (content) with structural complexity (form), defined by transformational grammar. A transformational grammar (TG) assigns a deep and surface structure to each sentence it generates. According to TG theory, the deep structure provides the semantic interpretation of a sentence, whereas the surface structure is phonetically determined. The procedure used to describe the relation between the structural aspects of language and its meaning and the assumption underlying this theory is what Hayes (1970) called the "correspondence hypothesis"—the hypothesis that sentence processing by the language user involves a sequence of psychological processes, and these processes correspond to the sequences in the transformational (directional) history of the sentence.

Studies have been made of the relation between the psychological level of complexity in the comprehension of specific utterances and the number of rules required by the grammar to generate these utterances (G.A. Miller, 1963a). Although these studies have not supported the thesis that performance mirrors the theoretical descriptions of grammatical complexity, and therefore indicate that this relationship alone cannot account for meaning, some materials in teaching language-disordered children are sequenced on the basis of transformational complexity, assuming that this complexity reflects the order of difficulty in content.

• *Feature Analysis.* Other linguists have employed semantic feature analysis to describe the structure of the relationship between grammar and its meaning. They believe that part of the understanding of language meaning involves comprehension of the characteristics of the word. A semantic analysis of the word *boys,* for example, might take the following form:

+ animate   + young
+ human   + plural
+ male

Word combinations can also be subject to semantic analysis. The utterance "the soldier's wife" is semantically sound while the utterance "the bachelor's wife" is meaningless because crucial semantic features of *bachelor* (− married) have been ignored in combining it with the word *wife,* which has the feature (+ married). This type of feature analysis involves an attempt to delineate all aspects of reality and to relate these to lexical and structural forms.

This approach has been used in studying the development of semantics in young children. Investigations were made of the features that appear first and the methods by which children discriminate among words. Some procedures for teaching vocabulary by identification of the feature boundaries of words have also been developed.

• *Case Theory.* Fillmore's (1968) case theory is of particular importance because it forms the basis of semantic interpretation of child language developmental behavior. It is upon this interpretation that assessment and intervention procedures in the semantic aspect of language disorders have been formulated. The basic notion in Fillmore's theory is that of *case relationships.* He viewed the basic structure of a sentence as consisting of a verb and one or more noun phrases, each of which is associated by case relationship with the verb. The basic sentence structure, which Fillmore refers to as the *proposition* (a tenseless set of relationships involving verbs and nouns), is viewed separately from the modalities such as negation, tense, mood, etc. Case notions identify certain types of judgments about events—who received the action and what was changed. For example, both sentences,

Jack broke the windshield.
A rock broke the windshield.

have a subject and predicate—a noun phrase and a verb phrase; also, the two sentences have the same surface construction. However, they differ insofar as in the first sentence, the subject (*Jack*) is an *agent* (an animate source of the action, which is identified by the verb) and in the second sentence, the subject (*rock*) is an *instrumental* (an inanimate object or force, which causes the action or state identified by the verb). The meaning of the construction is thus reflected in the verb case. Fillmore (1968) included other cases in addition to the agentive and instrumental cases described above. These include:

1. The dative, in which the animate is affected by the action or state identified by the verb (including possession). (Example: Susie gave the pencil to *Mary.*)

2. The factive, in which the being or object results from the action or state named by the verb. (Example: Mike polished the *car*.)
3. The locative, in which the place or position of the action or state identified by the verb is denoted. (Example: Robin is in the *house*.)
4. The objective, in which the role of a noun in the action or state identified by the verb is denoted by the semantic interpretation of the verb. (Example: Bill threw the *ball*.)

Fillmore's theory provides that every simple sentence is an array consisting of a verb together with a number of noun phrases. The verbs are subclassified according to the case environments that accept them; the semantic characterization of verbs relate them either to specific case elements in the environment or to elements containing specific features (such as animateness) that are obligatory accompaniments of particular cases. It was Fillmore's view that the case approach to syntactic analysis of deep structure provided a system of universal validity and was independent of such superficial differences as subject selection.

Bloom's approach (1971; Bloom and Lahey, 1978) to the relation between the form (surface structure) and its content (meaning) resembled that of Fillmore in the sense that she interpreted the form not on the basis of the relationship among external structure but on the basis of the semantic relations underlying the forms. Brown (1973) used Fillmore's cases to label children's two-word utterances on the basis of the semantic relations of the surface structures.

The linguistic approach to meaning, in which the correspondence between the grammar and its meaning is studied, has been challenged by Chomsky. He stated that nonlinguistic factors—beliefs and intentions of the speaker—enter into the interpretation of utterances in such an intimate manner that the attempt to discover a purely grammatic component of meaning is misguided (Katz, 1980).

Distinction Between Grammatic and Semantic Relations

Brown (1973) emphasized the distinction between the semantic relations described above and grammatical relations, such as subject and direct object, in his analysis of the language of children. His proposal of five processes that constitute the core of English sentence construction takes into account both types of relations, the semantic and the syntactic. These five major processes are as follows (Brown, 1973, p. 32):

1. *Semantic roles.* These include roles such as agent, instrument, and patient, which occur in simple sentences and have the surface form of word order, subject–object relations, prepositions, and postpositions.

2. *Semantic modulators.* These include forms that modify the basic sentence, such as number (e.g., the morpheme *s* added to nouns), tense (e.g. verb endings), aspect, and mood. These have the surface form of inflections or of free morphemes, which belong to small closed classes.

3. *Modalities of the simple sentence.* These include yes–no questions such as, Are you hungry?, questions that request specifying a constituent such as, Who is at home? (*Mary* is at home), negatives, and commands.

4. *Embedding.* This is characterized by a simple sentence that has a second one embedded in it in the form of a grammatical constituent or a semantic role. (The lady, who is standing by the window, is my mother.).

5. *Coordination.* This process is one by which two complete sentences or two sentences which are partially alike and partially different are joined by connector words such as *and* and *but.*

The search for a paradigm for charting the meaning of language continues. The most fruitful search will attempt to discover in all theories those elements that have validity and to reject all other elements only when the empirical evidence indicates *without doubt* that they are not valid.

The Function and Context of Language: Pragmatics

Definition of Pragmatics

Pragmatics is a term originally used by Pierce (1932) and further elaborated by C.W. Morris (1946, p. 217), who defined it as "the relationship between signs and their human users." The renewed interest in pragmatics came about through the realization that semantic and structural analyses of language did not provide an adequate and complete account of language and its development. The complete account is needed to understand the fact that "language is a social event carried out by human beings in realistic communicative contexts" (Bates et al., 1977). The application of principles of pragmatic analysis is not viewed as an ancillary or parallel aspect of the study of language structure but as an integral part of the nature and use of language by man. Bates (1976b, p. 426), states that "*all* of semantics is essentially pragmatic in nature."

The notion of pragmatics in language refers to the identification and description of factors and rules that affect the structure and use of the linguistic code. The particular choice of structures—their length, complexity, grammaticality—and the fluency and style (casual or formal) with which the structures are used are influenced by factors within the individual and his environment that are extraneous to the linguistic code itself. These factors, which are basic to the formulation of rules for the appropriate use of language, may be described under two major categories: function and context.

The Function of Language

One of the major pragmatic factors that influences language form is that of the function the language serves, both in society and in the individual, in general and at any particular time. The function most frequently referred to is the social one, that of communication; this should not imply "that the user is always and only communicating something to a listener when using linguistic signs" (Rees, 1978, p. 197). There are functions of language that are noncommunicative; these are self-directed functions (Rees, 1978).

The noncommunicative functions described by Rees are those of concept formation, self-direction, magic, and establishment of self-image. Others (Bates, 1976b) include among the functions of language that of being a tool used to (1) achieve potential and self-regulation (Luria, 1966); (2) develop the cognitive, emotional, and personality aspects of self; (3) develop relations with others; and (4) provide organization for cognitive structures.

An aspect of pragmatic development of particular importance in studying the language of children is *code-switching,* in which the function and style of the language used by the child is distinguished from the function of the language *addressed* to the child (K. Nelson, 1978). Bates describes the function of language in the young child as being associated with action—to be part of action, to accompany it, to indicate action, and to refer to it.

The basic unit in pragmatics is the speech act itself. In linguistic terms it is called the *performative.* Performative refers to the act that the speaker intends to carry out with his sentence—declaring, commanding, promising, asking questions, etc. (Bates et al., 1977).

In the adult, words may be events (Bates, 1976b, p. 427); the act of speaking is an event that has a specific intention or goal. Speech acts or *illocutions* comprise one division of utterances; the other two are *locutions* and *perlocutions.* An illocution is the conventional social act of ordering, advising, promising, etc.; it describes the intentions to command, question, etc. A locution is the actual production of the speech itself, i.e., the procedures or acts that underlie the pragmatics of reference. A perlocution creates the effects on the listener (Bates, 1976a; K. Nelson, 1978).

Oller (1978) describes some set–subset relations among speech functions. This framework begins with *acts* and identifies vocal acts (such as babbling) as a subset of acts. Conventional vocal acts serve as a subset of vocal acts and in turn have their own subset of communicative acts. A communicative act can be informative; one subset of information acts is requests. A function could be thus defined as an informal, communicative, conventional, vocal act. Oller believes that the classification of vocal acts in this manner would serve to clarify the description of linguistic functions.

The Context of Language

Context influences the form that language takes—both in comprehension and performance. It refers to factors in the environment or in the individual that influence the form of the linguistic utterance.

The environmental context may be social and/or situational. The social contexts that influence the form of language performance and comprehension are such things as (1) the listeners—the people present and the relationship between them and the speaker (kinship, age, and sex); (2) the shared intentions—the goal that communication is to accomplish and the topic; (3) the roles of the participants in the communication acts; and (4) the presuppositions that participants bring to the communication. The situational factors are such things as the time and place in which the communication occurs and the events that occurred just prior to communication (Hopper & Naremore, 1978; Hymes, 1967). The most obvious conventions occur in words that are part of a social greeting, and thus may not be interpreted literally. For example, the greeting, "How are you?" does not require an actual description of the listener's state of health. In fact, a literal response is considered inappropriate.

Individuals communicate nonverbally through gestures, eye contact, posture, etc. The form of communication is influenced by the cognitive and chronological level of the individual. In fact, each individual has a unique style of performance, which is related to intelligence, personality, and social experience.

There are rules governing the use of language for specific functions—for instance, conversation, discussion, or teaching—and for specific contexts—for instance, home, office, school, or public performance. Most individuals absorb these rules by observation and practice in real-life settings. Attempts have been made to make the rules explicit so that data may be collected and empirical judgments made on the role of pragmatics in language usage and development.

The rules for discourse within any language are highly conventional. All of these are learned by the child without official instruction. At a young age, the child learns the changing role of speaker and listener and the mutual sharing of information. The linguistic and nonlinguistic clues that signal that the listener now wishes to take part in the conversation are very specific, as are the rules that determine how many utterances must be semantically related to the topic under discussion before that topic may be changed by one of the other speakers in the group.

A LANGUAGE-AS-KNOWLEDGE MODEL

In this chapter, and in each of the subsequent three chapters, a theory or model will be presented to illustrate a specific interpretation of language, one that corresponds with the dimension discussed in the chapter. The model for this chapter will be one that describes language in terms of the linguistic code itself. Such a model reflects the linguistic point of view in defining language.

There are a number of linguistic models of language, but the one that has been most widely adapted for use in describing the nature of language disorders in children is that of Bloom and Lahey (1978). According to Bloom and Lahey (1978, p. 4), language is "a code whereby ideas about the world are represented through a conventional system of arbitrary signals for communication." The authors identified three major components of language: the content or meaning that is coded or represented, the form that codes the content, and the use or purpose of the code in a particular context. The knowledge of language is viewed as the integration of content, form, and use. Figure 2-5 illustrates this integration.

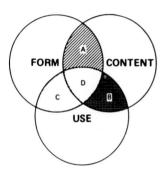

Figure 2-5
Bloom and Lahey's concept of the intersection of content, form, and use in language. (From Bloom and Lahey, 1978, p. 22. Used with permission of John Wiley & Sons.)

According to this theory, what the child acquires in learning language is a mental plan or system of rules. The rules include cognitive-linguistic rules for pairing sounds with meaning in messages, and social rules for pairing sound-meaning connections with varied types of situations. The development of language is the gradual and progressive integration of content, form, and use.

The underlying basis for speaking and understanding, according to this theory, is the knowledge of the integration of content, form, and use. Determination of the adequacy of knowledge that children have is determined by listening to and watching what children do.

The focus of Bloom and Lahey's theory, then, is language as knowledge of rules. Although they consider the rules governing content and use as part of language when they are integrated with form, content and use themselves are referred to as nonlinguistic. As stated, this model serves to illustrate the language-as-knowledge approach.

LINGUISTIC KNOWLEDGE IN AN INTEGRATIVE APPROACH TO LANGUAGE

The concept of language as being comprised of four major dimensions was introduced in Chapter 1. The present chapter has focused on the first dimension, that of the linguistic code itself. The major units that have been described are those of syntax or grammar, semantics, and pragmatics; it is the rules of these units that the child internalizes when acquiring language.

When dealing with a language-disordered child, the specialist includes as separate but related aspects of the linguistic structure evaluation (1) an analysis of the child's phonological sys-

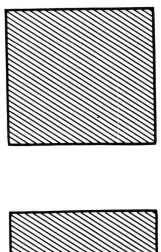

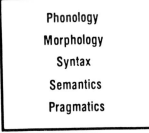

I. Units of the Linguistic Code

Phonology
Morphology
Syntax
Semantics
Pragmatics

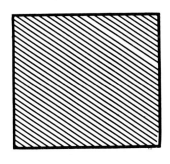

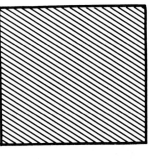

Figure 2-6
Components of the linguistic code dimension of a four-dimensional language model.

tem; (2) a study of his use of morphemes; and (3) the investigation of sentence construction and word order. Experience in studying the linguistic performance of the language-disordered child indicates that it is possible for a child to have a problem in one of these aspects of structure—such as phonology—but have no apparent problem in the other aspects. For this reason, phonology, and morphology will be listed as separate units from syntax, semantics, and pragmatics.

If the graphic code used in reading is considered to be part of the knowledge of a language (as it is in this text), the addition of graphemes (the characters used in printing and writing) is important to a complete listing of the linguistic code units. (The relationship between graphemes and phonemes will be described in Chapter 14).

The elements presented here (Fig. 2-6) form the first part of an integrative model that will be completed gradually as the subsequent three dimensions of language are presented in following chapters. This model will also be used as a construct from which to discuss theoretical and practical concepts regarding disordered language.

outline

COGNITION

External Objects of Cognition
The Cognitive Process
The Perceptual Process
The Memory Function
Conceptualization
Representation and Symbolization
Self-Regulation and Metafunctions

COGNITION AND LANGUAGE

A COGNITIVE MODEL OF LANGUAGE

COGNITION IN AN INTEGRATIVE APPROACH

the cognitive dimension

3

THE LINGUISTIC CODE is the only dimension of language that is invariant for a linguistic community; that is, each member of the community learns the same code. In order for an individual to be able to communicate with others in his linguistic environment, he must master the rules that govern the linguistic code. However, as the language code passes through each individual's unique cognitive filter, the resulting effect is a unique style of using language. Some cognitive systems permit language to reach the epitome of creative, symbolic, and logical performance, whereas other systems impede language use.

The multidimensional approach to language views cognition in language as having two roles: in the development of content and in performance. By means of the cognitive system, the child develops constructs through which percepts and concepts are formed. The cognitive system also provides the means of comprehension and producing linguistic data during language acquisition by the child and during language use by the adult. The development of meaning and the development of language performance are considered to be two separate dimensions of language in the integrative approach. This chapter will consider the cognitive processes related to the development and formation of language meaning—the percepts, concepts, and related abilities of representation and symbolization. The use of the cognitive system in the performance of language will be presented in Chapter 4.

COGNITION

Cognition has historically been considered the base upon which language develops. In general, it is believed that cognition precedes language and is a prerequisite for it. The multidimensional integrative interpretation of language considers the cognitive products of percepts and concepts to be more than a base for language; this approach views the meanings of language as an essential and integral part of it. Children who have difficulty learning the auditory vocal code because of severe hearing impairment, for example, associate another type of coded system—a manual system—with meanings. If only the auditory vocal linguistic code is considered language, those who do not use it will be considered as ignorant of language, which is inaccurate.

The relationship between language and cognition is of considerable interest to scholars. For specialists concerned with disordered language, an understanding of the types of interconnecting systems and subsystems that may exist between aspects of cognition and language is critical. Assessment and management decisions are based on the language specialist's position relative to the role of cognition in language.

In books on language development, cognition is often discussed with semantics and, in some instances, the terms are used interchangeably. If, however, the problems of the language-disordered child are to be understood, it is important to recognize the difference between the development of *meaning* and that of the *meaning of linguistic structure.* It is true that concepts such as object permanence, identity, etc., are often identified first by means of language, but these early concepts may develop prior to and separate from language use; the study of severely disordered children must take this into account. This chapter presents the development of the perceptual-conceptual system. Developmental aspects of the syntax, the semantics, and the pragmatics of language will be presented in Chapters 7–9.

External Objects of Cognition

Gibson (1971, 1972) has described three areas of knowledge about the world that serve as objects of cognition. The first area includes the distinctive features of things, such as books, apples, dogs, and voices, and the distinctive features of the external representations of things, such as pictures and symbols. The second includes knowledge of events, particularly those aspects that are invariant. Through perception of events in which one thing or person relates to or acts upon another, the common elements of these events are identified and abstracted. Gibson gave the example of the learning of size constancy, which is revealed through an event—the approach or receding of an object from the child or the child's approach or retreat from the object. The last area of information learned through cognition is structure, involving many levels of complexity. The discovery of this complexity proceeds, according to Gibson, in two directions, toward *superordination* (classification into broader or more abstract categories) or *subordination* (discrimination into more refined groups). At this point, the discussion leaves the external world and enters the internal processing system.

The Cognitive Process

The cognitive process is usually described in terms of discrete units of perception, memory, concept formation, and representation. This type of classification facilitates the understanding of the cognitive processing system but also oversimplifies it. It must be kept in mind that there is interaction among the activities (perception, memory, etc.) within the cognitive system, as well as temporal overlapping.

The Perceptual Process

Perception is a process by which an individual recognizes the features and qualities of objects, events, and relations in the external world. This process involves *discrimination,* which is the registration of differences and likenesses among things and events and the formation of primitive categories for grouping similar features and qualities. It also involves the ability to *generalize* the categories to apply to subsequent perceptions in such a manner that the new perceptions are recognized as belonging to a specific category. Implied in the functions of discrimination and generalization is the ability to abstract or identify the invariants as well as to filter out irrelevant factors in objects, events, and relations that are processed perceptually. This first level of perception is referred to by Church (1961) as participation, which he defines as an individual's organismically, reflex-like response to the physiognomic properties of a stimulus.

Decentering.   The formation of a perceptual category implies that the individual must have a series of experiences that are similar in one or more respects. Piaget (1969) distinguished between perception, which he defined as the quick, immediate view of the stimulus one gets at first glance, and perceptual activity, which involves experience, judgment, and correction of distorted first impressions. Upon exposure to a few encounters, the organism centers or fixates on the most compelling elements, thereby providing a possibility of error. Subsequent encounters *decenter* the perception to take in other details and thereby arrive at a correct perception. The need for perceptual redundancy is also reported by K. E. Nelson and K. Nelson (1978). K. Nelson (1973) found that children demand excessive redundancy for the recognition of members until the critical attributes of the category are well defined. This indicates that a significant repetition of tasks should be provided preschool children for the development of perceptual skills.

Although the individual is capable of making an almost infinite number of discriminations, they are performed on and limited to objects and events with which his society is concerned, and that have been made relevant to him. The child perceives only meaningful objects, and he perceives their meaning as much as, if not more than, the objects themselves (Church, 1961).

Perceptual Constancy. The ability to correctly classify the changing impressions of constan' objects is called *perceptual constancy*. Sizes, shapes, and colors snould be perceived correctly even when viewed from angles and perspectives that make them look distorted. This ability evolves from experience with moving objects. Movement seems to endow objects with qualities they lack entirely when at rest. According to Piaget (1969), perceptual constancy sets the stage for conservation, which is really constancy of quantity, number, weight, etc., despite changes in form. The importance of movement is apparent in children who cannot move because of physical impairment; ordinary experiences with touch, smell, vision, and proprioception are limited, and, consequently, so is perception and the development of related concepts.

Identity, Equivalence, and Object Permanence. Categorization at the perceptual level consists of the process of *identification,* which is the act of placing a stimulus input into a certain class by virtue of its defining attributes. Members of a perceptual category are not always exactly the same; they may represent different forms of the same event. A figure is perceived as having an identity when it is seen immediately as similar to some figures and dissimilar to others; this recognition is spontaneous and may occur on first exposure to the new stimulus object. The object that is perceived as having identity can be easily associated with other objects (or actions); lack of this capability will result in poor recall of the object, as well as poor recognition and naming (Hebb, 1949). A further distinction can be made between the *identity response* and the *equivalence response.* If a variety of stimuli are forms of the same thing (e.g., different sizes of triangles), their classification is called an identity response. An equivalence response classifies different things as the same (e.g., a rocker and a high chair are both chairs). According to Bruner, Goodnow, and Austin (1956), both responses depend upon the acceptance of certain properties of objects as being relevant and others as being irrelevant. This implies that both positive and negative experiences are necessary for developing categories.

Factors that determine the relevant characteristics of objects are the *permanence* of objects and the *movement* and change of objects. Ordinarily, objects and the events surrounding them are consistent and predictable (Gibson, 1966). Because of this object permanence, the consistent and inconsistent aspects of an event can be registered. Movement of objects also signals the important information to be perceived; the movement of a specific object in relation to other static objects, or in relation to the child, places the moving object in relief and thus calls attention to the object (Bloom & Lahey, 1978). The concept of object permanence also includes the understanding that objects continue to exist while they are out of sight. Research has indicated that the concept of object performance is a necessary development for the emergence of first words.

Perceptual Closure and Figure-Ground Perception.   Once perceptual categories have been formed, the categories are utilized in each subsequent perception by permitting *reconstruction* of a stimulus whose properties may be defective. The perceiver "fills in" features that may be absent or incomplete. This process is referred to as perceptual *closure*. The individual reacts to the stimulus as if it were complete.

Perception of a stimulus occurs in an environment; the perception of an auditory stimulus occurs in noise of some kind, and the perception of a visual stimulus takes place in a visual plane where there are numerous other colors, forms, etc., also present. The perceiver must be able to attend to the stimulus selected for processing and to ignore the irrelevant competing background environment. This ability is a special quality of perception. The relationship between the foreground and background is referred to as *figure-ground perception.*

Perception: An Active Process.   The organization of information received by the perceiver is a twofold procedure according to Piaget (1954, 1969). New information is either *assimilated* into existing structures or it is *accommodated.* Accommodation is the reorganization of existing structures or the creation of a new one to permit the incorporation of information that does not correspond to existing structures. This procedure is operating at all times during the reception of information and results in what Piaget refers to as *adaptive behavior.* Perception, therefore, cannot be thought of as a passive process. It involves strategies of exploring, focusing, and monitoring the external world as well as processing the input when it is received. The perceptual process, therefore, is made up of multiple stages, and at each level the perceiver is actively engaged either in selecting that which is to be perceived or in analyzing and synthesizing the input and reconstructing it in a manner suitable for storage.

This means that there is no such thing as a "simple perception." Perceptions are complex and additive; their apparent simplicity is only the end result of a long learning process (Hebb, 1949).

The Memory Function

Memory and Perception.   The perception function is basic to the memory function in that it provides the data upon which the memory operates. Memory is also basic to perception; the act of recognition of an even primitive categorization of a stimulus implies prior experience with the perceptual event and the memory of that event. Asch (1968, p. 217) stated that "the perception of motion or of auditory configurations, are instances of organization among immediately past and present stimulation. . . . the memory traces which participate in the process do not simply add their sensory content to the incoming stimulations; rather they impose a particular structure on a percept."

The formation of perceptual categories is dependent upon memory of the perceptual attributes of what is being perceived. When a pair of stimuli is perceived for discrimination and categorization, the individual can compare the two and judge their likenesses and differences. However, when a single perception is received and judged for categorization, it must be compared against a perceptual category that is reconstructed from the memory storage. This reinforces the importance of memory for adequate perception and indicates that perception involves experience, judgment, and correction of first impressions (Piaget, 1969).

Types of Memory.   Memory refers specifically to the power or ability to retain, revive, or retrieve past events that have been perceived or past thoughts or ideas about these events. The length of time between the event and its retention or revival is used to differentiate between long- and short-term memories. An operational definition of short-term memory was given by Olson (1973, p. 146) as the "limited capacity store within which the initial or terminal computations of reception or of productions are performed . . . largely oriented toward preserving transient features of the environment long enough so that relatively slow mental processes have a chance to operate upon environmental input." Thus, the primary function of short-term memory is to "hold information in momentary abeyance and possibly transform it somewhat to conform to one's long-term storage mechanisms (assimilation) or change one's long-term storage mechanisms to conform to the new information (accomodation)" (Muma, 1978, p. 58). Warrington (1971) stressed that subvocal rehearsal is necessary for the transfer of information into short-term memory storage. If this rehearsal is interfered with, the information held in sensory storage disappears and cannot be recalled.

Auditory and Visual Memory.   The auditory memory stores temporal events occuring in time sequence, and the visual memory stores spatial information that is received simultaneously. Not only do the auditory and visual memories deal with different types of events, they also differ in the manner in which events are processed. The visual and auditory short-term memory stores are similar in that they both hold information in a primitive or prelinguistic form; the stores differ in that the acoustic memory lasts for a second or two while the visual store is usually believed to persist only for a quarter of a second. Crowder (1972, p. 256) explained the superiority in *persistence* of the auditory over the visual storage: "The reception of stimuli in vision depends in large part upon the voluntary direction of attention (gaze) and thus the human being can often arrange for the persistence of the *stimulus itself* without needing a persistent stimulus trace." Furthermore, insofar as perception is dependent upon availability of contextual information, vision can capitalize on the parallel availability of context from a wide spatial array whereas audition is restricted to the temporal array furnished by memory.

Memory and Language.   The relation of memory to language is integral. Long-term memory participates in language by storing the categorical images of perceptions, which are the basic factors of conceptualization and meaning. Memory also assists in the organization and comprehension of images and retains the association between the arbitrary symbols of language and these images. The memory retention and revival systems are also utilized in maintaining the association between the perceived acoustic speech stimulus and its articulatory counter-parts. Wherever serial order is significant in language, memory allows this order to be maintained. The ability to comprehend sentences depends partly upon the ability to remember certain of the temporally presented constituents of the sentence while processing others. (This latter aspect of memory will be reviewed in Chapter 4.)

Although the relationship between memory and language is usually described as one in which memory aids the development of the linguistic code, Muma (1978, p. 58) has suggested that this relationship is more accurately described in reverse, i.e., that language facilitates both storage and retrieval processes.

Conceptualization

Concepts and Percepts.   The products of perceptual activity and memory functioning are called concepts. Concepts are an individual's categorical responses to a number of objects or events as though they were all the same. This process, by which cognitive skills are developed, involves, according to Neisser (1967), the reduction, transformation, and conceptual coding of experience so that it can be kept in memory.

There are two levels of categorization—perceptual and conceptual. As described previously, categorization at the perceptual level is accomplished by identification, the process of placing a stimulus input into a certain class on the basis of its attributes. Identification involves a "fit" between the perceptual attributes of a stimulus input (object) and the specifications of the category. In categorization at the conceptual level, however, the "fit" occurs between the abstract characteristics of the object itself and the category. Perceptual and conceptual categories are developed by the same process but by using different cues and materials. Developmentally, perceptual concepts occur first; children possess an *iconic* imagery orientation, in which they attend to perceptual properties such as color, size, shape, and number (Bruner, 1964). Only gradually are they able to integrate their perceptions to arrive at a functional wholeness of objects and events. Concepts develop slowly, from the specific to the abstract. The degree of abstraction is related to the degree of experience with an event or concept.

A further distinction between perception and conception was made by Piaget (1954, 1969). He believed that since perception is based upon immediate experience, it is subject to error. Conception, however, is dependent on thought, which can go back in time, review the evidence, and form a judgment strong enough to overcome the perceptual illusion.

Related to the distinction between perception and conception is the differentiation between nonverbal and verbal concepts.

Nonverbal concepts are known primarily through experience with referents, whereas verbal concepts are learned through verbal descriptions and explanations. Perceptual categories are usually nonverbal, whereas conceptual ones are usually verbal. A further distinction was made by Piaget (1954; Pulaski 1971), who defined knowledge about objects as figurative and operational. Figurative knowledge applies to information about the physical appearance of objects and the mental schema that made recognition of the object possible. Operative knowledge describes the mental schemas for acting that arise from children's actions and patterns of activity with objects.

Concept Boundaries.   The boundaries between categories are not always clearly defined. In many instances, particularly with respect to perceptual categories, the boundaries form arbitrary learned divisions for nondiscrete data. These boundaries will reflect, in many cases, the experience or experiences from which a concept was developed. Concept boundaries thus vary with individuals insofar as their range of experiences differ. This failure of concepts to correspond on a one-to-one basis from individual to individual indicates that the classes of categories do not exist in the environment. They are imposed on the environment. Bruner, Goodnow, and Austin (1956) said that the environment provides the cues for classification but that the same cues may be and are grouped differently by individuals. For example, a child raised in a rural area may consider the dog and the wolf as belonging to different categories, whereas an urban child unfamiliar with these animals may put them in the same category.

Rosch (1973), in a study of the internal structure of categories, agreed that concepts had ill-defined boundaries, but felt that other categories are highly structured internally. She defined the internal structure as the *core meaning* of categories. This core meaning consists of the clearest case or best example of the category. Furthermore, she proposed that the core meaning for concrete categories, such as form and color, is not arbitrary, but "given" by the human perceptual system; consequently, the basic content and structure of these categories are universal among languages. Rosch concluded from investigations of this theory that color and form categories develop differently from other categories because members of these categories are perceptually more salient than other stimuli in the same category domain. Supporting this conclusion are Rosch's findings that the natural prototypes—the perceptually salient members—were learned more rapidly than other colors and forms and with fewer errors.

Learning object categories differs from learning attribute categories, according to K. E. Nelson and K. Nelson (1978). The subordinate members of object categories (such as dog, cat, etc.) are learned before the superordinate object category (animal). With color, however, children respond more appropriately to the domain of color than they do to individual colors.

Types of Concepts. There are many concept types that a child must learn in his prelanguage period. The following form the basic nucleus upon which early language is formed.

•*Attributes.* Attributes of objects and events are received through the sensory channels to form early perceptual categories. E. Clark (1974) has listed the sensory-perceptual modalities employed for different categories of classification as follows: (1) shape: visual, tactile; (2) movement: visual, auditory; (3) size: visual, tactile, (4) sound: auditory; (5) taste: gustatory, olfactory; and (6) texture: visual, tactile. Data regarding body position, body movement, and body direction are received proprioceptively or internally from the body.

•*Body Concept.* The attainment of percepts and concepts about the real world is first of all dependent upon a stable body percept. The relations between the environment, the perception of it, and the body percept are reciprocal; that is, they rely on each other in their development, although they must remain separate and polar (Werner, 1965). The body concept itself has been looked upon in terms of a dynamic organization of essential centers of activity with more peripheral elements being superordinative (Merleau-Ponty, 1962). The functions of self-regulation and the awareness of "self" as a psychic structure should be related at some basic level of conceptualization. It is the integration and synthesis of the two that harmonizes the internal and external flow of events (Sander, 1977).

The central dimensions of body concept for development of percepts and concepts are those of posture and integrity of relation of body parts. Information that provides for this integrity, for the separateness of the body from the environment, and for awareness of the role of the body in comprehending the world comes from the proprioceptive mechanism whereby sensory data is sent from all parts of the body to its center and back, as well as from the movement of the body, which allows for various kinds of proprioceptive and exteroceptive data to be integrated. The concept whereby a child understands himself as a separate being is called *distancing.* Sigel and Cocking (1977) described distancing behavior as stimulus situations (social and physical events) that create distance (temporal, spatial, or psychological) between self and the object or environment.

•*Space Perception.* The self-concept is a prerequisite for the development of space perception. The concept of space is a relative one that uses the body as a point of reference for the development of dimension (size), position, location, direction, distance, etc. The three planes of space—horizontal, diagonal, and vertical—correspond to the child's positions during growth (pre-crawling, crawling, and walking). The knowledge of space as it refers to self is extrapolated to the relation of events and objects to each other in space. H. H. Clark (1973) stated that after the child learns perceptual space (p-space), he learns to apply spatial terms in his language to the p-space and so the structure of his space determines, in large part, the terms that he learns and how quickly he learns them (*big/little; near/far; up/down; north/south;* etc.).

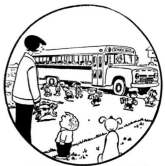

"Why does the driver sit on one side of the bus when she picks Billy up and on the OTHER side when she brings him home?"

A child's concepts of spatial relations are absolute until he realizes that shifts in the space direction/position of others are related to his own position. (The Family Circus, by Bil Keane, reprinted courtesy of The Register and Tribune Syndicate, Inc.)

• *Time Concepts.* The time schema seems to be more difficult for children to learn than the spatial one because the point of reference in temporal events is constantly changing. The future and the past vary with the present: today will be yesterday tomorrow. In addition to the seriation of temporal events, the child must learn the spacial aspects of time, the "length" of days and the shortness of minutes. If time concepts have not developed, the child will have difficulty with the parts of language that express time—with the terms "later," "now," "last month," and with the grammatical forms of "ed" denoting past, etc.

• *Relational Concepts.* Subsequent to the development of classifications for objects and their attributes is the development of relational concepts; that is, the relations of the child himself to other persons and to objects and the relations of these objects and persons to the child and to each other. These relations arise, according to Piaget (1970) and others (Leonard, 1976; Sinclair, 1971), out of the activity of children during the sensorimotor period and also from the integration of spatial, temporal, and self concepts.

As a result of such activity, the child will come to (1) anticipate the object (person) when not present; (2) nominate the object by performing in an abbreviated mode the action schema most habitually associated with it; and (3) cause the object to recur or preserve the events by first accidentally producing the event or effect and then deliberately repeating the action so that the event recurs (Brown, 1973; Leonard, 1976; Sinclair, 1971). These behaviors of anticipation, nomination, and recurrence are reflected in the early words of children.

Later relations involve the use of objects (including people) to serve the child's own goals (Bates et al., 1975). This is referred to as the child's use of means to attain an end. It may include the use of human agents to manipulate objects or the use of objects to manipulate people. In the child's perception, all things, events, pictures, etc., are equally real. The use of words as a means to an end is one of the first pragmatic functions of language. The development of self-perception, of relational concepts, and of the interaction between self and others leads to

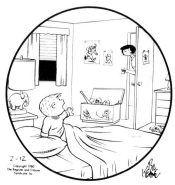

"Don't turn on the darkness yet."

The light switch is the cause of darkness in the room, since when it is flipped, the room is darkened. (The Family Circus, by Bil Keane, reprinted courtesy of The Register and Tribune Syndicate, Inc.)

verbal exchanges between a child and those in his environment. As the child becomes aware of the speaker–listener roles, he is able to use words that signal the shift in roles—the pronouns I, you, he, etc.

Cause-effect relations are at first built on perceptual and pragmatic effects. If two events occur in visual or auditory proximity, they are assumed to relate in a causal manner. Delayed or hidden effects are not recognized by the child. The child learns pragmatic sequences, however: a block tower topples if it is hit; milk spills if the glass is bumped (Church, 1961). He may relate the absence of one event with the presence of another. Children appear, however, to have little curiosity about causal connections—events are accepted on surface value.

Representation and Symbolization

To *represent* means to stand in the place of. A photograph is a representation of a real person or object; an ambassador represents a president at a political affair; a dove is used to represent peace. The representations may be concrete or abstract; in the case of the dove-peace representation, the dove is a concrete representative of an abstract idea. When the representation is used in the place of a real person, object, or event, it becomes a symbol of it. A photograph is not a symbol of a person, but a dove is a symbol of peace. Not all representations are symbols, but all symbols are representations. Figure 3-1 illustrates the differences between representation and symbols.

In the development of cognitive behavior, the individual learns to represent the world of events internally. He cannot place the actual persons, objects, or events inside of his brain so he deals with these reality events through representations; he

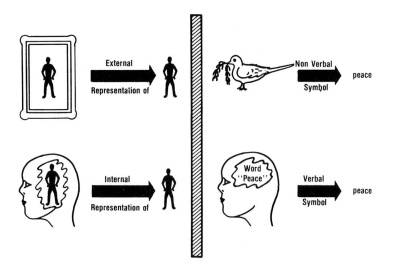

Figure 3-1
Illustration of differences among external and internal representation and nonverbal and verbal symbols.

develops a mental substitute for the real thing. Piaget (1954, 1962) used the term *image* to refer to the internal representations. If the mental image is a specific copy of reality, Piaget refers to it as a representative image. If the image is only remotely connected with what it represents, he calls it a symbol (Pulaski 1971).

Developmentally, representation appears to emerge in an intermediate stage between perception and conceptualization and continues past conceptualization into symbolization. Piaget proposed that everything past the stage of immediate perception is representation. Memories, images, concepts, and abstract symbols (such as words) are all forms of representation.

According to Piaget, imitation bridges the gap between sensorimotor behavior and symbolization. Instead of looking at and handling an object, the child begins to act like the object. The child's movements in imitation indicate that there has been an internalization of the object or its function and the child replicates this function in his own system. For instance, he hears a train whistle and makes a sound exactly like it.

Play, using a form of pretending such as imitation, suggests the use of representations. Piaget referred to this type of play as symbolic play. In symbolic play, the child uses substitutes for actual objects. A kitchen pan may be used for a crown and a spoon for a scepter. The pan and spoon are substitutes for the real objects, and, as such, are symbols for the mental image of these objects in the mind of the child. Children first use themselves and then other objects in symbolic games—as when pretending to use the telephone and then having a doll use it. The use of imitation and symbolic play is related to the development of mental images. Mental images are the form in which events are represented internally. They are personal and resemble the object or thing they represent. They may take the form of visual images, auditory images, or movement. Deferred imitation or play cannot take place unless there is an ability to remember events or objects through images.

The symbolic behaviors described above lead into the use of words as symbols and, therefore, into language. Morehead and Morehead (1974, pp. 153–154) stated, "Just as walking frees the child's upper body from gravity, so representation frees the child from the immediate present (i.e., perception and actions) and allows him to re-present reality (i.e., deferred imitation, imagery, symbolic play, language, etc.). . . ." The initial words of children are used as signs; they indicate and may even resemble that which they refer to. Once the child creates mental substitutes for things, the things do not need to be present in order for the child to deal with them. Then the child can begin to use words as abstract symbols—the shared symbols used in language.

Self-Regulation and Metafunctions

The development of psychological distancing and symbolization leads to the development of self-awareness and self-regulation. When a child is able to symbolize what transpires in his environment, he is no longer bound to his perceptions; he can represent what is occuring, can view it, and can regulate his own behavior. There is consequently a reduction of egocentric perceptions and an increase of social ones. From this ability to symbolize, the child develops a consciousness of his own mental operations. Vygotsky (1962) describes this change as a transference of mental operations from the plane of action to that of language. There is, according to Flavell & Wellman (1980) a difference between doing (unthoughtful response of an actor in a continuous transaction with his environment) and being aware of doing. In the latter behavior, the actor steps out of the flow of conduct and treats it as the subject of thought. The behavior in which one's own cognitive processes become the focus of voluntary, selective attention is called *metacognition.* The analysis and study of specific aspects of cognition as each is being performed are called metaperception, metamemory, and metacommunication or metalinguistics (Flavell & Wellman, 1980). The capacity to engage in metacognition and metalinguistics permits a child to take the role of others in viewing the events of reality. In taking the role of others, the child begins to construct a different level of ideas of things, of self, and of society (Mead, 1934). In a way, he becomes his own student, his own teacher, and his own parent.

The metalinguistic function is of particular importance in language pathology. In language intervention, the attention of the child being taught to speak or read is focused on the sounds of speech, on the meanings of words, and on syntactic patterns. Cazden (1973) described metalinguistic awareness as an ability to make language forms "opaque" so that they can be attended to in and for themselves. Metalinguistics is, according to Cazden, a special kind of language performance, one that makes special cognitive demands and appears less easily acquired than speaking and listening. One can teach children metalinguistic

Although Thomas Wolfe incorrectly viewed letters as symbols of speech, he realized the importance of language for putting order into the child's world.

... There he would crawl on the vast design of the carpet, his eyes intent upon great wooden blocks piled chaotically on the floor. They had belonged to his brother, Luke: all the letters of the alphabet, in bright multi-colored carving, were engraved upon them.

Holding them clumsily in his tiny hands, he studied for hours the symbols of speech, knowing that he had held the stones of the temple of language, and striving desperately to find the key that would draw order and intelligence from this anarchy.*

*From Thomas Wolfe: *Look Homeward Angel,* p. 39. Copyright 1929 by Charles Scribner's Sons; copyright renewed 1957 by Edward C. Aswell, Administrator, C.T.A. Reprinted with the permission of Charles Scribner's Sons.

functions by assisting them in developing a perceptual aware-ness of language—by talking about it and by allowing children to take the role of other students and of the teacher in language activities. Language needs to be made accessible to children, through methods such as word play and rhyming, for attention and playful manipulation outside of communicative contexts (Cazden, 1973).

COGNITION AND LANGUAGE

In some instances, the term cognition refers to abstract activi-ties that are engaged in when a person is "thinking." The rela-tion of thought and language has been of philosophical interest for decades and has consistently stimulated debate and contro-versy. On one hand, there are those who believe that language is the essence of thought. The others consider that language offers precision, stability, and economy of effort to thought, but is not absolutely necessary to thinking. They feel that mental activity can proceed without words and that language has a much wider function than serving as signs for thought.

The relationship between language and thought is of theoreti-cal and practical importance to the language specialist; the un-derstanding of this relationship is necessary for interpreting the order of acquisition of semantic and grammatic forms. Lan-guage specialists ask, "To what extent are cognitive factors re-sponsible for language disorders and to what extent should assessment and remediation take them into account?"

Jenkins (1969), in summarizing the literature on language and thought, identified three positions (Nos. 1–3 below) on the in-terdependence of thought (cognition) and language. Three more (Nos. 4–6) are modified from those proposed by Bates et al. (1977).*

1. Thought and language are the same.
   $$<L = T>$$
2. Thought is dependent upon langauge.
   $$<L \rightarrow T>$$
3. Language is dependent upon thought.
   $$<T \rightarrow L>$$
4. Developmentally, language and thought emerge as separate and independent functions.
   $$<L \quad T>$$
   $$\uparrow \quad \uparrow$$
5. Language and thoughts are derived from the same separate source.
   $$<L \quad T>$$
   $$\nwarrow_S \nearrow$$

*Modified with permission from Bates E et al. From gesture to the first word: On cognitive and social prerequisites. In Lewis M & Rosenblum LA (Eds): *Interaction, Conversation and the Development of Language.* New York: John Wiley & Sons, 1977, pp. 259, 263.

6. Language and thought, although separate, proceed through the same developmental sequences, which are basic to problem solving in complex cognitive systems.

$$\left\langle \begin{array}{l} S_1 \to S_2 \to L \\ S_1 \to S_2 \to T \end{array} \right\rangle$$

Positions 1 and 2 were accepted by early writers. Watson (McGuigan, 1966) supported the extreme position, the viewpoint that language and thought are synonomous. He described thinking as implicit movement of the speech musculature and seemed to consider thinking to be a form of subvocal talking. Position 2, that thought depends on language, was most widely accepted by Luria (1961); his thesis was that language is a second signal system, which controls and regulates all other internal and external responses. The linguistic relativity theories of Whorf (1967) would also fit into this second position. Whorf theorized that the world view held by members of specific cultures is determined to a large extent by the language they speak. Thus the individual's cognitive processes (the way he perceives reality) are influenced by language. Support for Whorf's hypothesis is provided by studies that show that the attachment of verbal labels to categories of events or objects can aid in remembering the categories (Brown & Lenneberg, 1954; Vygotsky, 1962).

Position 3 states that language is dependent on thought or cognition. This position is widely held by theorists in language development and cultural anthropology. Levi-Strauss (1963) proposed that thought determines the structure of language— an analysis of language yields categories of thought that are universal and characteristic of human logic. A strong supporter of the thesis that language is dependent on cognition is Piaget (1954, 1969). According to Piaget's theory, the development of sensorimotor behavior is necessary to, and precedes, symbolic behavior and language.

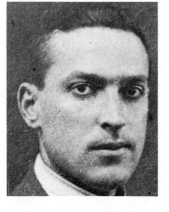

Lev Semenovich Vygotsky

Lev Semenovich Vygotsky began his systematic work in psychology in 1924, when he was 28 years old. With his students and co-workers (among whom was another well-known Russian psychologist, Aleksander Luria), Vygotsky launched a series of investigations in developmental psychology and psychopathology that terminated in the publication of several monographs on the psychology of the child and adolescent. Before he died of tuberculosis at the age of 38, he had acquired a nearly encyclopedic knowledge of psychology, philosophy, linguistics, literature, and the arts. At his death, he left close to eighty unpublished manuscripts. His most widely known book in the United States is *Thought and Language*, which appeared in Russia in 1934 and was translated into English in 1962.

Vygotsky's methods for studying the successive stages of mental growth have been widely used. He formulated a theory based on his studies that accounts for the development of specifically human functions. According to this theory, the child gradually internalizes cultural "tools" (including language), which mediate and guide his thinking. Vygotsky's arguments are still debated in literature pertaining to the relationship between language and thought; his position and writings with regard to this relationship reflected his criticism of Piaget's theories about cognition and language.

THE COGNITIVE DIMENSION

Position 4, the claim that language and thought have independent sources and sequences of development, has some support in the works of McNeill (1966, 1970), who has proposed a native, autonomous syntactic component in language. A modification of this position was held by Vygotsky (1962). He postulated a preintellectual period in speech and a prespeech period in thinking. He did not believe the connection between thought and speech to be a primary one, but one that originates, changes, and grows in the course of the development of both processes. Vygotsky further stated that there is a constant crossing between speech and thought; he considered the relation between the two to be a process. Vygotsky believed that once a child's speech becomes internalized, it serves to guide thought. Bates et al. (1977) suggested a modification of positions 2 and 4 to represent the ideas of Vygotsky.

$$<L \leftrightarrow T>$$
$$\uparrow \qquad \uparrow$$

Bates et al. (1977) described position 5 as one in which language and thought are derived from the same separate source. An interpretation of Lenneberg's view, in which categorization and extraction of properties (the perceptual system) are basic to both language and cognition, might exemplify this position. The formula would be written

$$< \, L \searrow_P \nearrow^T \, >$$

in which P is the perceptual system. Another advocate of this position is Pascual-Leone (1970), who suggested that increased information-processing capacity might affect the development of both language- and nonlanguage-processing skills, such as memory. Position 5 is considered by Bates et al. to be the most tenable model for the interaction among cognition, language, and social factors. The common factors are operative principles that are available to children at given developmental states.

Position 6 relates language and thought by analogy. Proponents of this position project a sequence of organizational development within thought and within language that is similar in process but not necessarily transferred from one to the other. In other words, language and cognition might go through similar sequences in development, not because of some shared source but because of the nature of problem solving in complex systems (Bates et al., 1977).

Although there is no agreement as to the relation between language and thought, there seems to be support for the contention that, once developed, language widely extends thought. The use of symbols shortens the process and extends the power of thinking. Black and Moore (1955) believe that language influ-

An insightful description of the role of language in thought, in behavior, and in society is provided by James Michener in his book, *Chesapeake.*

But always he lacked the essential tool without which the workman can never attain true mastery: he did not know the names of any of the parts he was building, and without names he was artistically incomplete. It was not by accident that doctors and lawyers and butchers invented specific but secret names for things they did; to possess the names was to know the secret. With correct names one entered into a new world of proficiency, became the member of an arcane brotherhood, a sharer of mysteries, and in the end a performer of merit. Without the names one remained a bumbler or in the case of boat-building, a mere house carpenter.*

*From James A. Michener: *Chesapeake.* New York: Random House, 1978, pp. 264–265. Reprinted with permission.

ences thought by providing the cognitive system with means of analyzing thinking, drawing abstract conclusions by inference, and conceiving the complex structure of the world.

If humans did not grasp events and objects in the environment according to the perceptual commonalities of the objects, each behavioral response would be unique, and there would be no need for language to "hold" the perceptions together. But humans do perceive commonalities and language assists them in retaining these perceptions. The symbolic process also helps to designate the points at which perceptual differences are distinctive within a culture. Language assists cognitive development; it mediates between the world and concepts. Concepts, in their turn, are the content of language, the meanings to which the words, phrases, and sentences of language are connected. Thus, the cognitive structures of humans permit them to acquire the knowledge of language and to internalize the association between the linguistic code and reality.

A COGNITIVE MODEL OF LANGUAGE

The model provided in Chapter 3 illustrated the interpretation of language from the point of view of the linguistic code and its form, content, and function (Bloom & Lahey, 1978). In this chapter, the model used to illustrate the cognitive approach to language is that of Piaget. Many theories of language describe language without reference to its cognitive dimensions (Chomsky, 1965; Skinner, 1957). Other theories allude to the cognitive system as a necessary prerequisite for language, but either omit it entirely from the language description (considering the concepts to be "nonlinguistic") or treat content in terms of linguistic structural meanings alone (Bloom & Lahey, 1978). A model of cognition that has integrated the process and products of cognition with language in the various stages of early development is that of Piaget (Inhelder & Piaget, 1958; Piaget, 1969).

Piaget described four cumulative stages of cognitive development that he considered to be essential parts of language development.

Stage One.   From birth to age two, the child's environmental adaptation is through the sensorimotor system. During this stage, the child's mental activity consists of establishing relationships between sensory experience and action by the physical manipulation of the world. As the child acts on objects through the sensorimotor system, he obtains knowledge of perceptual invariants of the environment. His internal representation of reality begins as does his use of symbols as a means of representation. This is the stage that Piaget considers to be an essential basis for learning to symbolize and, thereby, for learning language. The specific substages of stage one are as follows (Leonard, 1978; Morehead & Morehead, 1974):

1. *Substage 1: Birth to 2 months.* The infant is supine. Sensorimotor behavior is limited to reflexes, but even at this early stage the first modification of reflexes occur; for example, the sucking reflex is modified when the child searches for a desired object. All vocal or prelinguistic behavior is also reflexive and consists mainly of crying.
2. *Substage 2: 2–4 months.* The child begins to support his head. Coordinated sensorimotor behavior emerges as the child coordinates hand-to-mouth motions and coordinates looking with grasping and looking with listening. At this stage, the child is attracted by movement. Experience with observing objects from different perspectives lays the foundation for perceptual constancy. The child also begins to anticipate and will look at the spot where an object was previously. Vocal behavior consists of chuckling, gurgling, and cooing.
3. *Substage 3: 4–8 months.* The child has now freed himself from gravity and can sit alone and crawl from one spot to another. At this stage, the child begins to interact with the environment and discovers that he can act on objects with a limited number of actions, such as striking, rubbing, shaking, or swinging. The first awareness of self as separate from objects begins. Searching for objects continues, and the child now looks and grasps for the missing object. The child begins to babble and imitate sound production.
4. *Substage 4: 8–12 months.* The child now stands, creeps rapidly, begins to take steps, and can grasp. The child increases the motor patterns he can use with objects, and appears to understand that he has caused an action or was the agent of an action that occurred in some location in space. He continues to search for missing objects but in the place when he last found them—not in the place he last saw them. The child produces his first words.
5. *Substage 5: 12–18 months.* The child now moves freely with a stiff propulsive gait. He can throw a ball and stack several blocks. Now, as he handles objects, he tries to discover their

function and their properties. He constantly produces new behaviors and searches for missing objects where they "disappear," suggesting a degree of object permanence. Single-word utterances, usually associated with an ongoing event, predominate.

Stage Two.   From approximately age 2 to age 7, the child passes through the second major stage of development, the preoperational stage, in which he rapidly learns to represent objects and events by symbolic means. The symbols (images and words) are substitutes for the sensorimotor activities of infancy. He has acquired knowledge of spatial, temporal, and causal relationships and begins to use the language structure that symbolizes them. In this stage, the child begins logical thought. He discriminates and classifies, forming both subordinate and superordinate categories.

Stage Three.   Piaget refers to the stage covering the ages of 7–11, as the period of concrete operations. Operations (thoughts) are freed from physical performance and can thus be projected forward or backward in time and space. The term *concrete operations* refers to the child operating on concrete objects or that which represents them, through thinking. Existing mental structures are combined into new relationships by differentiation, extention, serialization, etc. The child produces hierarchical arrangements of objects. His language reflects these developments.

Stage Four.   The period of formal operations begins at 11 or 12 years and continues through adulthood. The adolescent can now "operate on operations," which means that he can think about thought. Formal operations concern the general laws or rules behind an array of particular instances. At this stage, the adolescent can develop a hypothesis and figure out what should follow, even if the hypothesis is false.

In each of these stages, Piaget has described cognitive behaviors that assist in the internal classification and structuring of the external world. Piaget regards these behaviors as nonlinguistic in that they derive from action and can develop without use of the linguistic code. He considers the use of the code as one aspect of the child's ability to represent and symbolize the world. In other words, language does not only depend on cognitive behaviors but is a part of these behaviors. Thus, he considers thought to involve more than language. It involves representations (visual images, auditory images, mental symbols, etc.) and operations (internalized actions such as combining and taking away).

The development of the content of language involves the translation of objects, events, and relations from their external existence to an internal representation of them. In the process of internalizing the world, humans group, classify, and organize objects and events so that the brain can store the information in an efficient manner and utilize the information for thinking, acting, communicating, and relating. The process by which this translation takes place is called cognition, and the units involved are sensation, perception, memory, conceptualization, representation, and symbolization. Adding the units of this second dimension to the integrative model introduced in Chapter 2 produces the second part of our four-dimensional language model (Fig. 3-2). It should be noted that there are arrows connecting the two dimensions, indicating a relationship between them and moving in a reciprocal manner. This reflects four types of relationships: (1) Development of cognitive elements is essential to the development of the linguistic code. (The extent to which cognition and language are related developmentally is discussed in Chapter 6.) (2) Cognition and language are related in that the structure and organization of meaning in language reside in the cognitive system; meaning is as essential to language as is the code. (3) Language provides the cognitive system with means for imitation, representation, and symbolization, which expand the means achieved through imagery and action. (4) Both cognitive and linguistic knowledge are used in the acts of comprehending and producing language.

COGNITION IN AN INTEGRATIVE APPROACH

Figure 3-2
Components of the linguistic code and the cognitive dimensions of a four-dimensional language model.

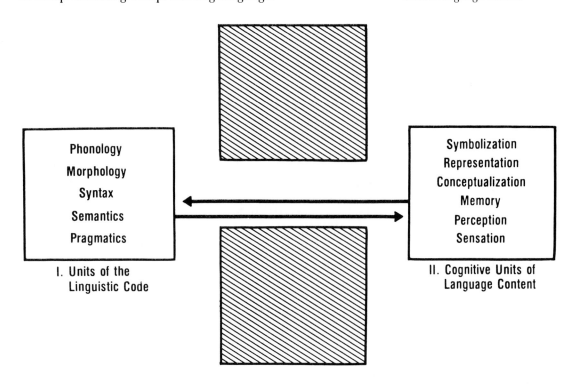

Phonology
Morphology
Syntax
Semantics
Pragmatics

I. Units of the
Linguistic Code

Symbolization
Representation
Conceptualization
Memory
Perception
Sensation

II. Cognitive Units of
Language Content

outline

COMPREHENSION

Stage 1: Speech Perception
Categorical Perception
Analysis by Synthesis
Memory and Speech Perception
Stage 2: Lexical and Syntactic Processing
Lexical Access and Syntactic Representation
Memory and Lexical-Syntactic Processing
Output of the Lexical-Syntactic Processing Stage
Stage 3: Representation of Meaning

PRODUCING LANGUAGE

Encoding
The Form of the Idea
Planning Units in Production
Coding Order
Phonological Coding
The Encoded Characteristics of Language
Language Production and Memory
Voluntary and Automatic Production

THE BRAIN AND LANGUAGE

The Brain and Speech Processing
Developmental Aspects of Dominance
Hemispheric Specialization

A PROCESS MODEL OF LANGUAGE

AN INTEGRATIVE APPROACH TO LANGUAGE PERFORMANCE

the dimension of language performance

4

 F OR LANGUAGE-DISORDERS SPECIALISTS, the focus of
interest in the past 10 years has alternated among three language dimensions—linguistic structure (the form), cognition
(the content), and the pragmatics of the communication system
(the use). The theoretical explications and research findings of
these areas of study have formed the bases for management of
the language-disordered child. These, however, are only parts
of the complex language system of humans. There is a fourth dimension of language that has not been given the same attention
as the others in linguistic theory. This dimension describes the
behavioral process that humans use to communicate. The
knowledge of language structure, concepts, and function needs
to be actualized. Once the linguistic, semantic, and pragmatic
rules have been internalized, there must be an integration of
these systems so that language can be performed. Bever (1970)
stated that although grammar is the epicenter of all language
behavior, grammatical structure has different functions that account for different aspects of linguistic behavior, e.g., talking,
listening, memorizing, etc. He suggested that the child's task is
to acquire concrete behavioral systems for actually talking and
comprehending.

Although usually referred to in a way that implies simple processes of language performance—reception/expression, input/
output, or passive/active—comprehending and speaking are in
fact complex. Comprehension and production involve stages
and strategies that are difficult to identify, not only because they
involve the interaction of a number of cognitive processes, but

also because direct measurement of internal cognitive activity is all but impossible. However, scientific studies have been made of specific behaviors from which comprehension and expression processes may be inferred and conditions under which these processes are modified (Crowder, 1972; Foss & Hakes, 1978; Lieberman, 1967). The findings of these studies have permitted the evolution of theories and models of comprehension and production. While there is some variation among the theories and models, there are specific aspects and explanations that are common to all of them. The experimental data that do exist permit a description of the behavioral processes of comprehension and production that provides insight into the normal system of language as well as to the possible disorders of that system.

Delays or disorders of the conceptual aspect of language are usually associated with impaired intellectual ability; impairment in the establishment of the interpersonal relations necessary to communication is most frequently associated with emotional disturbance. The performance dimension of language is frequently associated with clinical language disorders. The rules of the language code are invariant; that is, they are the same for all speakers of a dialect of a language. The behavioral system by which a person learns and uses language to communicate is the system most likely to be involved in a clinical disorder of language. In order to understand what happens when the behavioral system of a specific child does not effect appropriate comprehension or production, it is necessary to identify the components of adequately functioning processing systems.

In performance, a clear distinction can be made between the modalities through which the coded language enters and leaves the system. The description of stages in processing identifies the elements common to reading and writing and auditory comprehension and speaking, as well as the points of divergence. The physical symbols that make up printed and spoken words are interpreted into proper linguistic units and the sense of the units is the same whether the input is heard or read (Norman, 1972).

This chapter considers the processes of spoken language in detail. It also describes the various processes involved in and related to comprehension and production and outlines the theorized events that take place as part of these processes. (It should be noted that auditory perception and memory are components of both language development [see Chapter 3] and language performance.)

COMPREHENSION

A physics professor is giving a lecture in German. There are three students listening to the lecture: an American physics student who has no knowledge of German, a German literature major who has no knowledge of physics, and a German physics major. The American student hears the lecture but cannot decode any of it. The German literature major *understands* the language but can not comprehend the lecture. The German physics major hears, understands, and comprehends. The first student knows the meaning but not the code; the second student knows the code but not the meaning; and the third student knows the code and the meaning.

Comprehending language is a process by which meaning is attached to a code. Until the underlying message of the utterance is discovered, there can be no comprehension. The important point to consider is that comprehension involves understanding not the *literal* meanings of the words and phrases but rather the intended (*conveyed*) meaning of the speaker.

It appears that comprehension occurs quickly and easily. Yet, at a general linguistic level, comprehension involves analysis of complex grammatic structures: (1) vocabulary; (2) grammar; and (3) word order. To comprehend the Spanish sentence: "Al perrito le pego el muchacho," (The boy hit the little dog) an individual would need to know (1) the basic vocabulary; (2) that the "o" ending on the nouns means masculine; (3) that the suffix "ito" at the end of *perrito* (dog) means small; (4) that the stress on the "o" at the end of the verb *pego* (hit) means past tense; and (5) that the specific function words "al" and "le" make the dog the recipient of the action even though the word specifying the actor, *muchacho* (boy), is at the end of the utterance. In addition to decoding the linguistic utterance, the listener needs to understand the appropriate concepts that are signaled by the utterance, such as size, gender, and past tense.

Comprehension is a process with stages of events that overlap; there is constant, reciprocal, simultaneous processing within all levels of the system. The stages are described as discrete, sequential units, however, because at each stage there are transformations, each one changing the structure of the incoming utterance so that it more closely approximates the form in which it can be "understood."

A particularly good example of the breakdown in comprehension when conveyed and literal meanings are confused. (Beetle Bailey by Mort Walker, reprinted courtesy of King Features.)

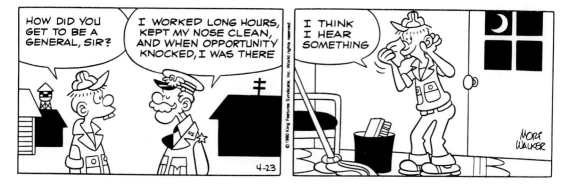

Foss and Hakes (1978) describe three stages of comprehension: (1) speech perception, which transforms a physical sound wave to an internal phonemic representation of it; (2) syntactic and lexical processing, in which words, morphemes, and word groups are "looked up" in a mental dictionary; and (3) transforming the representations of stage 2 into the meaning of the utterance.

Stage 1: Speech Perception

The first stage of comprehension occurs when the acoustic signal is perceived by the listener. The output of this stage, the phonological representation, serves as the input to the second stage.

Categorical Perception

The perception of most events is continous; that is, the perceptual mechanism imposes artificial categories on continuous data that are received by the sensory mechanism. The perceptual mechanism can therefore usually recognize differences within categories as well as differences between categories. Speech perception is unique in being *categorical* rather than continuous. Research by A. M. Liberman et al. (1967) has indicated that subjects discriminate between consonant categories but do not discriminate well between allophones of a consonant phoneme. This phenomenon, known as categorical perception, has been observed in the perception of plosive consonants, which differ according to the place of articulation and voicing. It appears that consonants are identified as language noises. Vowels, on the other hand, are perceived in a continuous manner, as musical tones. This is of particular interest to the language specialist, as the most frequently disordered sounds in articulation are the consonants.

The ability to discriminate consonant categories exists in the absence of phoneme boundaries when measured by a spectogram; the characteristics of the consonant boundaries are not clearly identified when viewing the acoustic signal. This means that the speech signal typically does not contain segments that correspond to discrete phonemes (Liberman et al., 1967). In fact, A. M. Liberman et al. (1967) have theorized that the relation between perception of the phoneme and articulation is more nearly one-to-one than the relation between phoneme perception and the acoustic signal. These researchers have concluded that auditory decoding for speech is accomplished by means of a special perceptual mechanism for speech, a species-specific "speech decoder."

Alvin Meyer Liberman

An internationally recognized scholar in the fields of linguistics and psychology, Liberman received his M.A. and Ph.D. from Yale University. In 1944, soon after he completed his graduate studies, he became associated with Haskins Laboratories in New Haven, Conn. where he served as director of research. Much of the research and theory in speech and language perception and in linguistics has been provided by Liberman and his colleagues at Haskins. Liberman's efforts have provided continued support to the study of the relationship between cognitive processes and language skills. The contributions of Haskins Laboratory to the understanding of the reading process are particularly significant. Liberman is the author of over 50 professional papers dealing with language and speech perception.

Speech perception is the first stage of comprehension; the output from this stage is phonological and does not provide syntactic or semantic information. Phonological restructuring of the input takes place by interaction between this stage and subsequent stages; analysis by higher-level processes is used to structure the input linguistically and to resolve uncertainties at the phonological stage (Foss & Hakes, 1978). Thus, the process of speech perception involves both analysis and synthesis; it is an active process that the listener uses to determine the phonological structure of what he hears.

Analysis by Synthesis

Analysis by synthesis converts the sound wave to a meaningful utterance. Analysis involves the identificaton of the features of the input speech signal; *synthesis* represents the integration of information from the speech signal with information from other sources.

Analysis.   In analysis, the listener's *feature detectors* permit the system to take the incoming speech signal, which is a continuous sequence of sounds made by the speech mechanism, and structure it to form a phonological sequence. There is often no segmentation in the incoming signal, yet the listener segments it appropriately.

Amazingly, this phonological structure can be created even when the acoustic signal is imperfect. Licklider and Miller (1951) commented on the ability of humans to comprehend when only the upper or lower half of the speech spectrum is perceived, when the wave forms are distorted, and when there are considerable changes in the intensity and fundamental frequency of the sound. This is due to the ability to fill in absent phonetic features.

Synthesis.   Lieberman (1967) described synthesis as that process by which hypotheses are formed and either accepted or rejected. The output of analysis forms a preliminary hypothesis about the phonological content of the signal. The hypothesis is tested against the information available. Lieberman (1967) theo-

The study of bird "language" provides interesting parallels to the development of speech in children (Marler, 1967).

1. Some bird species, such as the white-crowned sparrow, are predisposed to learn some sound patterns rather than others; this innate predisposition is similar to the predisposition for some aspects of human speech.
2. Auditory feedback, the ability to hear its own voice, is necessary for the bird to translate the memory of the parent's song into motor activity, i.e. into the production of song resembling that of the parents.
3. The song of the young bird develops gradually; it is preceded by subsongs, which are transitional stages in the development.
4. A bird group uses a common song dialect. These dialects distinguish bird groups. The dialectal patterns appear to be environmental rather than genetic.

rized that if the hypothetical meaning is reasonable and consistent with the communication exchange, the listener accepts the hypothesis, which then permits him to "hear" distinctly those parts that are indistinct. If the meaning is not satisfactory, the listener may try another phonetic hypothesis, or he may simply not understand what has been said.

In order to discover those features that are not available in the message, as well as to impose a phrase structure on the input, the listener uses his knowledge of the syntax and semantics of the language as well as of the social context in which the message is presented. Garrett and Foder (1968) stated, for example, that adjacent sounds and the acoustic context of the syllabic level will influence the perception of specific sounds.

In an attempt to determine the effect of grammatical structure and meaningfulness on perception, G. A. Miller and Isard (1963) asked listeners to "shadow"—to repeat aloud—exactly what a speaker said for fifty grammatical sentences, fifty anomalous sentences, and fifty ungrammatical strings of words, all formed by the same words. Eighty-nine percent of the grammatical sentences, eighty percent of the anomalous sentences, and fifty percent of the ungrammatical strings were shadowed correctly. Thus, perception of the stimulus is enhanced by the syntactic and semantic contexts in which the stimulus is presented. What is perceived is a phonological representation based on (1) an analysis of the signal itself; (2) an analysis of the signal's surrounding context; and (3) a synthesis of the two (Foss & Hakes, 1978).

Memory and Speech Perception

It has been pointed out that the decoding of speech presumably occurs in several stages, each of which is associated with a memory storage buffer that aids in the decoding process. This buffer provides the time needed to analyze, synthesize, and re-analyze (when necessary) in order to reexperience the acoustic signal and detect sound features, stress, and breath patterns (Norman, 1972).

The process of categorizing speech sounds so that they are translated to internal phonological strings takes some time. The physical properties of a signal need to be retained long enough for sounds to be categorized. Foss and Hakes (1978) described the memory involved in the initial activity as a *sensory register* or *echoic memory*. This echoic memory is similar to that described by Crowder (1972) and Gough (1972).

Crowder defined memory that retains acoustic signals in a prelinguistic form for a fraction of a second to several seconds as precategorical acoustic storage (PAS). PAS allows the listener to select items for the next level of memory and, according to Crowder, is at a relatively peripheral acoustic level.

Gough (1972) labeled the next memory level, the small-capacity buffer storage system, *the primary memory* (also referred to as short-term memory). He described four possibilities for speech items entering this system. (1) If the items are ignored, they will simply and rapidly decay; (2) The entire input or parts of it can be renewed through rehearsal; (3) The primary memory has a fixed capacity, and when the capacity is reached, the items in residence are displaced for incoming items; and (4) The items may be transferred into a more permanent store.

The immediate or primary memory holds the words of a sentence until the segment is interpreted; while the next sequence of words comes in, the first segment is being processed (Figure 4-1). Glucksberg and Danks (1975) have suggested that verbatim information is discarded to make room for subsequent incoming material after the interpretive process is completed. Limitations in memory processing can interfere with the early processing of a speech stimulus, and therefore with comprehension, when there is insufficient time for interpretation prior to the introduction of subsequent segments and thus the stimulus is discarded before it can be understood; there is a premature overloading of the processing capacity.

Limitations in memory are not restricted to limitations of the memory span, or the number of chunks of information the memory can hold, or the length of time the chunks can be held.

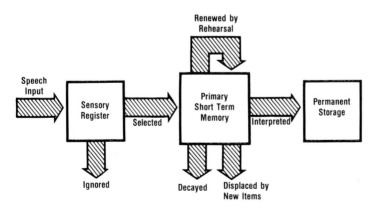

Figure 4-1
Possible fates of speech items entering the primary short-term memory.

There may be limitations in memory for the sequence in which input occurs. Cromer (1976) suggested that inability to reconstruct the order of occurrence underlies some types of aphasia. Language input materials that have a high probability of retention in short-term memory are (1) the initial words in sentences, (2) the vowel quality of the stressed syllables, (3) pitch and other intonational properties, and (4) the sequence of the material (Ervin-Tripp, 1973).

The memory used in speech perception is said to be a precategorical, prelinguistic memory of the echoic type. This seems to imply that the listener is capable of repeating the input exactly, whether or not the input is accurate or complete with respect to phonemic representation. In other words, it is possible to repeat almost exactly an utterance in a foreign language even when the phonemic categories of that language have not been learned. However, once the listener has learned the phonemic categories, "correction" of a distorted or inaccurate input may take place rapidly and possibly without as great a need for higher-level comprehension processes to aid in forming the phonemic representation.

Stage 2: Lexical and Syntactic Processing

The phonological representation that is structured during speech perception is the basis for retrieving the more permanently stored information necessary for synthesizing the input. In a way, the elements of the phonological representation resemble instructions to a computer for locating appropriate lexical and grammatic data. The final linguistic structure of the input is a result of the process that translates the phonological representation to a lexical and syntactic one.

During lexical and syntactic processing, the search for meaning begins. Stress and intonational cues are used to begin identifying meaningful units. Lexical gaps in the phonological representation are completed by using the context of the sentence (Foss & Hakes, 1978). For example, the completion of the following utterance is dependent on the verbal context if only the last two phonemes, /il/, of the missing word are heard:

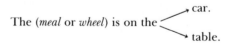

The (*meal* or *wheel*) is on the car / table.

The process by which meanings are "searched for" is the basis of this stage.

Lexical Access and Syntactic Representation

The lexical access stage involves searching through a mental dictionary or mental thesaurus (Glucksberg & Danks, 1975). It is hypothesized that one means of entering the mental dictionary is by using the phonological structure of words. Information about a word may be stored by its initial sound. As Norman (1972, p. 284) suggested, ". . . the sensory input itself helps determine the memory location of the lexical component of that input. . . ." According to Norman, the lexicon of language is organized partly around sensory features used to communicate the morphemes of language. Until the word is found, it has no meaning.

Glucksberg and Danks (1975) have suggested that multiple features of words are stored in memory: (1) morpheme structure; (2) part of speech (syntactic category); (3) information about how the word relates to others in sentences; and (4) semantic function. The input words may be segmented into morphemes for the lexical search (e.g., *un-consider-able*). The input words may also be constructed into syntactic groups. There is some evidence that the syntactic groupings resemble underlying base structures of the kind suggested by Chomsky rather than a structure that resembles a surface representation of the input.

The mental dictionary has been compared to a regular one in which each entry lists a number of properties, and access to these properties is gained through the spelling of the words (Glucksberg & Danks, 1975). The mental dictionary differs from the printed one in that the humans have other means of access— through rhyming words and through meaning. G. A. Miller (1978, p. 62) has provided a summary in the form of a minimal list* of the kinds of information a person must have stored in the mental lexicon in order to understand (and produce) a word:

1. *Pronunciation* (and spelling for written languages)
   a. Phonology (including stress features)
   b. Morphology (including inflected and derivitive forms)
2. *Syntactic categorization*
   a. Major category (noun, verb, adverb, etc.)
   b. Subcategorization (syntactic contexts)
3. *Meaning*
   a. Definitions (concepts expressed; relation to other concepts)
   b. Selectional restrictions (semantic contexts)
4. *Pragmatic constraints*
   a. Situation (relation to general knowledge)
   b. Rhetoric (relation to discourse contexts)

Ervin-Tripp (1973) suggested that speakers store prepackaged sequences in the form of phrases, idioms, and cliches. The normal sentence processing strategies are bypassed when these

---

*From Miller GA: Semantic relations among words. In Halle M Bresnan J, & Miller GA (Eds): *Linguistic Theory and Psychological Reality.* Cambridge, Mass: MIT Press, 1978, p. 62. Reprinted with permission.

prepackaged sequences are used in comprehension and production. The mechanism for processing utterances functions more efficiently with words that occur frequently. Other data (Ervin-Tripp, 1973) indicate that the recency with which a word has been heard also influences the efficiency of processing. Foss and Hakes (1978, p. 107) speculated that "information in the mental lexicon stays in a state of readiness or excitation for some time after it has been retrieved." It appears, then, that the internal representation of each word in the lexicon has a "threshold" of response and when the threshold is exceeded, the listener understands the word. The threshold of meaning is sensitive to input from the phonological representation as well as from semantically related words.

Memory and Lexical-Syntactic Processing

In the decoding process, the listener analyzes the input in parts, not in entire units. The memory buffer described in the first stage holds a limited number of phonological strings. New words can only enter the short-term memory storage when the ones already there have been removed. This is done by analyzing the meaning of each part and storing this meaning in a different form in a more permanent system, sometimes referred to as semantic memory (Glucksberg & Danks, 1975). If the listener has difficulty in decoding the first portion of an input, the last part either decays or is not decoded if it depends on the decoding of the first part. This presents problems in decoding ambiguous sentences and sentences that can be understood fully only when terminated (Glucksberg & Danks, 1975). Foss and Hakes (1978, p. 110) give an example to illustrate the need for *redoing* sentences as each additional bit of information is provided:

> The shooting of the prince shocked his wife since she thought that he was an excellent marksman.

The meaning of the sentence changes after hearing the last three words, which places a burden on the memory of the listener. What takes place in processing ambiguous sentences, according to Glucksberg and Danks (1975), is the need to generate two tentative interpretations instead of one. There is an increased burden on the memory if the interpretation is delayed until sufficient material is obtained to clarify the ambiguity.

Under ordinary circumstances, the exact phonological construction of a stimulus is forgotten immediately after having decoded it; by the time the decoding is complete, the memory retains an abstract representation of the utterance. A study done by Sachs (1967), in which an unrelated sentence was embedded in a paragraph describing a historical event, demonstrated that the listener recalled the sentence meaning but not its form. The type of representation the sentence meaning actually has in memory is not understood.

The lexical and syntactic data stored for reference in constructing grammatic strings out of phonological information seem to be available for use even without any specific meaning being attached to the linguistic structures. There are reports of aphasics in whom the higher level language functions are isolated from the perceptual ones. These aphasics demonstrate *echolalia,* the automatic and seemingly compulsive repetition of a verbal input in the absence of comprehension. Their ability to "parrot" the input supports the existence of the temporary storage buffer for phonological data. However, it has been reported that there is grammatical "correction" or completion of ill-formed input utterances by some echolalic aphasics (Whitaker, 1976). Whitaker described an aphasic who lacked auditory comprehension but who altered the grammatical structure input by providing or deleting a plural, by supplying missing verbs, by changing pronoun case, etc., where appropriate. In the same report, the aphasic demonstrated the presence of categorical phonological representation by correcting phonemic distortions or errors in the presence of the stimulus object.

Output of the Lexical-Syntactic Processing Stage

The output of the lexical-syntactic processing stage appears to resemble deep structure (described by Chomsky; see Chapter 2) rather than surface structure. In other words, as a listener reconstructs a sentence for himself, the reconstruction provides morpheme boundaries, pauses, word grouping, etc., which may or may not have been present in the phonological data. It is this reconstruction that provides the input for the representation of meaning.

Stage 3: Representation of Meaning

The input to stage 3 is the reconstructed underlying utterance structure that has been processed in stage 2. The underlying reconstructed segment is interpreted semantically; the output is a representation of the utterance meaning. At this stage the listener uses his knowledge of the world in general, the speaker in particular, social and linguistic conventions, and the particular situation to "comprehend" what has been spoken. At this level, a distinction is made between the literal meaning of the words and their conveyed meaning.

It is generally suggested that mental representation may be either in a verbal form, through imagery, through abstract conceptual representation, or perhaps in all of the above—depending on the meaning being represented (Potter, Valian, &

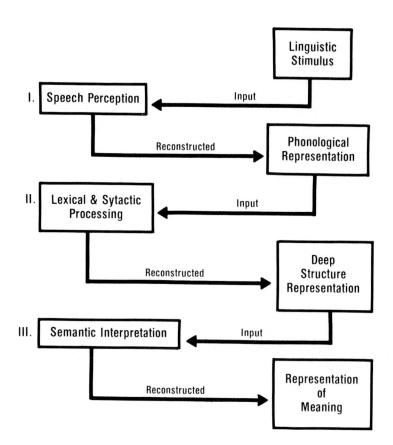

Figure 4-2
Three stages of processing in auditory comprehension.

Faulconer, 1977). Verbal representation involves the use of words to represent meanings; this is not, however, the acoustic form of a word—it is the mental representation, which is the common denominator of all written and spoken tokens of a given word type. Images or perception-like representations are most likely used with sentences about concrete events and objects. Glucksberg and Danks (1975) suggested that if material cannot be easily imaged, representation takes an abstract conceptual form. The input is translated into a conceptual format containing abstract elements and their relations (Potter, Valian, & Faulconer, 1977). There is some evidence to suggest that in this last type of representation, the sentence meanings are in propositional form, which is an abstract form that specifies relations among concepts. Figure 4-2 presents a diagram of the stages of comprehension and their corresponding outputs.

PRODUCING LANGUAGE

The production of language is a very complex process; articulating sounds and words is only a small part of language production. Many transformations occur between the act of ideation and the final act of speaking (Fromkin, 1972).

Each level in the progression from idea to expression involves restructuring input into that level, which adds, in a way, different elements of the coding system. The levels can be viewed as stages in which different types of encoding operations take place; the elements of the messages are transformed as they pass through each successive process (F. S. Cooper, 1972).

The translation of a message from idea to speech involves a sequence of encoding stages. First, the representation of thought is mapped into an underlying linguistic code by a series of encodings. The linguistic code is then transformed into an abstract physiological motor pattern code which is transformed to movement of the muscles of the speech articulators. Encoding can be said to be part of the language production process, while the transformation and movement are parts of the speech production process.

The description of the chain of events that occurs in language production is a speculative one (Gough, 1972). However, much of the information that has permitted inferencing these events is found in language performance itself. As MacNeilage (1972) pointed out, studies of speech errors have provided important clues to the organizing principles that underlie language production; these errors provide guidelines for the construction of explanatory models in both speech physiology and linguistic theory.

Encoding

The Form of the Idea

The original form of content is assumed to be nonlinguistic. It is speculated, however, that although this form is nonlinguistic, the content is coded (Foss & Hakes, 1978). The mental code that forms the message contains the information to be conveyed in the message. The most popular current view of the representational system underlying sentences is that, like comprehension, representation is based upon propositions (relations among concepts) and upon those processes that produce new propositions from old ones.

The concepts that form the elements of the proposition may be viewed as feature constellations made up of separate features combined in unique ways. These were described in Chapter 2 as semantic features. The example provided in that chapter was the feature constellation, of which the word is the symbol, e.g., the features that make up the concept of the word *boys* are those symbolized by the words *animate, human, male, young,* and *plural.* Foss and Hakes (1978) suggested that, in this first stage of production, the concept underlying *boys* is constructed from the feature components and that this construction is an early process in the production. F. S. Cooper (1972) concurred with this view; he stated that the semantic processor somehow selects and rearranges both lexical and relational information that is implicit in the nascent sentence in the form of *semantic feature matrices,* which are similar to the feature constellations described by Foss and Hakes.

Planning Units in Production

The observation of the act of speaking and of errors or "slips of the tongue" (involuntary deviation in performance from the phonological, grammatical, or lexical intent of the speaker; Boomer & Laver, 1973) that occur in speech indicates the necessity of distinguishing between the mechanism by which speech is programmed and that by which it is performed (Cohen, 1973). There are various approaches that describe the size and use of planning units in which the content is translated to linguistic structure (Foss & Hakes, 1978). These descriptions are referred to as models of production.

In the left-to-right model, the production unit is said to be the single word; each word is considered to be the factor that influences the choice of each subsequent word. This model does not take into account the hierarchical levels of syntactic structure and is not considered to be adequate for describing the planning unit. Foss and Hakes (1978) conclude from reviewing available data that the planning unit is larger than a single word and more closely resembles a phrase or clause. A second production model is illustrated by a tree diagram (Figure 2-3). This, referred to as the top-to-bottom model, specifies that the "higher level" units in the diagram are selected before those at the lower levels; sentences are generated, in general, according to phrase structure rules. A third model describes the selection order in terms of transformational grammar. The process begins with an underlying base structure. Subsequent operations are performed that resemble the application of successive transformational rules. This model is called the direct incorporation model because part of the grammar is directly incorporated. None of the models is universally accepted.

Coding Order

Once the basic underlying structure is selected for conveying the desired message, specific elements for further coding are added. One of the earliest elements is stress. Important words in a sentence usually receive greater stress than the others. Error data show that the stress remains in the same location in the syntactic structure even when the important word is transposed, indicating that stress is an early form of encoding, happening prior to the selection of the word that is to be stressed.

Early in the coding of the idea, a morpheme such as *ly* is incorporated and added to a word such as *love(ly)*. If an error is made and the stem *love* is separated or transposed (as when "I like things that are lovely" becomes "I love things that are likely"), the suffix does not move with the stem. This indicates that at least some suffixes are part of the syntactic structure rules rather than part of the lexical items (Foss & Hakes, 1978).

The next stage of coding involves the lexical search, which involves seeking morphemes among specific semantic constellations. It is possible to select a word having some but not all of the semantic features needed. This results in slips of the tongue such as saying *girls* for *boys;* the semantic feature of *male* is momentarily obscured. Errors in which two words having the same meaning compete with each other for coding and are therefore blended into one word (e.g., when *chair* and *stool* are uttered as *chool*) and errors in which an item adjacent to the desired item is substituted for it (the use of *likely* for *lovely*) occur at this stage of encoding. These types of errors also provide information about the methods of lexical storage available for language.

Next, items are arranged in a sequential order. Errors at this level occur among items that are in temporal proximity; these items don't necessarily have semantic or form-class relationships. The errors occur with phonologically similar words and include phonological anticipation (*faby face* for *baby face*); phonological perseveration (*happy hog* for *happy dog*); reciprocal change (these errors are sometimes called spoonerisms; *balking toy* for *talking boy*) (Foss & Hakes, 1978).

The last stage involves "last-minute" adjusting or repairing errors. A shift or substitution of a word may require a change in the article preceding it. Some errors may be edited out at this level, particularly those that contain nonsense words. From the last stage, syntactic encoding, the linguistic form is translated into a motor form and instructions are given to the musculature involved in speaking (or writing).

Phonological Coding

The message now enters the level of phonological processing. Here, an internal phonetic representation made up of discrete invariant units is transformed into the external continuous variable acoustic sounds of speech. F. S. Cooper (1972, p. 33) specified three subprocessors of the speech processors, each having its own function. First, "the abstract feature matrices of the phonetic structure must be given physiological substance as neural signals (commands) if they are to guide and control the production of speech . . ." (Remember that *phoneme* and *phonemics* are abstract concepts of speech sounds whereas *phone* and *phonetics* represent the actual variable utterance of the sounds.) Second, Cooper stated, "these neural commands then bring about a pattern of muscle contraction; these, in turn instruct and cause the articulators to move and the vocal tract to assume a succession of shapes; finally, the vocal tract shape (and the acoustic excitation due to air flow through the glottis or other constrictions) determines the spoken sound."*

The variability of articulatory events has been amply supported. Cooper stressed the importance of the encoding that occurs at the moment of articulation as a means of dealing with substantial quantities of information in spite of limited memory capacity. It is therefore inappropriate according to MacNeilage (1972), to view articulation as a discrete, static, context-free linguistic category of phonemes and distinctive features. Instead, it should be conceptualized in terms of its dynamic properties, which involve moment-to-moment coordination of the continuous flow of speech.

The Encoded Characteristics of Language

There appears to be progressive shortening of the message by means of encoding throughout the language production process. This permits the speaker to communicate large quantities of information efficiently. Encoding begins when the propositions are chosen, and underlying syntactic structures are selected to represent the propositions. The underlying structures are then collapsed into phrases, and stress, word order, morphemes, etc. are added. Finally, the phonological string is telescoped by producing syllables whose sounds overlap temporarily. The message has now been uttered.

The form and content of a message are dependent on information available to the speaker, and the level of difficulty of the message is unconsciously influenced by the listener's ability to understand as well as by the conversational and social contexts. A speaker can encode the same propositions in a variety of ways; no two speakers will use the same forms for encoding. Many individuals can utilize various codes in either separate languages or dialects of the same language. The process of encoding in various codes as circumstances dictate seems to be relatively easy for the bilingual speaker.

Language Production and Memory

Utterance length has been linked historically to memory. The primary techniques of measuring short-term memory have used repetition of random numbers or other unrelated words. The

*From Cooper FS: How is language conveyed by speech. In Kavanagh JF & Mattingly IG (Eds): *Language by eye and ear*. Cambridge, Mass.: MIT Press, 1972, p. 33. Reprinted with permission.

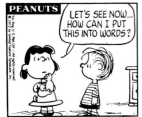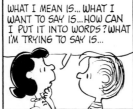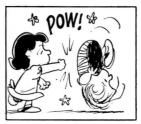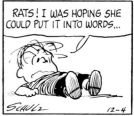

Sometimes actions speak louder than words, especially when the words do not flow easily. (Copyright 1972, United Feature Syndicate, Inc.)

inability to reproduce the verbal strings of words is frequently interpreted to mean that the individual has a short-term auditory memory. The use of shorter utterances by children in spontaneous conversation and in imitation may also relate to memory; it seems that children have shorter memory spans than adults.

However, Olson (1973) reported studies in which children do as well as adults in memory tasks employing nonverbal stimuli. He concluded that the change in memory span is indicative of something more complex and interesting than a simple change in capacity of a static mental object: it is an increase in the child's capacity to handle *verbal* material—an increase related to the change in the child's internal representations (nonverbal to verbal)—that permits the child to gradually approximate adult capacity and repeat language stimuli.

Similar conclusions were arrived at by using children's recall of approximations to English (E. Carrow & Mauldin, 1973). Approximations to English are various levels of synthetic sentences that represent degrees of grammatic approximation to "real" sentences. In adults, Tulving and Patkau (1962) found that free recall of orders of approximation improved as the level of approximation (degree of grammaticality) increased. This was interpreted to mean that increasing grammaticality increases the number of items in a chunk. Miller (1956) hypothesized an upper limit to the number of information units or chunks that can be retained in immediate memory. Increase in chunk size with increasing approximations to English apparently results from increased organization available from syntactic and semantic information.

As children's language develops, they are able to handle larger chunks (C. S. Smith, 1970). Carrow and Mauldin (1973) found that chunk size increased as approximations more resembled "real" sentences for 6- or 7-year-olds but not for 4- and 5-year-olds. The younger children performed significantly poorer than the older children and adults on the fourth-order approximations—the level most like grammatical English—but not on the other levels. These results indicate that an individual's capacity to remember increasingly longer units is more closely re-

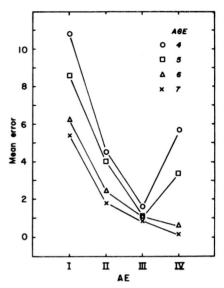

Figure 4-3
Mean errors in repetition for children as a function of approximations to English. Note the difference in performance between the 4- and 5-year-olds and the 6- and 7-year-olds in the fourth order of approximation, the one that most closely resembles English grammar. (Reprinted from E. Carrow and Mauldin [1973] with permission of *Journal of Speech and Hearing Research.*)

lated to his increased linguistic organization and knowledge of the language than his memory (Fig. 4-3).

Memory boundaries may be the same for children and adults. The strategies for coding data in the complex manner of language, as well as the perceptual knowledge that serves as a base for understanding the code, may be lacking in children's systems.

Voluntary and Automatic Production

Voluntary speech is the deliberate conscious expression of utterances of a symbolic nature. Automatic speech is largely the unconscious or nondeliberate production of semantically empty articulate speech. Early writers in the field of aphasia described a language behavior in which the higher-level semantic aspects of language were affected by complete dissociation from the control of oral speech production. An aphasic described by Whitaker (1976) could apparently perceive input segments of language, form a phonological representation of the segments, correct missing syntactic elements, and orally reproduce the corrected segment, without understanding it. This aphasics' auditory-vocal systems appeared to be connected at more than one level of performance.

The idea of an independent, automatic, auditory-vocal system is supported when an English-speaking person who knows no Spanish can imitate a Spanish utterance with a considerable degree of accuracy. The person may learn to read and spell Spanish words without any understanding, using the automatic perceptual-motor system through which these messages pass without the comprehension or formulation of language taking place. However, as soon as the individual learns some Spanish, he finds that as he attempts to evoke language meaning, he may begin to misarticulate words. The automatic system breaks down in the learning stages of language when the primary focus is to communicate meaning.

Similarly, Slobin and Welsh (1973) found that a child can imitate perfectly (parrot) ungrammatical and anamalous sentences if the length is within the capacity of his short-term memory. However, if the stimulus chosen for imitation puts stress on the child's immediate memory, and if he comprehends it, the imitation will reflect his level of syntax (Lenneberg, 1967).

Fay and Butler (1968), in observing the difference between pure echolalia (parroting) and mitigated echolalia (modified echoic responses) postulated the existence of two separate but parallel growth processes represented, respectively, by an audiomotor system and a syntatic-semantic system. They believed that a corollary of their hypothesis is that asymmetrical language status in children (performance difference between the audio-motor and syntactic-semantic systems) is evidence of the developmental nonconvergence of the two independent systems. It is also apparent that, in comparing the development of comprehension and production, the automatic and the deliberate aspects of processing language must be considered.

THE BRAIN AND LANGUAGE

The understanding of the relationship between the brain and language is relatively new compared to knowledge about other aspects of man's biological systems. Although the Egyptians observed that laterality was connected with the cerebral hemispheres, and Hippocrates wrote in the fourth century B.C. about the duality of the brain, it was not until 1861 that Broca (von Bonin, 1960) introduced the systematic study of the relationship between the brain and behavior. Broca presented a description of a patient who, as a result of a lesion to a specific area in the brain, developed a severe deficit in expressive language. This was followed in 1874 by a publication by Wernicke, who described a patient with severe deficits in language comprehension, which Wernicke ascribed to a lesion in the posterior part of the temporal-parietal lobe of the left hemisphere. These areas of the brain are still identified as Broca's and Wernicke's areas.

These reports by Broca and Wernicke initiated the study of *cerebral dominance,* the concept that one hemisphere of the brain is dominant for certain behavioral functions, and *localization,* the specialization of sections of the brain within each hemisphere for specific functions. The phenomenon of hemispheric asymmetry is also referred to as *laterality* when it describes the dominance of the left or right hemisphere in specific functions or skills performed by the eye, ear, foot, and hand, and in functions of language. Each hemisphere of the brain controls the activities of the contralateral side of the body.

The early data on cerebral dominance and localization was obtained from studies of diseased or injured brains. In surgical work with epileptic patients, Penfield and Roberts (1959) reported on patient responses to electrical stimulation of various areas of the brain. When appropriate areas of the left hemisphere were stimulated, the patient vocalized; however, the patient did not vocalize when the experiment was repeated on the right side of the brain. Large-scale studies of the results of head injury followed the First and Second World Wars. Head (1926), Goldstein (1948), and Russell and Esper (1961) cared for large numbers of soldiers with gunshot wounds to the head and their accounts of the effect of injury contributed to the understanding of the specific function of different parts of the brain. Their studies confirmed the dominant role of the left hemisphere in language. Injury to Broca's area was found to have a direct effect on the production of speech, whereas injury to the temporal lobe of the left hemisphere had a more diffuse effect on comprehension.

Early literature was devoted to studies of the disordered brain and language and the claims for left-hemisphere dominance turned out to be exaggerated (Kimura, 1975). As early as 1874, Jackson (cited in Taylor, 1958) had cautioned that cerebral dominance and specific localization of function in the brain were relative concepts, and that language was represented at many different levels according to a functional hierarchy. Although he associated the left hemisphere with speaking, he anticipated later demonstration of the importance of the right hemisphere in certain visual processes.

Over the past few years, studies of the normal brain's role in speech processing have contributed to the understanding of the relationship between the brain and language. Of particular value has been the research using dichotic listening techniques. Early researchers studied the brain asymmetry in speech production; newer researchers have studied the asymmetrical aspects of speech perception.

The Brain and Speech Processing

The primary procedure used to study the central aspects of speech perception is dichotic listening, which involves the simultaneous presentation of competing messages (phonemes, syllables, or sentences) to the ears. The rationale is that the message

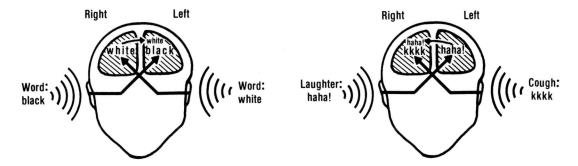

that is first or more accurately identified by the listener is the one received by the hemisphere that is dominant for speech in the individual being studied. The right ear input would have the advantage in individuals with speech represented in the left hemisphere since the input would have better access to that hemisphere (Kimura, 1975).

In experiments in which two different words were presented to the ears simultaneously, one word to the left ear and the other to the right ear, Kimura (1961) found that the words arriving at the right ear were more accurately identified. The significance of the dominance of the left hemisphere for *speech* sounds is further demonstrated by a variation of this experiment. When nonspeech sounds, such as a laugh and a cough, are presented to the two ears simultaneously, the reverse is true; the nonspeech sound presented to the left ear is interpreted more accurately. This so-called right-ear advantage (REA) for speech sounds is indicative of the superiority of the left hemisphere for speech language activity (Fig. 4-4). Dichotic studies have also been conducted with preschool children; children as young as 3 years of age can demonstrate a right-ear advantage (Kimura, 1975).

Studies analogous to those described in speech perception have been performed using visual stimuli. Vision is known to be subserved by the contralateral visual cortex. These studies have shown that linguistic material (letters, words, or digits) are more quickly and accurately seen with right-visual-field presentation than left. This again confirms the superiority of the left hemisphere for language (Neville, 1976).

Developmental Aspects of Dominance

The dichotic method has also proved to be very effective in studying the course of development of superiority of one hemisphere over the other. Speech discrimination has been tested in infants by measuring changes in sucking behavior as sounds are presented. Speech sounds to the infant's right ear produce more

Figure 4-4
Cerebral dominance for dichotically presented verbal and nonverbal auditory stimuli. From Fromkin V & Rodman R: *An Introduction to Language.* Copyright © 1974 by Holt, Rinehart, Winston. Adapted by permission of Holt, Rinehart, Winston.

changes in sucking behavior than sounds to the left ear. This demonstrates that even at a very early age there is a left-hemisphere superiority for the processing of speech sounds (Eimas et al., 1971).

The functional asymmetry of the brain is not only evident in early life, it is also more flexible then than in adulthood. Children who have had such extensive damage or disease that the entire left hemisphere has been removed develop better language than other children who retain an impaired left hemisphere. One explanation for this is that the damaged left hemisphere may inhibit the still intact right hemisphere from developing language. With the left hemisphere removed, the right hemisphere is free to develop language. These children recover their language skills or acquire language with fewer problems than might be predicted based on observation of adults. This suggests that during childhood the right hemisphere can develop language, although it is possible that the functions usually performed by the right hemisphere, such as visual-spatial tasks, may suffer in consequence (Kinsbourne, 1976).

Hemispheric Specialization

Studies of the areas of the brain have indicated that each hemisphere of the normal brain specializes in different tasks. With respect to motor functions, the left side of the body is controlled by the right hemisphere of the brain and vice versa. The left and right hemispheres appear to divide up other types of functions as well.

In general, the left hemisphere controls language, including not only speech but reading and writing and, to some extent, comprehension. In addition, the left hemisphere appears especially sensitive to temporal ordering. Verbal concepts and verbal cognitive tasks also appear to be controlled by the left hemisphere. (With this control of language and verbal cognitive tasks, it is easy to understand how some early investigators considered the left hemisphere the "major" hemisphere and the right hemisphere as a "spare" or "stand-by.")

The right hemisphere is concerned with visual-spatial tasks. In addition, the right hemisphere contributes to visual recognition, particularly the recognition of faces, and is especially concerned with musical ability. The right hemisphere has a capacity for imagery and is better able than the left to categorize nonspecific visual stimuli. In a right-handed person, injury to the right hemisphere is often especially destructive to musical or artistic ability and visual-spatial skills (Gazzaniga, 1974; Kinsbourne, 1976; Krashen, 1976).

The focus of description in a process model of language is on the internal processing system that controls the encoding and decoding of language as it takes place in a language exchange. Osgood and Miron (1963) and Wepman et al. (1960) developed similar theoretical models of language processing. Both models describe three major processes in the comprehension and production of language: decoding, encoding, and association.

The decoding (receptive) process begins with the visual or auditory sensory input of a linguistic stimulus and moves through perception and integration to the representational level where the linguistic stimulus is understood. The encoding (expressive) process begins with the intentional selection of semantic units and their grammatical integration and expression and continues through the motor systems of speech or writing.

The associative (Osgood & Miron, 1963) or transmission (Wepman et al., 1960) process deals with the central associations among words and their meanings (representational mediations), as well as the association between the input and output processes at the various stages from sensation to meaning. At the sensory level, the input-output association forms a reflex arc that has no relation to memory or recall. At the perceptual-integrative level, a linguistic input may be transmitted across the system from reception to expression without proceeding to the representational level where the linguistic signal is understood. When a crossover takes place at the perceptual-integrative level, the speaker is imitating without necessarily understanding what is spoken.

Osgood and Miron described the activities of the perceptual-integrative level as "automatic" and considered the grammatical and syntactic aspects of language to be formed, at least partly, at this level. Osgood and Miron referred to predictive integrations, which bring about the completion of patterns when the patterns have occurred with some frequency and temporal contiguity. For example, they considered the agreement between noun and verb and the ordering of word classes, once a particular construction has been selected, to be examples of predictive integration.

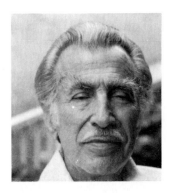

Joseph Wepman

Joseph Wepman began his academic work at the University of Chicago in 1936 and remained there throughout the span of his professional career. His academic degree was in psychology, but his primary research interest was in language disorders—first in adult aphasia and subsequently in child language disorders. His extensive writings were characterized by his efforts to classify disorders of language either on the basis of their linguistic characteristics or on the basis of their relation to cognitive functions. His integrative approach was evident in his comparison of five stages of language development to five types of aphasic disturbances. Wepman published tests of auditory and visual perception as well as numerous articles on aphasia. His most comprehensive work was *Recovery from Aphasia.*

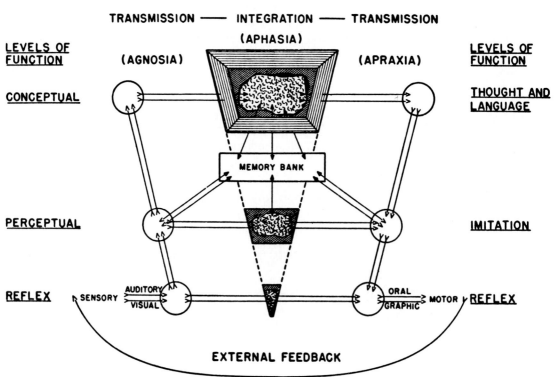

CENTRAL NERVOUS SYSTEM

TRANSMISSION — INTEGRATION — TRANSMISSION
(APHASIA)

LEVELS OF FUNCTION

(AGNOSIA)

(APRAXIA)

LEVELS OF FUNCTION

CONCEPTUAL

THOUGHT AND LANGUAGE

MEMORY BANK

PERCEPTUAL

IMITATION

REFLEX

SENSORY
AUDITORY
VISUAL

ORAL
GRAPHIC
MOTOR

REFLEX

EXTERNAL FEEDBACK

Figure 4-5
An operational diagram of the levels of function in the central nervous system. Note the interpretation of aphasia as a problem in the integration between the expressive, receptive, and memory processes. (Reprinted from Wepman et al. [1960] with permission of *Journal of Speech and Hearing Disorders.*)

The role of memory at the perceptual-integrative and the representational levels is apparent in both models. The description of recall at the perceptual level of Wepman and colleagues, resembles primary acoustic storage. Percepts that are transmitted across the system at the perceptual level in the form of echolalia leave a short-term trace on the memory bank but have no meaning for the individual. At the representational level, the linguistic input affects the memory bank by arousing associations with the past and forming a state of meaningfulness (Fig. 4-5).

AN INTEGRATIVE APPROACH TO LANGUAGE PERFORMANCE

Language is not only what a person knows but it is also what a person does with what he knows. The performance of language describes the sequence of events that take place from the time an utterance is received by the auditory system to the time it is understood and those events that take place when an idea is translated into speech. Although these stages in performance are neither independent nor discrete, they are considered so for explanatory purposes. The major processing stages in oral language performance are speech perception, lexical and syntactic

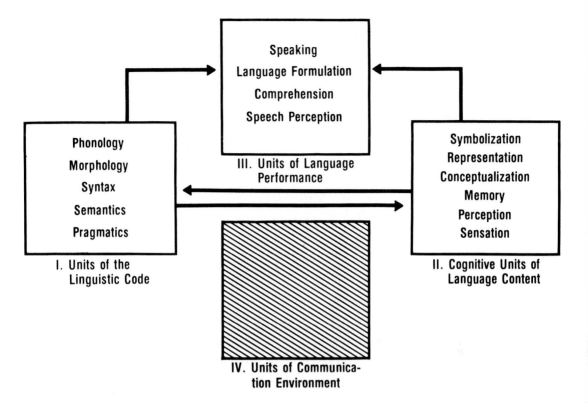

Figure 4-6
The dimensions of the linguistic code, of cognition, and of language performance in a four-dimensional language model.

processing, comprehension, language formulation, and speaking.

It should be noted that speech perception is listed here although there is a category of perception in the dimension of cognition. The interpretation given to the term perception in the cognitive dimension is a broad one that describes the activity of recognition of all sensory information as well as the products of this information as these contribute to the development of meaning. Speech perception in the performance dimension is an activity that is specially suited to the reception and processing of linguistic information as it occurs; i.e., it is a language-specific activity.

Chapters 2 and 3 presented parts of an integrative model of language: the linguistic code and cognitive content. Figure 4-6 is an expansion of the model to include the dimension of language performance. Language performance is related to both cognition and the linguistic code, and this is indicated in Figure 4-6 by lines and arrows showing the direction of the relationship. In order to perform language, the individual must have a knowledge of the rules of the code as well as a conceptual knowledge and the ability to symbolize. It is possible for the individual to engage in imitative activity using only the processing stages at the level of performance. This, however, is not language.

outline

the interpersonal dimension of language: the communication environment

5

Human language is only one aspect of the broad field of communication. In computer science, telecommunications, and information theory, communication refers to the transmission of information. Computers are programmed to store and process vast amounts of information, telecommunications systems beam messages throughout the world and into outer space, and electronics corporations market devices that allow machines to "speak" with human voices. These devices reflect not only the intelligence of the humans who designed and programmed them but also the powerful human need to communicate. Yet, while machines exist to provide information, no machine has concern for the receiver of this information; machines do not participate in a relationship between sender and receiver. In contrast, human language must include a relationship as well as content or message (Whatmough, 1956, p. 19). This relationship occurs whenever people are together, even if verbal information is not exchanged. For humans, the need to relate is more basic than the need to know. Speech is acquired in a social context, and interpersonal relationships precede verbal speech.

This chapter establishes the importance of the social context for language development. Within the social environment, the child is an active partner. Consequently the effects of the child on his environment are explored in this chapter. Next, the effects of the family and of society on language development are discussed. Since communication also consists of nonverbal behaviors, several types of these behaviors are reviewed. Finally, the interpersonal dimension of language—the communication environment—is presented within the integrative model of language.

THE SOCIAL CONTEXT OF LANGUAGE

Social knowledge is an integral part of the foundation for language development. As Lewis and Cherry (1977) have illustrated, individuals develop social, linguistic, and cognitive knowledge in interaction with each other (Fig. 5-1). This unified model emphasizes the social context in which language develops.

Humans are essentially social beings. At birth the infant is totally dependent upon others, and so an evolutionary perspective may develop that fosters the early establishment of strong social relationships (Lewis & Cherry, 1977). It has also been argued (Levi-Strauss, 1962) that all language represents a "social contract" in which members of a society agree upon the meanings of words. All knowledge is acquired through interaction with the social world; this incidentally acquired knowledge is crucial to the normal development of language (Lewis & Cherry, 1977).

EFFECT OF THE CHILD ON THE COMMUNICATION ENVIRONMENT

The environment of the infant or young child consists almost exclusively of his caretakers. The communication that occurs in this parent–child dyad is influenced by both child and parent. The communicative exchange is further influenced by whether the child is normal or handicapped.

The Normal Child

Infants and young children are sometimes depicted as egocentric, demanding creatures with no concern beyond their own comfort. Rees (1978), however, has suggested that they are actually sociocentric from birth. Observation of their behavior indicates that infants actively seek social interaction during their first year. Within weeks of their birth, infants attend to and are quieted by the sound of the human voice. Later they increase their own vocalizations in response to speech; still later they are motivated to imitate both speech sounds and human activity.

An important activity for infants and their caretakers is mutual gaze. During mutual gaze the eyes of infant and caretaker are focused on each other, on another person, or on an object of interest to the infant. Ninety-four percent of mutual gaze has been found to be initiated and terminated by the infant (Ramey et al., 1978). Mutual gaze tends to prolong visual attention for both the infants and adults. Infants also contribute to communication during the first weeks and months of life through the development of the social smile and the heightened activity that signals their excitement at the approach of an adult. Infants also engage in simultaneous and reciprocal vocalization with adults and in patterns of touching, reaching, looking, smiling, and playing (Lewis & Lee-Painter, 1974).

The infant's need for warm human interaction is well known. Studies of infants in institutions have shown that a child's failure to thrive during the early months of life may be accounted for by inadequate social stimulation, despite adequate physical care. Just as the infant needs adult attention, the normal adult appears strongly motivated to provide this attention. Apparently, infants' obvious needs and "babyishness" stimulate adults to pay attention to them. Adults make every effort to hold the young child's attention. They appear most successful in doing this by speaking to the child in a face-to-face manner, providing multisensory stimulation (visual, auditory, and tactile), exaggerating their vocal inflection, and using other verbal devices, which will be described later as "motherese." Caretakers apparently use a conversational model when dealing with infants. Parents take turns with their infants in reciprocal touch, in the exchange of objects, and in shared vocalization. They report that they play these imitative games because it gives them a feeling of contact with the infant (Snow, 1977).

During the first year of life the amount of language input the adult gives the child seems to be primarily a function of the adult's own interactive style, while after the first year it becomes much more the consequence of the child's own behavior. The speech of the young child appears to elicit adult response and expansion (Moerk, 1977). Adults are very adept in predicting what their own children can understand. The child in turn expresses his comprehension by increased attention to utterances that refer to concepts he possesses. The child further illustrates his attention by vocal acknowledgment that the message has been received and understood; however, it is not until about age 4 that the child begins to make the more adult comments of "mm," "humm," "uh huh," etc., to signal comprehension (Bates, 1975, p. 275). The adult in turn makes maximum effort

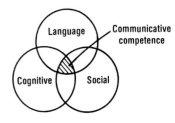

Figure 5-1
The interaction of social, linguistic, and cognitive knowledge. (Redrawn from Lewis and Cherry [1977, p. 231] with permission of John Wiley & Sons.)

to understand the child by interpreting the contextual cues, asking questions, and probing.

In addition to attention to parents, the normal toddler displays early sensitivity to the social environment. Studies of the affective responses of very young children are still limited in number—this area constitutes a serious research need (Yarrow, 1975). Preliminary observations of children between 10 and 30 months old contain various samples of behavior that illustrate the reciprocal responses of these children. For example, a 16-month-old saw her friend sobbing, walked over to the friend, patted him, then picked up a toy and gave it to him. A 12-month-old tried hard to "protect" her mother from having her throat swabbed by the doctor. A 22-month-old rubbed his own elbow after his mother responded to the pain from hurting her elbow. When a dog sneezed, an 18-month-old got a kleenex to wipe its nose (Yarrow, 1975, p. 302). These examples of reciprocal behavior show relationships out of which language emerges. They illustrate that the infant's behavior may occur in response to the behavior of others, but it is also clear that infants initiate actions—that they, as well as adults, know how to shape and modify the behavior of others. As de Villiers and de Villiers (1978) point out, most of the studies done so far have analyzed the speech of the adult or the child apart from the interaction between the two. Interaction studies are needed of normal children and their parents and of handicapped children and their parents.

The Handicapped Child

Some children have handicaps affecting language that are not apparent at birth, and it is difficult to study parental interaction with these children. However, some handicaps, such as Down's syndrome, are apparent, and the effect of the handicap on the parent–child relationship has been studied. Emde and his colleagues (1978) have investigated the interrelationships between a series of infants who have Down's syndrome and their parents. Based upon their review of the literature, the authors felt that there was good evidence that Down's syndrome infants were slow to develop interactive behaviors. They presented an in-depth study of one child named Dawn, to show the effect of this on the family.

Dawn was a first child. She ate well and gained weight during the first three months, but her mother expressed concern because she was "so content and placid." Around $2\frac{1}{2}$ months Dawn began to use her first social smile. When Dawn was 4 months old, the experimenters returned for a visit, expecting to find the social smile well developed and the parents playfully engaged with their baby. Instead, both parents displayed an air of heavy disappointment. The baby was not responding to them as they expected and did not show any sustained affection. Filming showed that at an adult's approach, Dawn smiled—but not normally. There was only a very slight upturning of the lips, her eyes did not crinkle or brighten, and she did not bicycle her arms and legs in anticipation (as do normal 3–4-month-olds). In addition, she did not maintain good eye contact and displayed minimal visual tracking of the activities of persons in her visual field. This behavior reduced the rewards her parents received from her: when an adult approaches a child, there is disappointment if the baby does not seem "glad to see them," and sometimes the adult feels ignored and rebuffed (Emde et al., 1978, pp. 354–357).

The experience of Dawn's parents has been replicated with the parents of other handicapped infants. Parents of autistic children report that their infants seem to actively want to avoid them. Deaf children initially respond appropriately but fail to engage in the expected reciprocal vocalization or to reinforce verbal behaviors produced by adults. Children with clinical language disorders are often silent and late to develop any words, thus reducing parental reinforcement for verbal stimulation. (Part 4 provides more information on how the communication environment differs for the child with various language disorders.)

The response of parents to the news that their child is handicapped may also affect the interpersonal relationship. No parent anticipates or desires having a handicapped child. When a handicap is diagnosed, the parents must mourn the loss of the "perfect" child. This period of mourning is similar to that following the death of a loved one (McNamara & McNamara, 1977) and seems to follow the stages of mourning that have been described in Kubler-Ross' (1975) influential book on the terminally ill. Kubler-Ross indicated that when faced with a crisis, such as the diagnosis of a fatal illness or the handicap of a child, the first reaction is denial. During this period, parents may take their child from one specialist to another in the hope of receiving a more favorable diagnosis. The next stage is anger, which may be directed by the parents at the specialists who made the diagnosis, at the child, or at each other. Following this is a "bargaining" period when the parents hope that if they do something extraordinary the child can be made normal. Eventual realization that this is not true and that the problem must be endured leads to depression, which later can become the type of constructive acceptance that results in habilitation for the child. Only after the parents have gone through this period of mourning can they learn to accept and love their child.

Although the stages of mourning have been studied in many

circumstances, they have only recently begun to be applied to language disorders (Tanner, 1980).

EFFECT OF THE FAMILY ON LANGUAGE DEVELOPMENT

Within the limited environment of the infant and young child, verbal and nonverbal communication begins.

The Adult–Child Relationship

Behaviorists

Latif (1941) described the development of language as dependent upon the establishment of a relationship between mother and child. The caring ministry of a mother to her infant, according to Latif, produces a state of comfort and well-being in the child. The association of physical comfort with the visual and auditory stimuli of the mother eventually causes the comfort state to occur in the presence of the auditory or visual stimulus alone. Subsequently, words spoken by the mother begin to have "meaning" for the child.

Mowrer's theory (1958, 1960) is similar to Latif's. Mowrer believed that a baby first learns to produce words because of an association of loving care with vocalization, which creates in the infant a predisposition to react with emotional satisfaction first to the mother's voice and then to his own, causing him to vocalize again, thus forming the basis for language.

Skinner (1957) felt that selective reinforcement helped the child to learn to talk. He assumed that parents would positively reinforce approximations of words. For example, as the child babbled "mamamam," the parent would respond positively, believing that the child had said "mama." Because of this reinforcement, the child would repeat the vocal pattern.

Psycholinguistic Theorists

Chomsky and Lenneberg described language acquisition as species-specific behavior. Other linguistic studies remarked on the great speed with which infants learned language with "no instruction" (McNeill, 1966); "baby talk" was considered an impediment to language learning (McCarthy, 1954; McNeill, 1966), and parents were counseled to avoid such speech. In contrast, more recent investigators have asserted that these parental adaptations are highly conducive to language acquisition.

The speech of adults to young children has many characteristics that distinguish it from their speech to other adults or to older children. This speech pattern, which is sometimes called "baby talk" (Gleason, 1973), "motherese" (Gleason & Weintraub, 1978; Newport, 1976) or simply "maternal or paternal language," has been extensively studied. It has been found that adults modify their speech in certain specific ways when talking to their children. When the speech of 24 mothers to other adults and to their 2-year-olds was measured (Gleason & Weintraub, 1978), the mothers' spoke in a higher pitch to the children than to the adults. The final pitch contours of many of the women rose when they were speaking to the children and fell when they were speaking to adults. The duration of words was exaggerated, and often there was double stress: for example, "PUSH the GREEN square." Also, they spoke more slowly to the children than to other adults and their speech was simplified, using the kinds of syllable duplication that children tend to use. Difficult consonant clusters were modified, as in calling a stomach a "tummy," or a rabbit a "bunny."

In motherese, names tend to be substituted for pronouns: for example, "Give Mommy a kiss" or "Where are Johnny's mittens?" The semantic relations in motherese consist most often of an agent plus action, object, or location, which are also the relations used most frequently by young children (Brown, 1973). The sentences addressed to young children in Brown's study were short, often repeated, and contained a greatly reduced number of inflections. Utterances addressed to young children were reduced in length and complexity, and so contained few clauses or compound words. Fully 16 percent of the adult–child speech consisted of phrases only such as "The red truck" or "In the box" (Snow, 1972). Apparently the child's lack of understanding influences the parent to reduce speech complexity (Ramey et al. 1978). Moerk (1977) and Ramey et al. (1978) have also suggested that the changes in the mother's speech is an adaptation to the continuous feedback of the child. This adjustment in complexity of input occurs primarily in speech addressed to children between the ages of 2 and 5.

There have been only a few studies of the speech of fathers to their children (Berko Gleason & Weintraub, 1978). Initial experiments indicated that the father's and mother's speech shared the features of simplicity and immediacy. However, certain differences were observed; these included distinction in speech addressed to male versus female infants. Essentially, the fathers tended to produce more imperatives than mothers to children of both sexes, but they used more threats and joking names with their sons than with their daughters. The fathers also used more complex words, such as *aggravating* or *complicated.* Despite these differences, fathers and mothers clearly adjusted their speech to their infants. More research is needed before the differences and similarities between maternal and paternal speech addressed to male and female children can be clarified.

Moerk (1977), Bowerman (1978a), and de Villiers and de Villiers (1978a) summarized the literature of parental speech to children and listed common modifications, a few of which are characteristic:

1. Parental speech is higher and more variable in pitch, with exaggerated intonation.
2. It is slower, with distinct pauses after each utterance.
3. It contains many short and well-formed utterances, which are often repeated.
4. There is a preponderance of questions, imperatives, and directives, with fewer declaratives.
5. There are fewer modifiers, pronouns, and functors.

These differences appear to be uniform across a number of languages studied and suggest that the speech of mothers and other caretakers to their children is ideal for teaching language. There is an almost universal tendency for adults to assist children in learning language (Berko Gleason & Weintraub, 1978, p. 190); parents apparently have a strong need to understand and be understood by their children. Consequently they continue to adapt their speech input to the linguistic and cognitive level of their children even after the usual stage of "baby talk."

The Child–Child Relationship

There has been much less study of the role of child–child speech in the acquisition of language. The consensus appears to be that the speech of peers is less conducive to learning language than adult speech (Berko Gleason & Weintraub, 1978; Moerk, 1977; K. Nelson, 1978). The most extreme example of peer language has been observed in twins, but folklore about a "secret" language shared by twins has not been borne out by research. Dales (1969) studied 14 pairs of twins and found them retarded in both motor and language development between 33 and 36 months. Another study (Svenka et al., 1972, quoted in Bates, 1975) suggested that what appeared to be "impoverished" language was actually a shared deep structure. Each twin was contributing a portion of one complete sentence rather than producing fragmental utterances, as had previously been thought.

Studies of birth order show that first-borns and only children score higher on language measures than other children. Many of the authors of these studies have suggested that this results from the greater share of adult attention these children receive. (Bates, 1975). This suggests that older children are not an adequate substitute for adults in teaching language. McCarthy (1954) found that the mean length of utterance (MLU) was highest in children who associated primarily with adults. K. Nelson (1973b) reported a negative correlation between the time children spent with other children and measures of language during the ages of 10 to 24 months.

The above studies would indicate that in cultures where infants are cared for primarily by siblings and somewhat older peers, language development should be markedly delayed. Slobin (1972), in his review of cross-cultural studies of language, found that these children still begin to speak at about the same time and have the same general course of language development. Nevertheless, in American middle-class culture, the differences between adult–child and child–child speech are important, and it is not surprising that there have been an increasing number of analyses of the characteristics of child–child speech.

A first observation was that young children, like adults, simplify their speech when talking to a younger child or an infant. Bates (1975) found that the speech of a child speaking to another child is shorter, syntactically simpler, and more restricted lexically than the speech of the same child to an adult (p. 267). These same criteria also characterize motherese, yet these speech characteristics are apparently not as conducive to language learning when used by a child as when used by an adult. This has been explained by Bates (1975) as resulting from two factors. The first is the more egocentric focus of the child on his own interest. In speaking with a child, the adult is most often guided by the interest of the child, or, at least, is careful to illustrate to the child what the topic of the conversation will be. Also, children have difficulty in signaling comprehension. Even when they perceive that their message is not understood, they have poor techniques for correcting the conversation.

Between 2 and 5 years of age, children become very fluent and engage in frequent social play with peers. This fluency is characterized by verbal and social play. Garvey (1977) describes verbal play as the noises and sounds children produce, often in chantlike routines. She illustrates this with a soliloquy of a 3-

Even children as young as four years will adopt the special code known as 'motherese' when addressing infants. (The Family Circus by Bil Keane, reprinted courtesy of The Register and Tribune Syndicate, Inc.)

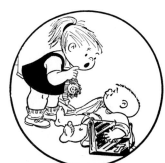

"Understand, honey? Mommy won't be home tomorrow — she'll be here the NEXT tomorrow."

year-old girl who repeated "yesterday," "yester," "yes," "ter," or "day" in varying combinations for almost 15 minutes as she explored the room and looked at the various toys. This type of verbal play was also recorded by Weir (1962) in the presleep monologues of her son. Garvey (1977) has noted that verbal play may also be engaged in as a mutual game by two children.

Other social play has been recorded as characteristic of preschool children. A common game is naming combined with misnaming. For example, one child may say to another "that's my mouth," while pointing to his nose and both children will laugh. Another type of social play is "make-believe," in which children assume different roles (Garvey, 1977).

The Electronic Media–Child Relationship

The influence of the mass media, particularly television, on the development of children has been extensively studied. Much of this study has concerned the possible effects of violence and stereotyping on the attitudes and actions of young viewers. Whatever these effects may be, it appears that the rate of both intellectual and linguistic development has accelerated during this century (Moerk, 1977). In studies of the role of socioeconomic factors on child development, a negative correlation was observed between the levels of ambient noise and cognitive development. Ambient noise ws considered to be the presence of radio, television, and varied conversation and verbalizations in the background. High levels of ambient noise were common in poor homes. K. Nelson (1973b) found that the amount of television viewing by young children was negatively related to the rate of their language growth.

The young child's need to relate to others as a part of the communicative process is apparent from observations of children answering the television, waving to the television screen, and in other ways attempting to establish an interpersonal relationship. With the electronic media as with child–child speech, the language model is reduced in effectiveness because the speech is neither adjusted to the child's level of comprehension nor does it effectively involve the child in interaction. (Moerk, 1977).

EFFECT OF SOCIETY ON LANGUAGE DEVELOPMENT

No language can be properly understood without a knowledge of the social and cultural forces that shaped it. Like language, social structures are systematic and highly coded; they concern interpersonal relationships, terms of address, and kinship terms. They also concern the cultural rules of the members of each social group. (Brown, 1965). The influence of socioeconomic status (and to some extent education) on the language spoken is crucial. *Sociolinguistics* is the study of the differences in the linguistic structure of socially defined groups and of rules of langauge used in different situations or contexts (Ervin-Tripp & Mitchell-Kernan, 1977).

The Role of the Social Group: Dialects

A speaker's region of birth can often be ascertained simply by listening to speech patterns. Differences in vocabulary, pronunciation, and grammer can mark the speaker as coming from the Deep South or the East Coast, for example. Such regional differences used to be ascribed to a lack of mobility; most people lived most of their lives where they were born and associated with few people outside their immediate environs. It was predicted that following the Second World War, with increasing mobility of the population and improvements in mass communication, these regional differences would tend to disappear, as would the problem of language variation.

It is true that geographic and regional differences have lessened; however, the problems of language diversity have increased. There is currently less difference in the speech of educated professionals coming from different parts of the country than between middle-class and ghetto residents of any large city in the United States. Dialects, and their implications and possible remediation, constitute a major educational and social concern.

Among speakers of English, the educational and social level of individuals become apparent as soon as they speak. George Bernard Shaw used this knowledge as the basis of his play *Pygmalion,* in which Henry Higgins, a speech professor, launches Eliza Doolittle, a poor flower girl, into London society as a duchess by changing her manner of speech.

Variations among speakers tend to be referred to using qualitative terms. Certain forms are considered "correct," others "incorrect." By implication, the people who speak "good" language seem somehow superior to those who speak "bad" language. The explanation that the linguist Bloomfield offered for this situation years ago still appears relevant. He (Bloomfield, 1964) indicated that the reason that language is described in terms of good or bad is that some people are felt to be better models of conduct and speech than others; the behavior and speech these persons use is felt to be better. This perception seems true of every group and applicable to all languages. In fact, a study of two forms (called high and low) of several non-English languages, including Greek, Swiss-German, Arabic, and Haitian Creole, showed that in each language all speakers could agree on the usage that constituted the high form (Ferguson, 1964). The high form was used in religious services, literature, lectures, news broadcasts, and official business. Even those people who had some difficulty following the high form were upset at the idea that religious services, for example, should be conducted in the low form. Some speakers denied that a low form of the language existed, even though their denial was stated using it.

In English, various dialects have been identified and described. A *dialect* is a variety of language used by a group of speakers of a particular geographical region and social status (Halliday, 1978). In Britian, dialects include those characteristic of Glasgow and Edinburgh, as well as Cockney speech. The standard, which is called the Queen's English or RP (for Received Pronunciation), is that form of speech acceptable in the royal court.

In American English, dialects include Black English (BE), Appalachian English, and Nonstandard Southern White English (R. Williams & Wolfram, 1977). The most common and best described of these is Black English, also sometimes called Negro English (NE) or Nonstandard Negro English (NNE; Fromkin & Rodman, 1974), which is spoken by large numbers of black people living in urban and ghetto areas.

The standard of any language is the normal speech of the educated and of those who conduct the important affairs of the country (Bloomfield, 1964; R. Williams & Wolfram, 1977). Until fairly recently, the American people were accustomed to hearing their President speak with an Eastern or Midwestern accent—obviously the standard. However, within a ten-year period, one president spoke with a distinct Southwestern accent and another with a Southeastern accent, both of which initially provoked amusement and clever books of "translation." However, once the speakers attained sufficient national and international prestige, the accents themselves became more accepted.

The language specialist is seriously concerned not with re-

Regional accents are the source of local color. Three of the major accents in the United States are Eastern, Southern, and Midwestern, and there are a score or more minor variations described by linguists (Pei, 1965).* Humorous "guides" to these pronunciations have been written. A guide to the speech of South Carolina provides the following definitions: "abode" is a wooden plank; "rah chair" refers to where you are; and "sex" is "one less than seven, two less than eh-et, three less than noine, foe less than tin." Not to be outdone by this, a guide to Brooklyn has the following clarifications: "fodder" is a male parent; "earl" is a lubricant; "oil" is an English nobleman; "tree" is the numeral preceeding four; and, of course, "Long Guy Land" is the island on which Brooklyn is situated (Long Island).

Immigrant dialects tended to disappear very quickly, with the exception of Pennsylvania Dutch.† This dialect, which is used primarily in several regions of Pennsylvania, is not Dutch at all but a variation of a 17th-century German, heavily influenced by French. Some Pennsylvania Dutch expressions are most picturesque, such as "outen the light" (put out the light); "the paper wants rain" (the paper predicts rain); and "his off is all" (his vacation is over). The unwary traveler might receive a direction such as "Go the bridge over and the street a little up."

*Mario Pei: *The Story of Language.* New York, Mentor Books, 1965, pp. 57–58.
†Penna. Dutch booklet. Available from Dutchcraft, Inc., Gettysburg, PA.

THE COMMUNICATION ENVIRONMENT

gional accents but with dialects, of which Black English (BE) will be discussed here in more detail. In considering BE, the contribution of two researchers is fundamental: Bernstein, a sociologist, described the social structure and its effect on language; Labov, a linguist, described the structure of language and how it varied according to social class.

Bernstein began by looking at social structures; he particularly studied what he called the middle and lower or working classes. He then analyzed the language produced by members of both and determined that there were two distinct styles of speech, which he called codes: the Elaborated Code and the Restricted Code. Speakers of the Elaborated Code tended to be middle class. Their speech suggested that they assumed that the listener would not understand them unless they provided a rather full explanation. Speakers of the Restricted Code tended to be lower class, and tended to assume their listeners would know what they meant despite a lack of explanation. People of the lower class were considered members of a subculture by Bernstein (1970) and Edwards (1979)—adolescents and prison inmates are other examples of subcultures; like all members of subcultures, they assumed that the listener shared the same contextual information as the speaker, so less explanatory information was provided.

Bernstein illustrated these two codes by providing transcripts of picture descriptions produced by two different 5-year-old boys living in London (Bernstein, 1970, p. 26). The stimuli consisted of four pictures showing boys playing football, breaking a window, being threatened by a man, and running away while a neighbor woman watched from her window. The middle-class boy described the picture by specifying that three boys were playing football and one boy kicked the ball through the window. He went on to explain that when the ball broke the window, a man came out and yelled at the boys, who then ran away. During this time a woman was looking out of the window. The lower-class boy, using the Restricted Code to tell the story, replied with a series of uncertain referents. This boy said only that "they" were playing ball and "he" kicked it through "there." The boy went on to say that "he" came out and shouted at "them," so "they" ran away. A person listening to the second telling of the story could not be sure who was playing ball, who broke the window, or who was yelling.

Bernstein was a supporter of the *difference theory* between styles or codes of speech. However, Bernstein's work was used to support those educators who, during the 1960s, espoused the *deficit theory*. The deficit theory evolved following the observation that children from lower socioeconomic classes were not succeeding in school. This failure was associated with a supposed lack in language skill, and rigorous programs were devised to "teach language" to lower-class children. The deficit theory hypothesized that ghetto children received little verbal stimulation and heard little well-formed language and so they could not speak complete sentences, did not know the name of common objects, and could not form concepts or present logical arguments verbally (Halliday, 1978; Labov, 1970). During the 1960s Labov started the first really serious research of the speech patterns of the cities—specifically in the ghettos of New York. He was motivated in part by a conviction that educators who proposed remedial language programs lacked any real knowledge about either language or black children (Labov, 1970, p. 153). His work demonstrated that the notion of "verbal deprivation" was a myth. Labov outlined the systematic way in which the English of the urban ghetto was different from the English of the middle class, including middle-class blacks. Neither English was more simple or illogical than the other. Just as there are no primitive languages, there are no primitive or simple dialects. Examples of some differences between standard and Black English are listed in Table 5-1. There are also many other detailed examples (Dale, 1976; Edwards, 1979; Fromkin & Rodman, 1974; Labov, 1972; F. Williams, 1970; R. Williams & Wolfram, 1977).

The Role of Context: Codes

Probably the most serious charge brought against speakers of Black English was that the children tend to communicate primarily nonverbally and have few means of verbal communication. Again, Labov (1970) explored and refuted this myth. Labov quotes an interview with an 8-year-old black boy named Leon from Harlem. In the first interview, Leon was brought into a small room in a school where a large, friendly, white interviewer put a toy on the table and asked Leon to tell him all he can about it. Following each 10 to 12 seconds of silence, the interviewer asked another question. All of these questions were re-

William Labov

William Labov combined his interest in linguistics with his understanding of sociology to provide a series of detailed analyses of the systematic variations among dialects. The most significant example of this work was his study of Black English. To accomplish this study, Labov and his colleagues gained the trust of several different gangs in the Harlem area of New York City that permitted them to tape-record and transcribe their spontaneous conversations. His analysis of various dialects was reported in *The Social Stratification of English in New York City* and in *Language in the Inner City,* among numerous other publications. The work on Black English, in particular, was instrumental in establishing that this dialect represented a rule-governed variation of standard English and did not reflect errors, simplifications, or impoverished language.

After obtaining his undergraduate degree from Harvard University in 1948, Labov worked for a number of years as an industrial chemist. He then obtained a Ph.D. in linguistics from Columbia University in 1964. Labov served first in the departments of linguistics and psychology at Columbia University and then at the University of Pennsylvania. His current work focuses on conversational interaction. In 1979, he served as president of the Linguistic Society of America.

Table 5-1
Some Differences Between Standard and Black English

	Black English	Standard English
Pronunciation		
• Word-final consonant clusters are reduced.	tes' des'	test desk
• After a vowel /l/ becomes /uh/.	steauh sistuh	steal sister
• Before a consonant /l/ is absent.	hep	help
Grammatical features		
• A copula that can be contracted is deleted.	He nice. They mine.	He is nice. He's nice. They are mine. They're mine
• If the copula cannot be contracted, it cannot be deleted.	Here I am. How beautiful you are.	Here I am. (*Not* Here I'm) How beautiful you are. (*Not* How beautiful you're)
• Nouns following numerals need no plural marker.	Two pound Twenty year ago	Two pounds Twenty years ago
• Verbal tense. The form "be" provides additional information in Black English.	He busy (momentary) He be busy (habitually)	He is busy. He is busy.

warded by one- or two-word answers. Labov concluded that this response represented a particular code that the child used when he perceived that he was in an asymmetrical situation where everything he said might be used against him. When Leon was brought back with one of his friends and the two boys sat with the interviewer eating potato chips and discussing the kind of insults and taboo words used on the streets, Leon competed actively for his turn to speak and proved to be highly verbal and imaginative (Labov, 1970, pp. 157–164).

A code, or register, is often defined as the type of speech each speaker chooses as appropriate for a specific circumstance. This choice depends upon the age, sex, and social position of the listener, as well as on the environment of the communicative exchange. Among bilingual speakers code-switching refers specifically to the alternation of different languages. Among monolingual speakers, a particular code is chosen according to the situation. In the example above, Leon was using what has been called a school code. This consisted of frequent "I donnos" and single-word responses, with which he attempted to protect himself from what he perceived as a hostile environment.

Implications for the Language Specialist

For the language specialist, an understanding of the variations that are normal aspects of language is essential. When it is understood that a nonstandard dialect is primarily a social disadvantage, then it will be obvious that an educational or linguistic solution cannot solve the social problem. As Halliday (1978) has noted, the problem in dealing with dialects is with the social value system, not the linguistic system.

Bidialectal instruction, in which children in the early grades are taught the grammar of both their native dialect and standard English, is currently being tried. The hope is that children may become fluent in both dialects. In practice, however, it is rare that speakers of standard English become fluent in Black English, and minority children are still expected to learn society's dominant dialect—the dialect spoken by people with whom they seldom associate. Apparently, the strongest motivation for change is the desire for upward mobility, and those children who decide it is to their advantage to speak both dialects usually master standard English rather quickly. Regardless of the approach adopted by schools, it is important that educators remain open to linguistic pluralism and refrain from penalizing the abilities children bring to school. If the children are expected to switch dialects, their teachers should also be able to switch to, or at least understand and respect, the dialect their students speak. Halliday felt that a speaker who was made ashamed of his own language suffered basic injury as a human being.

THE RELATIONSHIP OF NONVERBAL BEHAVIOR AND COMMUNICATION

Nonverbal communication follows highly systematic rules that differ from culture to culture, are essentially untaught, and are often unconscious. Kinesics and proxemics are two forms of nonverbal communication. Studies of these forms illustrate that two people engaged in a conversation are doing much more than speaking. Their eyes and bodies move, and their demeanor and appearance carry subtle messages.

The language specialist has a particular need for information on nonverbal communication; because children with language disorders tend to have as much difficulty learning the nonverbal as the verbal rules of language. Such children speak loudly in church, stand so close to the listeners that they tread on their toes, etc. Nonverbal rules often must be consciously taught to these children.

Nonverbal communication speaks loudly in social exchanges. To pass an acquaintance on the street without speaking, to catch

THE COMMUNICATION ENVIRONMENT

a stranger's eye and smile, or to turn away from a speaker all deliver clear messages. Psychologists have found in studies of prejudice that some students who have previously been identified as being prejudiced against racial minorities or homosexuals will talk to members of these groups using all the appropriate verbal politeness. However, analysis of nonverbal behavior such as eye contact, distance between speakers, and minute facial expressions indicated the students' distaste (Snyder, 1980). This finding has obvious implications for language specialists, who must realize that their feelings of impatience or disappointment may be conveyed to a child or adult even though their words are appropriately reinforcing.

Kinesics

Kinesics is the study of body movement, including facial expression, eye contact, tone of voice, and posture, used with communication (Birdwhistle, 1970). Like language, kinesics tends to be rule-bound, culturally specific, and learned developmentally. There is some evidence, however, that the significance of several basic facial expressions expressing emotions such as joy, fear, surprise, and anger may be the same in many cultures. People from such diverse places as New Guinea, Brazil, Japan, and the United States can correctly identify certain basic emotions from pictures showing facial expressions (Ekman, 1975). Some facial expressions may be universal because of common neuroprogramming linking facial muscles with particular strong emotions. However, the face is capable of thousands of modifications, and, not surprisingly, many expressions are specific to certain cultures; some are specific to a certain age group or sex within the culture (Birdwhistle, 1970).

An important means of nonverbal communication is eye contact, which is established between infants and their caretakers well before 1 year of age and remains important throughout life. By 2 months of age, the stimulus that most often produces a smile is a pair of eyes (Argyle & Cook, 1976). Eye contact signals a willingness to communicate, and lack of eye contact is taken to be evasive in some cultures. The rules for eye contact differ from culture to culture, however, and what may be considered evasive in one culture may signal attention in another, and what appears bold and aggressive in one culture may seem polite in another. In addition to cultural variations, eye contact varies within the same culture based upon the social status, age, and sex of those engaged in conversation. Thus, eye contact helps to clarify the nature of the relationship between the two communicators. Matters of social dominance, sexual availability, kinship, and aggression are all made evident nonverbally (Morain, 1978; Starkweather, 1977).

Proxemics

Proxemics is the study of how people use space. Four regions of space have been described by E. T. Hall (1959). The first is intimate space (0 to 18 inches), which occurs in intimate relationships between adults and between infants and their caretakers. Personal space (2 to 5 feet) is that distance at which good friends feel comfortable talking with each other in soft voices. Social space (4 to 7 feet) is that distance at which casual friends or acquaintances talk with each other in a conversational tone of voice. Anything over 8 feet is considered public space, and at that distance the speaker tends to use a raised voice and to employ more formal platform manners. Awareness of both intimate and personal space has been shown by children under 7 years old, while the use of social and public space is acquired in the school years (Hopper & Naremore, 1978, p. 109).

E. T. Hall (1959) has pointed out that the boundaries of space differ from culture to culture. Certain Mediterranean cultures operate in a casual or business space that is much closer than is comfortable for Americans. Lack of understanding of this difference leads some people with a Mediterranean heritage to consider Americans to be "cold" or "standoffish", whereas

Figure 5-2
The integrative model of language, showing the dimension of the communication environment.

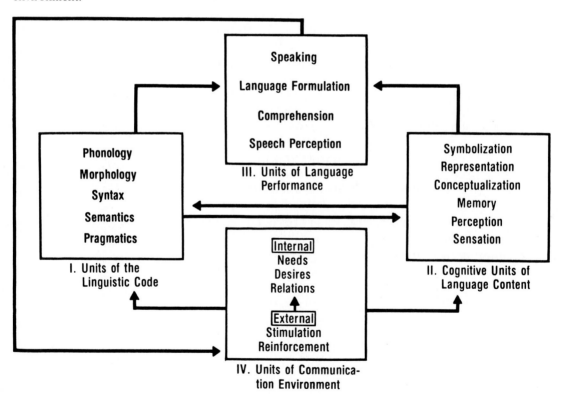

Americans may consider Mediterraneans "pushy." Other examples of this awareness of space abound. Some adults state that they immediately stake out their territory when sharing a hotel room. Family members report that they have "their" chair at the dining table and often "their" chair in the living room; finding a guest in that place may be so upsetting that they ask the guest to move. Families have "their pews" in churches that have no assigned seating. Even preschool children verbalize how they would fight to preserve their right to sit in "their" chair at nursery school (Hopper & Naremore, 1978).

Chronimics

Another less well-known branch of nonverbal communication is *chronimics*. This refers to the use of time and includes the timing of entrances (particularly tardiness), the rate of speech, and the duration of silence (Starkweather, 1977). As E. T. Hall (1959) has stressed, the use of time is culturally bound, and tardiness, which may be considered an insult in one culture, is not even noticed in another.

THE DIMENSION OF THE COMMUNICATION ENVIRONMENT

A model of the interpersonal dimension of language is presented in Figure 5-2. This model shows that internal needs and desires for interpersonal communication form the central core of the communicative process. (It is the authors' contention that social interaction is as significant as cognitive development in the learning of a language.) When the internal need to relate to others is impaired (as, for example, in autism), the communication process is also impaired. These internal needs and desires are stimulated and reinforced first by parents and then by peers. As the model illustrates, the interaction between the child and his parents and his peers is reciprocal, with the child affecting his parents and peers almost as profoundly as they affect him. The child's relationship with society is different. Society, in this case meaning the socioeconomic class into which the child is born, tends to have a unilateral rather than a reciprocal effect. The cultural rules of a society are arbitrary and exist apart from the child, just as the linguistic rules are arbitrary and constitute a type of knowledge the child must acquire. These linguistic and social rules are not modified for handicapped children, and every child is expected to acquire these rules or his performance will be judged defective. Although these rules are arbitrary, they are not uniform. Children who are born into a culture where a nonstandard dialect is spoken, for example, will learn that dialect. The use of that dialect reflects socioeconomic status, not cognitive or linguistic proficiency.

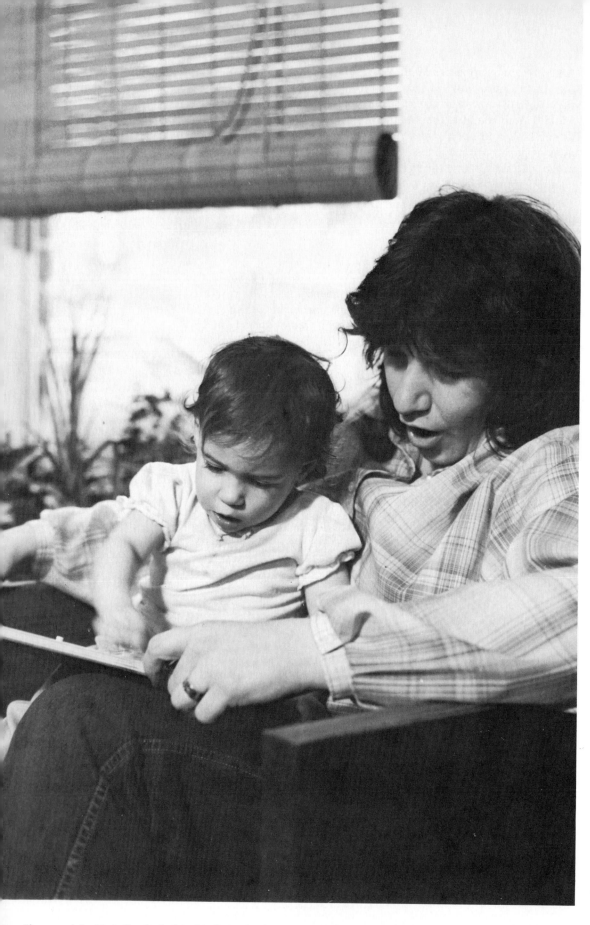

Photograph by Linda Stanford of the Media Production Center, University of Texas Health Science Center at Houston.

part two

normal language development

outline

ASPECTS OF EMERGING LANGUAGE

Order and Variability
Stages of Development

BASES OF LANGUAGE DEVELOPMENT

Acquisition Versus Learning
  Behavioristic Theories
  Innate Theories
  Critiques and Integration of Theories
Maturation
Imitation
  Types of Imitation
  Developmental Stages of Imitation
  Role of Imitation in Language
Conditioning
  General Aspects of Conditioning
  Role of Conditioning in Language
  Mediation in Language Theory
  Conditioning in Language Teaching
Linguistic Input

DEVELOPMENTAL SEQUENCES IN LANGUAGE

Order of Emergence: Cognition Versus Language
  Reciprocal Relationships Between Cognition and
  Language
Order of Acquisition of Words and Structures
  Cognitive and Semantic Complexity
  Linguistic Structure Complexity
  Frequency and Order of Acquisition
Order of Emergence of Comprehension and
Production
  Opposing Positions
  Evidence from Observation and Experiments
  Comprehension Redefined
Order of Syntactic and Semantic Relations

issues in language development

6

Q UESTIONS REGARDING HOW and in what sequence children learn language are among the most difficult and complex to answer. There is a constant accumulation of facts on language development through research and consequent changes in theoretical constructs. The periodic changes of emphasis seem to be influenced by the research being done at the time and by whether it is done in the linguistic or psychological tradition. There are numerous areas in child language development for which there are no facts available, and there is little commonality in the methodology used to obtain the facts that exist. The task, then, is to interpret, integrate, and compare an inadequate number of facts, and place them in a theoretical construct. However inadequate, each attempt at theorizing identifies the issues more clearly and assists in ferreting out the similarities and differences in interpretation. The language specialists who attempt to bypass theory lack a basis for making clinical decisions.

Awareness of theoretical themes and their historical sources allows language specialists to evaluate current methods and procedures and to choose among them judiciously. Although the extreme points of view may no longer be held by theorists, these positions continue to influence thought and application. For this reason this chapter includes a brief review of the psychological and linguistic positions in a language development, in addition to a discussion of general issues that are critical to the understanding of this development.

Order and Variability

Language is a process that most children learn without "conscious tuition" (Slobin, 1971a) and that most parents observe with love and interest and usually without interference. The rate of acquisition of language differs markedly from child to child. The major observable changes in the language of most children take place between the ages of 2 and 4. Language continues to develop throughout the elementary school years, and some aspects of it, particularly vocabulary, continue to expand throughout life.

The emergence of language in children is orderly and hierarchical. The various language dimensions follow broad sequences of appearance in children's speech. Order is present in phonemic and semantic development, as well as in syntactic structure development. Early stages are basic to the development of subsequent stages. The developmental stages are characterized by rehearsals and approximations. For the child to be in error—by adult standards—is considered normal. Children practice language as they struggle to match their adult models or, perhaps, as the adult models accept and reinforce those aspects that are most like their own language. Children's errors may result from the communication demands placed on a system that is not fully developed. They will mold their ideas into the forms they have assimilated as a means of saying what they wish. Thus, the syntax may be simplified in an effort to make language an instrument of their own intentions.

At times in the developmental sequence, it may appear that the child is regressing; he begins to make errors in structures that he had appeared to have mastered. Bowerman (1978b) explained these errors as reflections of an important advance in development rather than of a loss of knowledge. The early "correct" use of words may be habitual and specific to certain situations and contexts. Later the words are given a wider application and overlap with similar concepts, and the child begins to make errors. Bowerman (1978b) believed these errors to be an indication of an appreciation that the child did not previously have of the underlying relationship and regularities in the language structure.

Children differ in the ease with which they learn language. Some variation is normal. Bowerman (1978b) suggested that children may even follow different paths to adult language. Huxley (1970), Bloom, Lightbown, and Hood (1975), and Dore (1974) have described differences in the way children start using the linguistic code, which are reflected in the function the language has for a child—for labeling and practicing, or for an instrument to obtain needs and information (Dore, 1974)—and in

*PJ's sister recognizes that learning to speak is a developmental task. (*The Family Circus *by Bil Keane, reprinted courtesy of The Register and Tribune Syndicate, Inc.)*

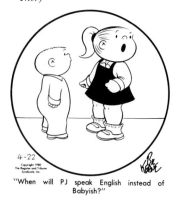

"When will PJ speak English instead of Babyish?"

the type of constructions used. The fact that there is variation among children in acquiring language makes it difficult to distinguish between normal variation and variation that reflects a language disorder. This is particularly true if we observe the output only, since there is no single standard to use as a guide for judgment.

Bloom (1978) has pointed out that the variation observed in child language has its own regularity, so that both the variation and consistency exhibit orderly and predictable patterns. This signifies that, in addition to differences among children in the development of linguistic skills, there are differences within each child; that is, development is not linear. K. E. Nelson and K. Nelson (1978) refer to the uneven quality of the child's advances as a pendulum which moves from creativity in language to inflexibility and systematization. According to Nelson and Nelson, the shifts occur in the acquisition, application, stabilization, tightening, and integration of the rules. They describe the system in terms of stages as follows (1) idiosyncratic first steps; (2) general rule stage (few, generally broad rules); (3) many-rule stage (rapid change, additions, revisions); (4) integration and consolidation (stable, coordinated rules); and (5) flexible extension (adaptive, conscious rule use). They characterized the growth process as change from a relatively open to a closed stage, and then, in some cases, to a new openness defined by a "higher-level understanding of the system as a whole and its potential usefulness."

Stages of Development

Because of the variation in the attainment of specific linguistic abilities, Brown (1972) has suggested the use of stages of development instead of the traditional reference of chronological ages. A stage model has also been utilized by Piaget (1954, 1955, 1970) in describing cognitive development. Piaget discovered that behavioral changes in cognition emerge in a sequential manner in children. He found the stages to be hierarchical, i.e., structures defining earlier stages become integrated into subsequent stages (Flavell, 1963). As Prutting (1979) noted, Brown's stages are not true stages in the sense of those described by Piaget, but are more or less arbitrary dividing points along a continuum of development data.

The stages developed by Brown were structured on the basis of the mean length of utterance (MLU). He believed the MLU to be a good index of grammatical development because it is simple to compute and is reflective of every new kind of linguistic knowledge. According to Brown, children matched for MLU are much more likely to use the same level of constructional com-

Table 6–1
Brown's Stages of Language Development

Stage	MLU	Major Development	Upper Morpheme Boundary
I	1.0–2.0	Semantic relations	5
II	2.0–2.5	Grammatical morphemes	7
III	2.5–3.25	Modalities of sentences	9
IV	3.25–3.75	Sentence embedding	11
V	3.75–4.25	Coordination of sentences	13

Adapted from Brown R: *A First Language: The Early Stages.* Cambridge, Mass.: Harvard University Press, 1973.

plexity than are children of the same chronological age. These stages provide "way stations" that describe the developmental sequences preceding the stage and the linguistic constructions typical of the stage (Table 6-1).

A basic factor in language development, viewed from the reference point of stage of development, is change or movement in the direction of the target language through the established stages. The rate of change is not as important as its existence and direction. The amount of change required of a child at any stage corresponds to the distance the child's approximations are from his adult models, but his performance must be measured against himself at a previous stage. The child's motivation to reach the models is the basis for change. If for any reason the child stays at the same level of approximation for any sound or grammatic structure, the probability that he will remain at that level increases with the time he is at the level and with the frequency of occurence of the approximation. If the child's language is not changing or if his changes are not orderly—if they are significantly out of phase with established developmental sequences of language or with non-language aspects of his own development—he may have a clinical language disorder.

Although the stage model process appears to reduce the child's role to a passive acquirer of language, this is far from the truth. The active, dynamic role of the child has been described and emphasized by Piaget and others (Bloom & Lahey, 1978; Muma, 1978). Bloom and Lahey described the development of operative knowledge in children based on the work of Piaget (1954) and Gratch (1975). Children form mental representation or schemes for acting with objects. By moving objects from place to place, infants see them in relation to one another and in relation to their own actions. This activity forms a basis for subsequent stages in development and ultimately for the development of language (see Chapter 3).

Prutting (1979) cautioned against the absolute interpretation of a stage model. She stated that, since the stages highlight the differences between stages, the overlapping aspects and similarities are frequently overlooked. Bruner (1975) also stressed that development takes place through continuity and gradual "ritualization" of schemes rather than by reorganization into stages through qualitative changes. Thus, the stage model is a useful means of classifying developmental information, but it cannot be interpreted as an absolute system of categorization.

Acquisition Versus Learning

The literature that describes the bases for the development of language by children provides two labels for this process: *language acquisition* and *language learning.* Superficially, these terms appear to by synonymous, and in some instances they are used interchangeably. Strictly interpreted, however, they represent divergent points of view.

Behavioristic Theories

The older term, language learning, describes a process whereby a child is taught to speak by means of principles, described in learning theory, that emphasize such events as stimulus-response (S-R), conditioning, and reinforcement strategies. The behaviorists, who are proponents of this viewpoint, believe that the S-R approach can account for novel sentence generation from past experiences, particularly if studied within the framework of response hierarchies, word association, and complex environmental stimulus control (Staats, 1971). The behaviorists describe language learning as a passive process in which properties of verbal strings, and correlations between these properties and other events, are registered and accumulated (Braine, 1971).

In 1957, Skinner, the foremost proponent of behavioral psychology, published *Verbal Behavior,* which many psychologists

BASES OF LANGUAGE DEVELOPMENT

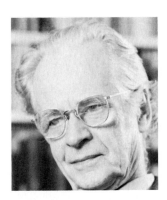

Burrhus Frederick Skinner

Seven years after receiving his doctorate from Harvard, Skinner wrote his first book, *Behavior of Organisms,* which set forth an interest in and dedication to behaviorism that was to last throughout his professional career. In 1948, he wrote a provocative novel, *Walden II,* which described a behavioristically designed Utopia. More recently, he became a prophet of behavioral engineering in his book, *Beyond Freedom and Dignity.* Students of psychology know Skinner for the precise science of behavior that he developed. His approach was characterized by emphasis on observing physically measurable properties of responding and on developing a practical technology for controlling observable responses. Skinner's interest was not only theoretical, however; he pioneered efforts to apply his theory to the improvement of education and to the modification of the abnormal behavior of mental patients and delinquents. Of particular interest to language specialists is his theory of language development described in his book, *Verbal Behavior* (1957).

felt would be the definitive document on language learning. (Even now, Skinner's single-stage model may be considered the prototype of the behaviorist theories.) In his book, Skinner stated that language was a type of stimulus-response association and so could be fitted into S-R terms. The basic mechanism in Skinner's theory was the verbal operant, which he defined as a dependency relationship between a verbal response of some sort and an antecedent condition. This behavioral explanation of language formed the basis of subsequent psychological theories of language.

Innate Theories

The behaviorist theory of language development is in direct opposition to the nativist theory. The term acquisition is used by the nativists, who describe the development of language in children as a process in which the children, having innate capacities for linguistic knowledge, interact with experience and develop language automatically, naturally, effortlessly, and quickly (McNeill, 1970). Language, according to this theory, is regarded as a biological phenomenon—the product of evolutionary specialization (Lenneberg, 1967)—and so a child requires only a certain amount of language input to activate this inborn knowledge.

The "language acquisitions device" (LAD) proposed by the innate theorists was first described by N. Chomsky (1957, 1965), and was later elaborated by McNeill (1966, 1970). It is a theoretical construct that describes an internal structure possessed by children that is capable of taking a corpus or body of linguistic input and converting it to an internal grammar. McNeill (1971) hypothesized that children acquire language by discovering the relations that exist between the surface structure of sentences and the universal aspects of the deep structures; the deep structures are manifestations of children's own capacities.

The nativists arrived at the concept of innate language because of the regularities in language behavior, the complexity of language, the universal features across language, and the creative aspects of language (Staats, 1971).

Critiques and Integration of Theories

Staats (1971) and others have objected to the nativist's explanation of language. Staats stated that information and observation about behavior does not explain language, nor does it give evidence of internal structure. He recommended that since language is composed of repertoires of skills (speech, imitation, comprehension) that are functionally combined, a credible theory of language must specify these repertoires and the learning principles by which they are acquired. Ervin-Tripp (1971), in response to the nature/nurture controversy, suggested that processing models be substituted for description models; such models would account for real-time events and psychological concepts as well as for speech and sentences.

In the eyes of some theorists (Garrnett & Fodor, 1958), the differences between the nativist and behaviorist positions are more apparent than real. They claim that empiricists accept inborn principles implicitly, in the form of properties that lead to the perception and integration of stimuli, and that they therefore believe that part of language is learned and part is acquired through inborn principles.

Fodor (1966) wrote of an ability by which children could "project a unique correct grammar on the basis of exposure to a corpus." He stated that the characterization of the child's intrinsic information suggests a process for the induction of the base grammar. Piaget (1970), in reinforcing this dual influence on language learning, stated that the establishment of cognitive behavior consists neither of a simple reproduction of external objects nor of the unfolding of structures inside the subject, but rather involves progressive building of structures by continuous interaction between the subject and the external world. Although Fodor's and Piaget's approaches are essentially different, both attempted to integrate the innate and environmental contributions to language development. It appears that a combination of Piaget's and Fodor's positions is the most likely to be true. Prutting's statement (1979, p.5) succinctly summarizes the integrated viewpoint: "Development does not seem to commence according to a prior timetable within the genetic code nor according to arbitrary reinforcement schedules provided by society. Linguistic and communicative behavior seems to be determined simultaneously by maturation, the continual reorganization of internal schemes as well as the behavior of society."

Maturation

Maturation is the term used for the process by which the child's physiological and psychological systems gradually change toward completion, full potential, and full capability. Certain levels of maturation are said to be required for the accomplishment of specific tasks; the phases when these levels are reached are called *readiness periods*. Lenneberg (1967, p. 126) presented signs of maturationally controlled emergence of behavior: "(1) regularity in the sequence of appearance of given milestones, all correlated with age and other concomitant development facts; (2) evidence that the opportunity for environmental stimulation remains relatively constant throughout development . . . (3) emergence of the behavior either in part or

Eric H. Lenneberg

Eric Lenneberg's interest in all of the scientific domains that related to the study of the mind led him first to graduate degrees in linguistics and psychology at Harvard and then to postdoctoral work at Harvard Medical School specializing in neurology and children's developmental disorders. He was born in Germany in 1921 and lived in Brazil during his youth. When he came to the United States to pursue higher education, he was already embued with the European tradition of an organic, holistic theory of the brain.

Lenneberg is thought to be the first to propose that the human capacity for language can be explained only on the basis of the biological properties of man's brain. He applied his biological concept of critical or sensitive periods to the study of language. Lenneberg's contributions have been particularly powerful in the integration of concepts regarding the brain, behavior, language, and the disorders of language. His integrative skills are demonstrated in his major publications, particularly in *Biological Foundations of Language.* The science of neurolinguistics, and the series of volumes and conferences in his memory, testify to his influence as a researcher and, more importantly, as a teacher. His concept of language is best expressed by the statement "Children begin to speak no sooner and not later than when they reach a given stage of physical maturation."

entirely, before it is of any use to the individual; (4) evidence that the clumsy beginnings of the behavior are not signs of goal-directed practice."* Language, he believed, satisfied these requirements. Consequently, according to Lenneberg, language cannot begin to develop until a certain level of physical growth and maturation is attained.

Lenneberg (1967) proposed that the maturational changes in the child between the ages of 18 and 28 months account for the beginning of speech at that age. However, it is not the general maturation factors that are responsible for language, according to Lenneberg, but a language-specific factor. The strongest support, in fact, for the nativist's theory has been provided by the work of Lenneberg, who traced the universality of language development and correlated it with other forms of emergent and largely untaught behavior and stages of brain maturation. He observed that children in all cultures learn to walk, and also to say words, at similar ages. Also, cross-cultural studies of children learning to speak indicate a great commonality among the early utterances in all languages so far studied.

Moerk's (1977) interpretation of maturation and nativism was that there are innate structures and tendencies for behavior and perception. However, these structures are not solely responsible for the emergence of language. The structures interact with the environment and result in cognitive and behavioral functions; a wide variety of these functions (discrimination, vocalization, etc.) develop before, and help to produce, verbal behavior.

It is not obvious which factors of physical growth and maturation are related to language capability and which are not. Chase (1966) argued that the understanding of the correlation of physical and chemical parameters with language is imperfect, and

*Reprinted with permission from Lenneberg EH: *Biological Foundations of Language.* New York: John Wiley & Sons, 1967, p 126.

that language might develop at an earlier stage of maturation if environmental contingencies were different. Chase offered a counterproposal, which stated that stages in the development and interaction of phonological and syntactic organization correspond with specific junctures in the development of specific *needs* for information-exchange systems.

There appears to be disagreement regarding the exact roles of maturation and environment in language development. Both the nativist and the behavioral points of view concede to a combination of both factors; the difference is in the extent, timing, and level of interaction between maturation and environment.

Imitation

The role of imitation in child language development has been disputed throughout the history of the study of child language. The behaviorists considered that imitation played a significant role in language learning by forming an important base for the stimulus-response-reinforcement paradigm. Since psycholinguists considered language acquisition to be a specifically human and innate function, they gave imitation a negligible role in its development. As has been true of other issues, part of the disagreement resulted from a failure to define what exactly is meant by imitation. Moerk (1977) proposed that denials of the possible effects of imitation may result from restrictions arising from definition of the term employed.

Types of Imitation

In general, according to Piaget (1962), there appear to be two kinds of imitation: (1) imitation that is an immediate repetition of a model (in the case of language, a model utterance); and (2) deferred imitation, which is delayed and produced in the absence of the model. Piaget's definition specifies that the first type of imitation occurs in situations where the models are immediately available to perceptual activities. According to Bandura's interpretation (1971) of observational learning (learning through imitation), the acquisition of a skill can be removed in time from its application or performance, even though the performance is clearly a result of observation of the model, as is deferred imitation.

Developmental Stages of Imitation

Piaget (1962) considered imitation to precede and form one of the bases for language learning. He proposed that imitation itself goes through developmental stages, and considered it an example of what he referred to as *accommodation.* In accommodation, internal structures are modified in accordance with environmental influences.

During the early stages of imitation, the infant will only imitate what he is already capable of producing and auditorily monitoring. The next stage finds the infant attempting to establish a correspondence of "shared features" in imitation, the shared features serving as mediators between new behavior of the model and his own familiar action schemas. At a subsequent stage, the imitation involves active discovery and systematic attempts to modify the action schemas in order that more exact correspondence exist between the child's behavior and the behavior of the model. Representation, the appearance of symbolic function, is seen in imitation at the next stage—behavior is imitated without the model being immediately available to perceptual activity. Imitation in this deferred form, according to Piaget, is the first indication of internalized accommodation or representation; this internalization forms images that function to designate objects or events not immediately available to perception. Deferred imitation thus has a role in identifying form as separate from content and establishing a basis for symbolic behavior (see Chapter 3).

Role of Imitation in Language

Moerk (1977) stated that the child learns about the structure of verbal and nonverbal behavior from adults whom he observes and imitates. This imitation leads first to the selection of sound patterns of the mother tongue, then to single words, and later to the acquisition of the complete adult language skills. R. Clark (1974) also believed that early sentences are unanalyzed, imitated sentences. She suggested that the first "novel" sentences are not the products of true syntactic rules; rather they are simple modifications of imitations. This is accomplished by internal analysis of memorized sentences. Clark refers to the copying and alternation strategies as *performance without competence.*

Other functions of imitation in child language are reported by Schuler (1979) in a review of literature in this area: (1) to contribute to the acquisition of lexical items; (2) to serve as requests for elaboration or explanation; (3) to serve as an aid in processing material by prolonging what is seen and heard; (4) to serve the linguistic functions of labeling and affirmation; (5) to maintain communicative interaction and social rapport; and (6) to assist in the acquisition of discourse rules.

In a grammatic study of imitation in six children, Bloom, Hood, and Lightbown (1974) concluded that imitation is not necessary for language development. In the children who used imitation, however, Bloom found that their imitations were developmentally progressive and involved an active and immediate processing of utterance; i.e., they imitated patterns of which they did not have complete mastery.

Slobin (1968) reported that at 18 months, 13 percent of one child's utterances were imitative, while at 35 months, only 2 percent were. This finding was supported by Bowerman (1973a), who reported that as language age and mean length of utterance increase, the percentage of imitative utterance decreases.

The fact that many of the early utterances of children are dissimilar to adult speech is given as evidence for discounting the role of imitation. It is argued that in cases where children appear to imitate adult speech, the output is reduced to the level of the form of the child's own grammar. Early in language development, children do not imitate sentences more successfully than they spontaneously produce them (Slobin, 1973). Ervin (1964) found that children's imitations (under the optimal conditions of immediate recall) were *not* grammatically progressive and concluded that the imitations cannot account for children's rapid progress in acquiring grammatical structures.

Insight into the role of imitation in language development emerged from a study of the different *styles* children use in acquiring language. Bowerman (1978a) described children who analyze sentences covertly, so that they have some understanding of the internal structure of what they are saying when they begin to talk. Other children plunge directly into production, appearing to use stored sentence fragments not yet analyzed. Bowerman reported on studies that found children who spoke sentences before the onset or completion of Piaget's appropriate sensorimotor stage, as compared to other children who were advanced in imitative skills and heavily reliant on modifying imitated sentences. Bowerman concluded that there are probably important differences among children and within children with respect to the uses and functions of imitation.

Distinctions in evaluating the role of imitation have been pointed out by Schuler (1979). She stated that the level of automaticity of the echoing behavior needs to be judged as well as the immediacy of the response. The degree of actual similarity between echoed and model phrases may be significant. Another important factor is the choice of echoed responses in terms of who is imitated or which discussion is imitated. The level of complexity of linguistic imitations should also be considered.

Prutting and Connolly (1976) concluded that the evidence regarding both spontaneous and elicited imitations as they relate to language acquisition is inconclusive, and suggest that the use of clinical procedures involving imitation be used with caution.

Conditioning

General Aspects of Conditioning

Conditioning is a behaviorist term, used primarily in literature pertaining to S-R learning theory, and refers to a process by which stimuli and responses are associated. Behaviorists view the learning of language in the same manner as they view learning in general, so that the general principles of learning would apply to language, except that language is probably more complex. In fact, their criticism of Chomskian psycholinguistic theory is that it does not provide a method of studying how the child learns his various repertoires of language or how these repertoires function in the individual's behavior and in social interaction.

Role of Conditioning in Language

Palermo (1971), a proponent of the conditioning theory, stated that the acquisition of the child's first word is a function of simple conditioning or paired-associate learning, and that sequences are developed through chaining, and word classes through equivalences. Skinner (1957) considered verbal behavior to be subject to the same sets of variables that influence nonverbal behavior. His functional approach stipulated that the emission of verbal responses is shaped and maintained by a verbal environment—people respond to behavior in specific ways because of the practices of the group of which they are members (Skinner, 1957). The emission of a response followed by reinforcement serves to strengthen the dependency of the response upon any and all antecedent conditions. Chomsky (1967), however, attacked the concept of reinforcement as having no explanatory force. It is commonly observed that children speak at approximately the same age even when exposed to the most adverse environments, as long as they have the opportunity to hear language. Children are observed to speak often and voluminously even when alone or in play with peers who give no verbal or nonverbal reinforcement.

Mediation in Language Theory

The current view in psychological circles is that single-state learning theory models are insufficient to account for the learning of language by children. Criticisms of the use of S-R theory in understanding language behavior state that this theory cannot account for both the accounts of the structure of language and the reflection of that structure in actual behavior (Bever, 1968). Braine (1971) and Osgood (1967) have suggested mediation theories instead. Although the mediation theories differ, they essentially describe a mediating factor between the stimulus and response; the aspect of conditioning, however, remains (see Chapter 2). In some instances, the mediating factor is associations within classes of words, in other cases it is the word meaning (Osgood, 1967), and in still other cases it is the position or temporal location of the word in an utterance (Braine, 1971).

Conditioning in Language Teaching

It is difficult to completely ignore the contributions of conditioning to language development if conditioning is interpreted to include the rewards and reinforcements that serve to strengthen language behavior at least in its function. Hundreds of children have been taken to language disorder specialists because they have not started talking by the age of 3½ to 4 years. Extensive study of many of these children has revealed normal intelligence and normal development in every aspect of growth other than language. It may happen that the environment of the child has not provided a need for the child to talk. In such cases, a regime of providing rewards (giving the child what he requests verbally) and punishments (denial of desires until verbally requested) usually brings about the initiation of verbal communication. This is not to say that he acquired the grammar of the language through conditioning, but that he acquired the behavior of using language to communicate through conditioning.

Reinforcement behaviors make up a considerable proportion of the child's language-learning environment. Modeling and expansion serve, among other things, as means of supporting the verbal output of the child. Verbal responses to a child's input are forms of reinforcement. On the other hand, to consider relations between words and their meaning as conditioned association would limit the change in breadth and specificity that occurs with language development.

The degree to which the internal structures of children or the external factors in the environment provide the means whereby children abstract the rules of the language they hear, and use the rules to comprehend and produce language, is not yet understood. The complexity of language belies a simple explanation. This complexity also dictates that no theory be totally rejected, since it may explain at least some part of the language-acquisition process.

Linguistic Input

The effect of material linguistic input on language acquisition is an issue that has been of considerable interest in the history of child language development (Chapter 5). The only period in which the interaction between mother and child was not considered a significant variable was during the time when the nativistic philosophy of language was prevalent. Nativists, primarily Chomsky (1965) and McNeill (1966, 1970), stated that the language input to the child was disorganized, disfluent, ungrammatic, and haphazard and consequently could not serve as a primary basis for child language acquisition. This theory empha-

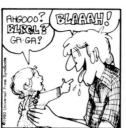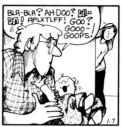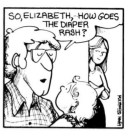

Linguistic input to children is adapted to their level of comprehension—that is, if no one is looking. (Reprinted courtesy of Universal Press Syndicate.)

sized the induction process as a means of acquisition, and therefore, according to the proponents, the child could not induce order from disorder. Instead, they suggested that since the child is equipped from birth with certain information about linguistic structures and operations, the child processes the input he hears in accordance with his knowledge of the language.

The behaviorist position, on the other hand, relied heavily on input in describing the language-learning process. Since the notion of "stimulus" is essential to the S-R theory, the input of the parents, particularly the mother, is of paramount importance to the learning of language. Recent studies have given credence to the importance of the role of maternal speech input to the child's acquisition of language. To begin with, the assumption that the speech children hear is of poor quality is false (Bowerman, 1978a). The speech parents use when speaking to their children has been found to be not only fluent, but free from error (Brown & Bellugi, 1964).

As described in Chapter 5, adult-to-child speech differs from adult-to-adult speech. Parents adapt their speech input to the linguistic and general cognitive level of their children, particularly while the child is 2 to 5 years of age. As the child grows and improves in using language, qualitative changes in input seem to predominate over quantitative ones.

DEVELOPMENTAL SEQUENCES IN LANGUAGE

Order of Emergence: Cognition Versus Language

As the philosophical positions relating language and thought differ (see Chapter 3), so do positions regarding their developmental sequence. There are two primary viewpoints regarding the order of development of cognition and language in children. One side considers that concepts are first introduced to the child by means of language; the early concepts are based upon the first words acquired in the language development process. The second position considers that concepts develop before the comprehension and expression of the first word. The child "brings certain meanings to the task of language acquisition, and these meanings affect even his very first word" (Cromer, 1976, p. 295). The child is thus viewed as coming to language-

ISSUES IN LANGUAGE DEVELOPMENT

learning equipped with a stock of basic concepts that he has built up through his interactions with the world.

Many investigators have studied the relationship between cognitive stages and corresponding language milestones. They have been particularly interested in Piaget's account of the sensorimotor period and its relationship to the linguistic structure of first words. Sensorimotor schemata that account for subsequent linguistic abilities have been described by Sinclair (1971): (1) the ability to sequence temporally and spatially corresponds with the sequence of sound and word elements; (2) the ability to categorize objects or to use them in action corresponds with the classification of linguistic elements into major categories (noun phrase, verb phrase); (3) the ability to relate objects with actions, permitting the grammatic relations of "subject of," "object of," etc. Other investigations proposed a clear relationship between the child's cognitive development and advanced syntactic constructions, namely, conjoining, embedding, passive voice, and certain transformational operations (Leonard, 1978).

Ruder and Smith (1974, p. 575) summarized the Piagetian interpretation of cognition as a prerequisite to the language acquisition process as follows: "(1) the infant brings to the acquisition task, not a set of innate linguistic universals, but innate cognitive functions which ultimately result in universal structures of thought of which linguistic universals are a function and (2) since intelligence exists phylogenetically and ontogenetically before language, and since the acquisition of linguistic structures is a cognitive activity, cognitive structures should be used to explain at least the initial stages of language acquisition rather than vice versa."*

Not all researchers and theorists are in agreement with respect to the interpretation of this relationship between cognition and language. Leonard (1978) suggested that the interpretation should be limited to the view that cognitive and linguistic development are "related" in some general way, the extent of the relationship varying with the nonlinguistic task and the feature of language studied. Other researchers have found "correspondence" between sensorimotor stages and productive language characteristics to be a better term than "prerequisite" for describing this relationship, because of inconsistent findings relative to the prior emergence of one or the other (Ingram, 1978; Dihoff & Chapman, 1977; and Miller et. al., 1980).

Bates et al. (1977) also took issue with the concept of cognitive prerequisites to language and offered in its place a model that emphasizes interdependence of cognition, language and social development. Their studies have led to the position that developmental skills arise from shared inputs or common origins.

*Reprinted with permission from Ruder KF & Smith MD: Issues in language training. In Schiefelbusch RL & Lloyd LL (Eds): *Language Perspectives—Acquisition, Retardation and Intervention.* Baltimore: University Park Press, p 575.

They borrowed the term *homologue* from culture anthropology and have applied it to describe the nature of the interdependence of the developmental tasks. ("A homologue is a structural similarity between diverse species or cultures which is the result of common origin" [Bates et al., 1977, p. 273].) They concluded that both the linguistic tasks and the cognitive ones are dependent on underlying operative schemes shared by the two domains.

Reciprocal Relationships Between Cognition and Language

The lack of definitive findings in the relationship between cognition and language may be related to failure to specify the aspect or level that is being studied. As indicated in Chapter 3, cognition may refer to the processes of perception and memory as well as conceptualization; the perceptual and memory aspects of cognition assuredly precede language. Concepts may be concrete categories or abstract classes, and the relationship of concepts to language may depend on the types of concepts under investigation. Furthermore, language may be considered in its signal use or in its symbol use; language as signal may precede specific concepts whereas language as symbol may not. Language in turn can be mediational or representational and communicative, and the function may influence the order of development of concepts and language. There are forms of signal and symbol behavior other than those of language that are reflective of cognitive behavior, and these may precede the emergence of linguistic structure.

The cognitive process of concept formation, which includes perception and memory, begins in infancy. The child uses physical actions such as arm gestures and object manipulation, which indicate the presence of concrete perceptual concepts in the absence of learning. The young deaf child can function meaningfully, without language in the world of relations. The prelanguage child and the deaf child do use signs, however, to point to or indicate their needs, feelings, desires, etc. In this sense, they are communicating and may indicate their knowledge of color, form, and other perceptual concepts. They may show knowledge of the concepts of objects by using them in the correct manner—sitting in a chair, drinking from a glass. Young deaf children who neither comprehend nor use linguistic forms can match color, size, shape, and like objects according to visual configurations and function. Even some of the early words of children function as signs. These words are used to point to or indicate, not to designate, and they illustrate the signal use of words (see Chapter 2). Words used by prelanguage children are thus functional and mediational; they serve to gratify their egocentric and immediate needs. They are not used symbolically and may not be considered by some specialists to be true language. In studying the relationship between cognition and language, the differences between using words and signs and symbols must be taken into consideration.

Although it is possible to develop concepts without language, the presence of language influences the further development of concepts, particularly abstract concepts that have no sensory referent and those that are conveyed by the grammatic structure itself. Words point to distinctions that have meaning; e.g., a small glass with a handle is a cup. If a child does not understand cup as a concept separate from glass until the label or word is used in his environment, it might be said that the word preceded the concept. The child perceives the difference, but does not consider it significant until it is labeled. There are many differences that exist in reality that are not significant and are consequently not labeled. While some of these are perceived, others are not recognized until they are pointed out (labeled). A deaf child who learns neither visual symbols nor spoken language does not develop concepts in the same way as a hearing child. Language of some kind (spoken, written, or signed) is essential to the acquisition, elaboration, and oral refinement of certain abstract concepts. But language cannot cause words to have meaning, because meanings of words can and often do change.

Order of Acquisition of Words and Structure

It is a fact of language development that the understanding and production of some words and constructions appear before others. The sequence of emergence may be due in part to (1) the relative difficulty of the cognitive underpinning among words and structures; (2) the complexity of the manner in which the content is expressed formally in the grammar, i.e., the complexity of the linguistic markers; (3) the type and frequency of the verbal environmental stimuli to which a child is exposed in learning the language; or (4) all of these.

Cognitive and Semantic Complexity

There are two aspects to be considered in the cognitive complexity of linguistic structures: The first is the relative complexity of the concepts that form the meaning of language—i.e., the supposition that it is more difficult to understand some concepts (space, time, numerosity, etc.) about reality than others. A second aspect, dependent on the first, concerns the manner in which the words and structure of language reflect this cognitive complexity, and consequently are "more or less difficult" insofar as they represent more simple or more complex functions.

The first aspect is referred to as *conceptual complexity,* the second as *semantic complexity.*

An example of semantic complexity was described by Cromer (1976), who reported a study of the development of words that expressed time relationships. The words representing the less complex aspects of time (naming of points of time) developed together and earlier than those representing the more complex categories of relevance from the past and timelessness (*never, always,* and *sometimes*). Cromer reported that this difference existed even though the frequency of use of the words in the environment appeared to be about the same. He concluded that children did not acquire common structurally simple forms until they had the cognitive capacity to understand the concept to which the forms referred.

There are two similar hypotheses delineating rules for categorizing the semantic complexity of words themselves and their consequent order of emergence: (1) the complexity hypothesis, stated by H. H. Clark (1973); and (2) the semantic feature hypothesis, described by E. V. Clark (1973). In these hypotheses, complexity is related to the word meanings but not in the same way as the relationship described by Cromer. Cromer's study involved words that expressed meanings that were more or less complex. The linguistic structure complexity refers to the number of ideas or features that a word contains making it more complex than another.

H. H. Clark's system involves cognitive marking of lexical items in such a way as to designate the level of difficulty of the words. His complexity hypothesis is stated as follows: "given two terms, *A* and *B,* where *B* requires all the rules of application of *A* plus one or more in addition, *A* will normally be acquired before *B*" (H. H. Clark, 1973, p. 54). He suggested that a preposition such as "in," when used in its spatial meaning, expresses a single notion such as location; a preposition such as "above" expresses two notions—location and relation (the location of one object is related to another). Therefore, "according to the complexity hypothesis, "above" is more complex than "in" and is learned later by children.

E. V. Clark's (1973) semantic feature hypothesis specifies that the adult lexicon has features or components of meaning, and the child has only partial aspects of the total adult meaning of a word. The child's development is accomplished by adding features to approximate the adult meaning. This hypothesis predicts that general semantic features are acquired prior to specific ones. E. V. Clark's theory, which is similar to H. H. Clark's, also predicts that if two words share a set of semantic features, but one has an additional feature, the meaning of the less complex word would be learned first.

Semantic complexity has been said to also account for the order of emergence of grammatic inflections and other grammatic notions. Slobin (1973) stated that the earliest grammatic markers appearing in a child's speech encode the basic notions available to the child's mind. He illustrated this with the semantic relation of verb-object, which is developed early cognitively and also expressed early either by word and order (e.g., in English) or by inflection (e.g., in Finnish and Russian). Additional support to this position was given by Brown (1973), who found that the verb inflections that are marked in children's speech are those whose meaning is evident in comprehension and implied in expression, indicating that the early forms are semantically simple for the child. Slobin (1973) suggested that the awkward or ideosyncratic forms used by children also indicate their knowledge of a meaning for which they do not have a form. In summary, Slobin (1973, p. 184–185) suggested a principle to support these conclusions: "New forms first express old functions, and new functions are first expressed by old forms." For example, a newly learned grammatic structure such as the plural morpheme may be used to express an already known concept of plurality, or a new concept of size relationships may be first expressed by an old form, *more big,* and then by a new form, *bigger.*

Linguistic Structure Complexity

Most of the support for the notion of surface complexity is provided by Slobin (1973). In his study of the acquisition of language by children learning different languages, he found, for the most part, that basic meanings were expressed in surface structure at about the same developmental period regardless of the language spoken. However, there were examples in which the developmental stage of the expression of certain semantic relations varied among languages. In the two examples he provided, the yes/no questions in Finnish and the noun plurals in Arabic, the *form* coding the meaning in the structure of the language was extremely complex, and therefore, the reported delay of acquisition was attributed to surface complexity.

Slobin also compared the acquisition of constructions reflecting the same semantic notions in the language of bilingual children. He reported the case of two bilingual girls who had learned to encode semantic relations (locative) in Hungarian that they were barely developing in Serbo-Croatian. The manner of encoding the indicated meanings was more complex in the latter language and consequently the emergence of this form was delayed.

A description of grammatic complexity similar to that of the semantic complexity hypothesis of Clark was described by Brown and Hanlon (1970). Brown (1973, p. 407) stated "In our *cumulative* sense of complexity a construction x + y may be regarded as more complex than either x or y because it involves everything involved in either of the constructions alone plus something more." Brown added that the primary determinants of acquisition order would prove to be semantic and grammatic cumulative complexity. Brown and Hanlon (1970) illustrate cumulative deviational complexity with the negative passive, which they consider more complex than either the negative active or the affirmative passive equivalent.

When Brown (1973) applied the concept of cumulative complexity to morphemes, he found a relationship between the degree of complexity and acquisition order and concluded that semantic complexity is one determinant of order of acquisition and a demonstration of the law of cumulative complexity.

Frequency and Order of Acquisition

The frequency of occurrence of certain structures in the environment of the child might also influence order of acquisition. Brown (1973) examined the hypothesis that the more frequently a morpheme is modeled by a child's parents, the earlier it is acquired. He studied samples of parent speech that occurred immediately prior to stage II in the children's level of development. Brown did not find a relationship between parental frequency and order of acquisition, and therefore concluded that frequency is not a significant variable.

Order of Emergence of Comprehension and Production

Opposing Positions

The literature in child language has traditionally reported that children comprehend language earlier than they produce it (McCarthy, 1954). Lenneberg specified that the lag time between comprehension and corresponding production to be a matter of a few months, particularly between the ages of 18 and 36 months (Lenneberg, 1967). This position has been supported by the observation that children in natural language situations give evidence of comprehension of sentences that are considerably more complex than their own speech (Sachs and Truswell, 1978). Results of experimental studies also support this order of emergence (Fraser, Bellugi, & Brown, 1963).

The validity of this view has been seriously questioned by Bloom (1974) in view of findings that placed production ahead of comprehension. Bloom (1974, p. 286) believed the issues to be more complex than formerly considered and suggested that the "developmental gap between comprehension and speaking probably varies among different children and at different times and may be more apparent than real." Her position was that speaking and understanding are mutually dependent but are comprised of different underlying processes; the direction of influence of one on the other shifts throughout the developmental period of language. D. Ingram (1974a, p. 316) in a response to Bloom's theories and conclusions, reaffirmed the essence of the traditional position but restated it: "*Some* comprehension of a specific grammatical form or construction occurs before it is produced." Ingram (1974a) proposed that the issue was not one of the priority of comprehension or production but rather of the nature of comprehension and production and the extent of the gap between them.

Evidence From Observation and Experiments

The need to define more clearly the terms *comprehension* and *production* is manifested in the interpretation of the observations and experiments that have been used to defend the various positions described above. There is also a failure to delineate clearly the hypotheses that are being studied and the premises that underlie them. Bloom (1974) pointed out additional factors that make it difficult to evaluate the findings in the reported studies. She noted that the presence or absence of nonlinguistic cues, which would alter the performance of subjects in studies, particularly in comprehension, are frequently not identified. The redundancy in the structure and in the environment are also important considerations in the evaluation of the responses of children. D. Ingram (1974) suggested that conclusions from observations of spontaneous situations may not be equivalent to those from controlled observations in experimental studies. A final point made by Bloom was that the data on the comprehension and production of single words should be viewed separately from that on multiword utterances. A few studies and reported observations will be provided to illustrate the problems that occur when a study fails to define exactly what is meant by comprehension and production.

A report by Huttenlocher (1974) indicated that children at 10 to 11 months of age looked for objects when the objects were named. Two of the children she studied could respond, by 14 months, to the query, "Where is X?" by going to the spot where X was ordinarily located, even though the object was out of sight at the time of the study. The active vocabularies of the children being observed were either nonexistent or limited to one or two words, even though there was positive indication of mental representation. This report seems to indicate that these children understood more language than they could produce at this period. The implied interpretation of "comprehension" was that of recognition of the signal relationship between the word X and the object. There was no indication of the children's knowledge of the word as a symbol, as referring to other members of class X, nor of the features of the word that the children "knew."

Bloom (1974) wrote of her daughter, Allison, who toward the

end of her first year responded to the words *birds* and *music* by arrest of attention and shifts of gaze toward the objects. Allison did not respond to these words in any other manner for many months. Three months after "recognizing" these words she started producing speech. When she began speaking, the early recognized words and the spoken words did not correspond (Bloom, 1974). Bloom's report seems to indicate that Allison responded to the words as signs and not as symbols. Although Allison seemed to recognize more language than she produced at this particular period, she did not produce words in the same order as they emerged in recognition; she did not know all the features of the words she recognized; she did not respond in the absence of visual cues; and she did not respond to the words in varied situations. If these factors are essential to comprehension, then in this case, comprehension could not be said to have preceded recognition.

Werner (1948) gave a description of a child who used *afta* to designate a drinking glass, a pane of glass, a window, and also the contents of a glass. Bloom (1974) interpreted this behavior to indicate that the child "did not understand the word used in each situation before using it himself because there is little likelihood that he heard the word in the same situation...." Bloom's implications are not clear. It seems that she believed either that children must comprehend all the features of a word and *only* those appropriate to the word before it can be said that they truly understand it, or that children must hear a word in each and every situation before producing it in that situation, in order to say that comprehension precedes production. If these implications are valid in defining comprehension, then comprehension will never be said to precede production in children because it is unlikely that children will have heard a word used in every situation in which they use it. The ability to generalize is an integral part of the language-learning ability of children.

A study by Keeney and Smith (1971) reported that 4-year-old children did not understand the verb inflexion markers corresponding to subject-verb agreement in nonsense pairs such as "The snup jumps" or "The snups jump." These authors interpreted this finding to mean that production is ahead of comprehension since children this age produced these constructions correctly. The problem with comprehension test situations of this type is that a forced choice is required, one in which the semantic feature boundaries of morphemes, as well as all members of the class, must be clearly identified and distinguished from similar grammatic constructions. The use of this construction in production, however, can occur without the child's "knowing" the rules for subject-verb agreement, or the agreement in syntactic forms in utterances may well be a result of automatic speech production. This automatic speech may reflect the frequency of occurrence of certain constructions that are in temporal contiguity to each other. Evidence for this may be drawn from the speech of children or adults with severe comprehension disorders who echo what they hear either immediately or in another inappropriate situation (see Chapter 4). The syntactic structure of these children is often correct in reference to the adult standard.

Comprehension Redefined

It appears that this controversy will continue unless the terms used are specifically delineated and the hypotheses are clearly stated. As stated above, D. Ingram (1974a) attempted to specify the traditional position as follows by stating that "*some* comprehension of a specific grammatical form or construction occurs before it is produced." Other possible statements of position may take one of the following forms, which are more specific than the general statement that comprehension precedes production or vice versa: (1) children understand more language than they produce at each specific period during development; (2) children understand most vocabulary items (single words) before they can produce them; or (3) the sequence of the words children learn to understand is the same as the sequence in which they learn to express them. The following statements about comprehension and production are even more specific: (1) children must comprehend all the features of a word and only those appropriate to the word in order for it to be said that they truly comprehend the word; (2) there must be a one-to-one relationship between the features a child uses in comprehension and those he uses in production for comprehension to be said to precede production; (3) a child must respond to words and to all situations in which words occur consistently for it to be said that the words are comprehended; (4) a child must respond without nonlinguistic cues to indicate that comprehension is taking place; that is, words must be understood as symbols, not as signs; (5) automatic speech production of a specific syntactic construction is possible without comprehension and without generative, semantically based production of that construction; (6) comprehension of grammatic markers is more complex than using the markers in automatic speech production; and (7) com-

A word can mean so many things; it's no wonder we have difficulty in defining comprehension. (Copyright 1968, United Feature Syndicate, Inc. Reprinted with permission.)

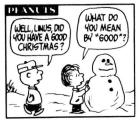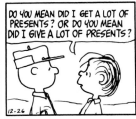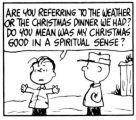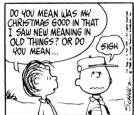

prehension precedes production of generative language expression of a specific linguistic form but not always of automatic speech using the same form.

The preceding lists have been presented in order to emphasize the complexity of comprehension and expression and the danger of using the terms broadly without specifying exactly what is meant by them. If specific questions are asked, it is more likely that specific answers will be found.

A final comment regarding the use of the word *comprehension:* comprehension depends on the formation of a relation between a word or structure and its meaning. It appears that *comprehension* is often used to describe *both* the knowledge of the relation between a word and its meaning *and* the evocation of a meaning when a word is heard. Unless there is a distinction made, there will continue to be considerable disagreement.

Order of Syntactic and Semantic Relations

Linguistic theory as proposed by Chomsky considers the relational concepts underlying child language as grammatic in nature; that is, the relations are the essence of the deep structure and are identified by the subject and object of the sentence. I. M. Schlesinger (1971) suggested that the relational concepts that form the basis of child speech are semantic in nature (rather than grammatic) and reflect the manner in which the world is perceived by the child. Schlesinger added that the child learns grammar by associating the adult expression of the relations with the context of the child's perceptions of the relations. He denied that there were any specifically linguistic relational concepts hidden away in deep structure.

Bowerman (I. M. Schlesinger, 1974) agreed with Schlesinger's idea of the validity of semantic relations. She pointed out that a syntactic concept like "subject of" in deep structure does not correspond with any single semantic concept; instead, "subject" may represent a number of semantic relations. The subjects in the following sentences "John wants bread," "John cuts bread," and "The knife cuts bread," play different semantic roles. According to Bowerman, the early concepts and relations learned by the child are semantic ones, and it is these semantic relations that he learns to express. Eventually, the child realizes that nouns expressing semantic relations follow similar rules with respect to position in the declarative sentence. This then leads to the abstraction "subject," which, from that time, functions in the child's system of rules (I. M. Schlesinger, 1974). In general, then, word position rules in sentence construction are specified on the basis of semantic roles as agent, action, etc., rather than on syntactic roles as subject and predicate. Brown (1973) stated that the syntactic relation of subject and direct object is the major syntactic means of expressing semantic relations.

Bloom, Lightbown, and Hood (1975) disagreed with Bowerman's interpretation and argued that the child's ability to use the same sorts of words in the same position in the sentence to express a variety of different semantic functions is indicative of the prior development of the superordinate grammatic categories—subject, predicate, and object. They suggested that the grammatic system is learned first, and the variety of semantic distinctions are encoded within the system. Bowerman (1978a), however, did not consider the fact that a given position in a sentence is shared by words with different semantic functions as proof that the speaker regards these words as equivalent in syntactic function. Furthermore, the fact that inconsistent or incompatible word orders do occur (Braine, 1976) offers positive evidence, in the opinion of Bowerman, that children do not have an understanding of higher-order syntactic relationships such as subject and predicate.

outline

learning words: semantic development

7

OVER 20 YEARS AGO, Roger Brown (1958) called the process of learning words the "Original Word Game." To play this game, at least two players are required—one who knows the language and is the tutor, and one who is learning the language (very often a child). The game is not complete until the child has discovered the stimulus attributes governing the tutor's verbal behavior; since the child does not understand the metalinguistic terms that describe language, the rules cannot be explained by the tutor, but must be discovered by the child (Brown, 1958, p. 210). This chapter describes the ways in which children begin to discover these rules. What is most significant about this process is that children appear to progress unfailingly through each succeeding stage. Although the age at which each stage is accomplished may vary, the order of development appears invariant across both individual children and different languages.

Early investigators of semantics were forced to content themselves with counting the number and types of words used by children at different ages. With recent advances in psycholinguistic techniques, a number of in-depth studies have explored the particular styles and strategies individual children have used to learn words. The cognitive precursors of vocabulary development and the semantic intentions of the young child, have also been analyzed. The material chosen for discussion in this chapter is designed to increase the language specialist's awareness of how children discover the relationship between words and their referents and the order in which they make these discoveries.

The focus of this chapter is on the period when children are developing single words, and beginning to express semantic relations requiring several words. This chapter begins prior to Brown's stage I and ends at the point when the child enters stage II. (See Chapter 6 for a more complete discussion of Brown's stages.)

This chapter provides information for the language specialist, who must decide whether a particular child is developing an adequate vocabulary, and who also may be in the position of choosing a curriculum to teach a first vocabulary to children with language disorders.

KNOWING A WORD

The concept of "knowing" a word appears obvious, yet there are complex behaviors involved, and knowledge of even simple words is a cumulative process that results from gradual development. For an adult, knowing a word implies a conscious or unconscious understanding of the critical attributes included in a dictionary definition, such as the part of speech, how it can be combined in a sentence (selectional features), and which words have similar meanings (synonyms) and opposite meanings (antonyms). For some technical words, the definition is likely to be very specific, while for many common words, such as *run*, there can be many different meanings. *Run* is used primarily as a verb and would be expected to follow an animate noun or agent as in "boys run," "dogs run," and "horses run." Synonyms of the word include *jog, sprint, gallop,* or *race*, while antonyms include *walk* or *stroll.* The verb *run* may also be combined with inanimate noun subjects to yield fragments such as "the machine runs" or "his nose runs" without violating the selectional features for the combination of the verb *run. Run* may also be used as a noun and may function as the subject or object of a verb in utterances like "a run of luck" or "a run on the bank." The adult language user knows that still other meanings are possible. The presentation of new words in a college course signals to the student that this is an empty category that will be filled as the course progresses; thus, when the professor speaks of *running subjects* in a beginning psychology course, the student immediately recognizes that her previous attributes for that word most probably do not apply, and so she waits to learn new attributes. This sense of collecting attributes or categorizations is crucial to the learning of words. Native speakers also recognize that *run* may occur in an idiom like "run of the mill," where the meaning has nothing to do with either the action of running nor the condition of a mill.

PRECURSORS OF SEMANTIC DEVELOPMENT

The majority of psycholinguists accept that children acquire language by mapping words onto the knowledge they already possess about their world. The contribution of psychologists like Piaget to the specification of cognitive behaviors which have particular significance for the emergence of speech was discussed in Chapter 6. Other cognitive precursors of semantic development have been suggested by Moerk (1977), who has identified the following:

1. *Attentional capacities.* These may be observed by 5 to 6 weeks of age. The infant begins active scanning in response to a stimulus. There is evidence of especially prolonged attention to the human voice.
2. *Discriminatory ability.* By 2 months, the infant can discriminate the mother's voice from that of a stranger. By 3 to 7 months, the infant reacts to intonation, and by 7 months actual words are comprehended.
3. *Classification abilities.* The infant's manipulation of objects appears to lead to an understanding of "thingness" and "classes of events." Further experiences lead to categorizing of spatial, temporal, and action structures, which must all precede the use of words for these concepts.

In addition to these cognitive precursors, there are functional or pragmatic precursors to semantic development. Bruner (1974–1975) identified certain behaviors requisite to the process of naming. These include:

1. *Indicating behaviors.* The first of these is mutual gaze, in which both infant and caretaker share attention directed toward a single object or event. Somewhat later, the infant can further direct the adult's attention by pointing toward an object. In Bruner's opinion, the child's first words express some aspect of *who* does *what* to *which* object, and may also indicate to *whom* the object *belongs* and *where* the object is *located.*
2. *Communicating behaviors.* Initially, the infant communicates exclusively by crying. These cries are interpreted very early by the adult caregivers and may be classified. At first, the cry has the communicative function of demanding. This may be expressed by a "fretting" cry or a scream. Next, the infant expresses what has been called the "request mode." This is followed by shared and reciprocal vocalization.

Once the standard meanings of words have been mastered, some speakers are able to use simple words to express images that go much beyond the dictionary definitions. Such imagery constitutes the artistic use of language and is illustrated by the following excerpt from Virginia Woolf, which attributes physical characteristics to words themselves.

"Those are white words," said Susan, "like stones one picks up by the seashore."
"They flick their tails right and left as I speak them," said Bernard. "They wag their tails; they flick their tails; they move through the air in flocks, now this way, now that way, moving all together, now dividing, now coming together."
"Those are yellow words, those are fiery words," said Jinny. "I should like a fiery dress, a yellow dress, a fulvous dress to wear in the evening."

Virginia Woolf: *The Waves.* New York: Harcourt Brace Jovanovich, 1931, p. 188. Reprinted with permission.

It is apparent that while all of the meanings of a word might be known to any adult, the word might be used productively by that person in only one or two senses. This dichotomy between comprehension and expression is intuitively accepted. Infants and even domestic animals demonstrate ability to follow directions, especially when the directions are appropriate to the environment. On a more abstract level, children can identify objects they cannot name, and adults understand certain commonly used terms, such as GNP (gross national product) in context, although many of them cannot accurately define such terms.

Differences Between Comprehension and Production

Certain of the differences between comprehension and production have implications for the study of the acquisition of first words. These include the following observations: (1) the first words comprehended are not necessarily or usually the first words spoken; (2) the number of words comprehended depends upon whether or not the child is allowed to use context to assist in understanding; (3) the type of feature errors the child makes may differ in comprehension and expression; and (4) there are differences between comprehension and expression in the rate of acquisition of words.

The difference between the words first comprehended and expressed was noted by Leopold (1939), who reported that while his daughter first understood *no-no* and *daddy,* these were not her first spoken words. Bloom (1973) [in the example already referred to in Chapter 6] indicated that her daughter first recognized the words *birds* and *music,* but that this recognition was specific to her bird mobile and to her record player and that they were not among her first spoken words. Huttenlocher (1974) and Benedict (1978), who both studied the development of comprehension, verified differences between the first words comprehended and the first words spoken.

In both children and adults, comprehension is enhanced by context. Young children are especially dependent upon context. One interesting experiment demonstrated that an infant's ability to differentiate *bite* from *throw* was dependent almost entirely on whether the child was tested in a highchair or a playpen. If the child was in a highchair, the response to the verbal command was always to *bite,* while if he was in a playpen, it was always *throw* (Lewis & Freedle, 1973, p. 150).

Another contextual variable is the children's tendency to choose the object that is most attractive. If presented with candy, a block, and a stick, most children will take the candy regardless of the instruction. Finally, children tend to respond with what they consider the most likely occurrence. Knowing that a dog may bite a boy, but probably not the reverse, children may give only the "likely" response. In a nontest situation, this use of context facilitates communication for both parents and children. Children are expected to grasp the intent of the overall situation and behave appropriately. Parents may therefore correctly report that their children seem to understand "everything." Yet in a test situation in which context and previous experience are of no help, children may fail to correctly identify a referent or follow a command three out of four times. They may also fail to distinguish the referent from a similar foil. Both the real-life situation and the test measure comprehension, but the criteria for demonstrating comprehension differ.

The gradual acquisition of the features of words is important to the acquisition of both receptive and expressive vocabulary. Apparently, however, the same features are not acquired with equal ease in both processes. Huttenlocher (1974) found that the overextension of words, which is almost universal in expressive vocabulary, was uncommon or nonexistent in comprehension. (See Theories for Extending Words, p. 140, for a more detailed discussion of this concept.) For example, the toddler who commonly overextends *daddy* to refer to all men, shows no confusion in identifying *daddy* as one special person distinct from all other men. Huttenlocher (1974) also studied errors in comprehension as children were tested for recognition of body parts. Even though there were errors, those errors were within the same general class of object; for example, when asked to show *eye* the child might point to a nose or hair, but not to a bottle or a ball that was also available. The nonrandom nature of the errors demonstrated the gradual accumulation of features despite the differences observed between receptive and expressive vocabulary.

Differences have been observed in the rate of vocabulary acquisition of comprehension versus production. The children in the Benedict (1978) study learned to understand twice as many new words as they produced. On the average, these children mastered twenty-two words each month in comprehension but learned to say only nine new words. Huttenlocher (1974) reported unpublished studies showing that receptive noun vocabularies were several times greater than expressive vocabularies in three subjects, while in three other subjects almost as many nouns were produced as were understood.

Although several researchers have discussed the time lag between comprehension and production, this was of particular interest to Benedict (1978) who conducted a longitudinal study of the development of comprehension in eight children. During the period when the children were between 9 and 15 months old, lists were generated of the first one hundred words understood and the first fifty words produced by the children. Analysis revealed that they understood an average of sixty words *before* they produced their first ten words. The data further revealed a 3-month time lag between comprehension and production at the level of ten words. There was a 5-month lag at the fifty-word level. Bloom (1974) also noted a 3-month lag between her daughter's first sign of comprehension and her first spoken words.

Development of Comprehension

As a result of her study of comprehension, Huttenlocher (1974) noted certain developmental stages. When testing her subjects, who were less than 1 year of age, she found that the first step was to attract the infant's attention. Attention was demonstrated by the infant establishing eye contact. The next evidence of increased comprehension was that the infant would begin a random search of the whole visual field for the object requested. At this early stage, the infant always engaged in random search even through many trials. As the level of comprehension increased, the infant could look or go directly to the object requested if it was in view. The next level of comprehension was when the toddler was able to get an object that was out of view. Next the toddler could get an object that had been placed out of view at some previous time. Once the child could identify an object or person or follow an action command such as *bye-bye* (wave) or *bang-bang* (hit an object), the next levels of comprehension were directly related to increases in the grammatic complexity of the utterance.

Despite the serious, unanswered questions regarding comprehension, D. Ingram (1974) felt that there is still support for the assertion that comprehension preceeds production. More important to the language specialist is the realization that a time lag between comprehension and production is expected. Variation in development among individual children is also to be expected. While some children appear to say the majority of the words they comprehend, others have comprehension that is far in advance of their productive skill. This appears especially true of children with language disorders.

LEARNING TO SAY WORDS

Strategies for Learning Words

Through studies of the first words of children, it has become increasingly apparent that children are not taught to say *bottle* or *ball* by hearing that object labeled by an adult; rather, they learn appropriate words to express concepts they have already developed. Children *bring* meaning to the symbols they use, they do not *get* meaning from the words. The child's prelinguistic organization of the world forms the foundation for the development of words. Various complimentary theories contribute to our understanding of the process of word acquisition.

Activity Theory

According to Piaget, the onset of first words occurs during the sensorimotor period, when the infant learns to act on his environment. Piaget felt that experience in interacting with people and things is a necessary condition of development during the first 2 years of life. Apparently, the similarity in infant concepts accounts for the great similarity in the first vocabulary acquired by young children around the world. Some researchers (Sinclair-deZwart, 1973) feel that the closest links between language and cognitive activity occur during this initial language-learning period.

Piaget stressed that knowledge about the world is acquired through action. As action patterns become established, extended, and combined with other patterns and differentiated under the influence of experience, knowledge of the world is built up. Through repeated experience with the objects in his environment—by grasping them, holding them, shaking them, dropping them, seeing them appear, disappear, and then reappear—the child discovers the properties of objects and their functional relations (Morehead & Morehead, 1974). During the first 18 months of life, the child also begins to realize that he is an active person distinct from the objects he acts upon. At this time, the child differentiates himself from others as a separate person, and it is as a separate person that he has need for language.

The importance of action for the child is well illustrated by first vocabularies of infants (K. Nelson, 1973b). Early noun vocabularies suggest that children choose to speak about objects upon which they can act, not simply about objects that exist in their environment, no matter how prominently. Of all their articles of clothing, children speak of shoes, socks, and hats—the only articles of clothing most infants can independently manipulate. The one universal article of clothing for this age group is *diaper,* but that word did not occur among the first 50 words in Nelson's study. She suggested it may constitute an infant taboo word (K. Nelson, 1973b, pp. 32–33). The toys and personal objects that infants find important enough to name include ball, key, block, book, bottle, juice, milk, and cookie—all objects over which a small child has some control. Infants also name some objects that they cannot control, but these objects tend to display movement. These include dog, cat, car, clock, and light (which goes on and off). Most early verbs also refer to movement or change. Verbs like *broke, fell,* and *open* describe changes in objects while other early emerging verbs refer to the child's own actions such as *jump, run,* and *throw.* These first verbalizations show the importance of the child's activity and involvement with objects and people in his environment.

Theories for Extending Words

During the time when a child has a limited repetoire of words, these words may not have the same range as they would for an adult. There are several theories concerning how children make the decisions as to which objects or events will be included in a single word. E. Clark (1973), in her semantic feature theory, postulated that a child attends primarily to the perceptual qualities of objects and so gathers the attributes that he will group under a heading of a single word. A semantic feature (see Chapter 2) is a shorthand method of specifying the conventions for using a word. Common perceptual features that Clark felt that young children attended to include shape, movement, size, sound, taste, and texture. Since no child can explain why he forms a category and labels it, this information has been gained by analysis of the first words produced by young children. Clark observed that objects that were referred to by the same word were perceptually similar in some way, particularly with regard to shape, and to a lesser extent to size, texture, movement, and sound. For example, any object having four legs might be labeled *dog*.

K. Nelson (1974) contended that children first classify objects not in terms of perceptual features, but in terms of the actions associated with them. Thus, if objects function in a similar manner, they will be called by the same name. For example, all referents for the word *ball* might share the functional feature "can be rolled." In her review of differing theories, Bowerman (1978c) observed that both theories had relevance but that each was still too restricted to account for all of the diversity illustrated in the over- and underextensions of early speech.

Over- and Underextension. Overextension refers to the child's application of a word to a referent that an adult would regard as belonging outside of that semantic category. *Dog* is one of the most frequent first words, and for many children *dog* or *doggie* may apply to all four-legged animals, both alive and stuffed. A child using this overextension appears to be attending to the perceptual feature of shape and is grouping everything with that feature together. Other common overextensions based on shape include the use of *car* for any type of vehicle and *daddy* for all men.

According to E. Clark's semantic feature theory (1973), children eventually learn to attend to additional features; they begin to separate dogs from horses on the basis of size; dogs from cats on the basis of sound; dogs from rabbits on the basis of movement; etc. Bowerman (1978c) provides examples of overextension from data obtained from her study of her daughters Eva and Christy. Eva not only used the noun *moon* to refer to the actual moon, she also overextended it by using that same word in sixteen other circumstances. These overextensions included

Eva's name for the circular dial on the dishwasher, for a crescent-shaped scrap of paper, and for a lighted floor lamp. Another word Eva overextended was the verb *kick*, which she used not only to refer to kicking a ball and a floor fan but also to a moth which was fluttering, to turtles 'dancing' on television, and to hitting a ball with her kiddicar. The importance of overextensions in early language development is indicated by the results of a recent study (Rescorla, 1980) that indicated that one third of the first seventy-five words learned by the children studied were overextended.

Overextension is only one of the ways in which children use words differently than adults. A child may underextend words, from the adult viewpoint, and so use a word for only a subset of the items an adult would include. Bloom (1973, p. 72) gave the example of her daughter, Allison, who used *car* at 9 months of age to refer only to cars observed from the window of her high-rise apartment. She did not use the word for any cars seen at street level, nor when she was in a car, nor when she saw a picture of a car. Subsequently, this word disappeared from her vocabulary and did not reappear until approximately 5 months later, when it included the usual range of features. Another example of underextension was provided by Bloom (1973), who noted that her daughter at first used *dog* only to refer to dogs she saw in the country.

In another example of underextension, M. M. Lewis (1959, p. 74) described the gradual broadening of the term *fa-fa*, which meant *flower*. At 16 months, his son used the word only to apply to jonquils growing in a pot. He next applied it to the same flowers in a bowl. A month later, the same word was applied to flowers of another type in a bowl and pictures of flowers in a book. Finally, 8 months later, he correctly identified embroidered flowers on bedroom slippers and sugar flowers on a cookie. This slow accumulation of knowledge was necessary to reach proper understanding of the word.

Relational Terms.   Relational terms do not attain all their complexity until a child is 4 or 5 years of age or older. (Since relational terms illustrate the role of features in extending words, they are discussed in this chapter.) According to E. Clark (1973), a relational term is a set of paired words that may operate as an adjective, a noun, an adverb, or a verb. The study of the acquisition of these words not only lends support to Clark's theory of first-words acquisition, but also clarifies common errors in the speech of children. Relational adjectives include antonyms such as *more/less, big/little, tall/short, same/different,* etc. (H. H. Clark, 1970; Donaldson & Balfour, 1968; Donaldson & Wales, 1970). E. Clark (1973) reported studies showing that the 3-year-old children she studied gave no indication that they could differentiate the word *less* from the word *more.* Although

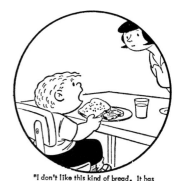

"I don't like this kind of bread. It has FRECKLES on it."

Overextensions, such as this use of the word freckles, *account for some of the charm of the speech of young children. (The Family Circus by Bil Keane, reprinted courtesy of Register and Tribune Syndicate.)*

they were correct in identifying *more* 91 percent of the time, they identified *less* correctly only 27 percent of the time. Obviously, there was a great lack of similarity in development of these terms. Further experimentation suggested that the children had overextended the word *more* to include *less;* at that stage of development, the children considered *more* as a synonym rather than an antonym of *less.* When semantic features of these words are analyzed, it is seen that both *more* and *less* contain the feature ± amount. Initially, it is apparently the feature of + amount to which the child responded, disregarding other features.

Similar confusion was found with other words expressing dimensionality. Children responded correctly more often when the adjective belonged to the positive set (*more, big, tall, fat,* and *high.*) Further studies seem to support a developmental order of acquisition of this knowledge involving not only the acquisition of the positive set of words before their opposites, but also the acquisition of more general adjectives such as *big* prior to more specific adjectives such as *tall, high, broad, thick, long,* and *wide,* with *thick* and *wide* being the last to be acquired. The hypothesis is that *big* is the first to be acquired because it applies to all dimensions of size.

E. Clark (1973) described a relevant experiment conducted by Piaget of the emergence of relational nouns such as *brother* and *sister* and *boy* and *girl.* Piaget asked a 5-year-old boy and two 7-year-old boys to explain what was meant by *brother.* The 5-year-old replied that a brother was a boy and insisted that all boys were brothers just as all girls were sisters. The first 7-year-old confirmed that he believed that all boys were brothers but denied that his father could be a brother because he was a man. The second 7-year-old indicated that he believed that his father could have been a brother when he was a little boy.

It is apparent that these children treated *brother* and *boy* as synonyms with only the following features being considered: + male, − adult. As the children got older, other features (± male, ± adult, ± sibling, and ± reciprocal) were added until the word attained the adult meaning.

Considerable study has also been done on children's knowledge of relational verbs, such as *give/take,* that express a transfer of possession, as well as *buy/sell* and *ask/tell.* Carol Chomsky (1969) found that children under the age of 8 years consistently interpreted the verb *ask* as if it meant the same as *tell.* These studies suggest that the task of learning words is continuous.

Typical First Words

It is possible to predict, within certain boundaries, which words a child will say first. These predictions seem to hold true regardless of what language the child is learning or what developmental disability the child may have. First words can be divided into two general classes: substantives and function forms.

Substantives

Substantives, also called content words, refer to object and person names (nominals or nouns), action words (verbs), and attributes (adjectives). This class of words figures heavily in the first lexicons of many children. As previously discussed, the early substantives refer to objects like shoes and keys, which children can act upon, and to objects that show action, such as dogs or cars. Most children talk about objects, their location in space, and the people associated with the objects. The most common first words of the eighteen children studied by K. Nelson (1973b) were *mommy,* and *daddy,* (specific nominals); *dog,* and *ball,* (general nominals); and *up, push,* and *run* (action words). K. Nelson (1973b) found differences between the characteristics of the first ten words and the first fifty words acquired by her subjects. Within the first ten words, animals and food were the main categories, accounting for 48 percent of all words. When vocabulary increased from ten to fifty words, the most obvious change was an increase of specific nouns. As the number of words increased, it was found that the category of animal words significantly decreased in importance and was replaced by body parts, which ranked with the category of food, together accounting for 56 percent of the words used. The words learned by these children represent selective choices that were for the most part action-related.

The most frequent verbs were calculated for four children in the initial language-learning period (Bloom, Miller, & Hood, 1975); the most common action verbs were *get, do,* and *make,* whereas *put, take,* and *go* were the first words commonly used to express locative action. These verbs are very general and can be used with many different objects in a great variety of circumstances.

The attributes that children initially use reflect an interest in change. Most children do not initially learn adjectives describing permanent attributes, such as *round* or *red*—instead they learn adjectives describing changeable qualities such as *hot, wet,* and *dirty* (Bowerman, 1976). Other common attributes are those of size and those of description (K. Nelson, 1973b).

Function Forms

Function forms express relationships between objects or ways in which objects change. It is impossible to understand a function form without evaluating the context in which the word is used.

Bloom (1973) indicated that the following function forms were used by her daughter between 10 and 18 months: *away, all gone* (expressing *disappearance*); *again, more, 'nother* (expressing *recurrence*); *uhoh, this, that* (expressing existence or calling attention to an object); and *no, all gone* (expressing *nonexistence*). It is apparent that these words did not make specific reference to any particular class of objects or actions; rather they expressed intentions beyond the meaning of the word itself.

Semantic Intention

Semantic intention refers to the meanings intended by a child's verbal expression at this early, single-word stage of language development. The relationship between a child's utterance and his intended meaning is his semantic knowledge. Semantic knowledge goes beyond the adult definition or use of word classes. When a child's total vocabulary consists of only a few words, the child needs to use the same word to express a range of semantic concepts. Bloom (1970, 1973) and I. M. Schlesinger (1971) were among the first to stress that the major meanings of utterances at stage I were composite meanings—the totality of the meaning the child intended to convey by the utterance.

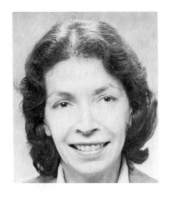

While studying the use of single words, Bloom (1973) noted that Allison first used *more* at the table when she wanted a second portion of food. Allison next used *more* to ask to be tickled again. Here the word *more* does not fit the adult definition of comparative adjective; instead it expresses the semantic intention of recurrence. At 10 months of age, Allison was using *away* to accompany the gesture of throwing an object into the trash, out of her sandbox, etc. Within several days she used *away* to indicate the disappearance of objects and people, and as an accompaniment to *bye-bye*. She also used *away* in reference to finishing her food. Thus, in all of these contexts the word *away* conveyed the semantic intention of disappearance.

Lois Bloom

Lois Bloom's doctoral dissertation at Columbia University was completed under the direction of William Labov and was subsequently published as a book, *Language Development: Form and Function in Emerging Grammars* (1970), which was responsible for moving the field of child language from its focus on syntax into the domain of the cognitive and semantic aspects of early language. In discussing her work, Roger Brown (1973) said that Bloom contributed to the introduction of what he called the *rich interpretation* of grammar.

Bloom began her professional career as a speech pathologist and after having worked as a speech clinician, she obtained her doctorate in psycholinguistics. In addition to her longitudinal studies, Bloom is also a parent-linguist. Analysis of the single-word utterances of her daughter, Allison, was reported in *One Word At A Time: The Use of Single Word Utterances Before Syntax* (1973). Bloom's professional interests came full circle with the 1978 publication (with Margaret Lahey) of *Language Development and Language Disorders*. This book combines reports of significant research in normal acquisition of language with application to language-disordered children.

At present, Bloom is a professor of education and psychology at Teachers College, Columbia University, where she continues her research on language development.

In contrast to the use of a single word to express the same semantic intention in different situations, there are examples of a single word expressing several different semantic intentions. Bloom (1973, pp. 99–100) illustrated this from Allison's early vocabulary. The word *daddy* was used as a greeting, to note the presence or existence of her father, and as an agent meaning "Daddy fix it."

It is possible to list typical single words, or chained words, and the semantic intention they frequently express (Bloom & Lahey, 1978; Bloom, Lightbown, & Hood, 1975; Bowerman, 1976; J. Miller, 1978).

Between 12 and 18 months, the semantic intentions that are often verbalized include the following. (They are listed according to the general order in which they tend to emerge and the approximate age ranges during which expression of the semantic intention may be expected.)

1. Existence (nomination): *this, that, mama, papa, juice, cookie, doggie,* (or name of pet).
2. Nonexistence (disappearance): *gone, no-more, all-gone.*
3. Recurrence: *more, 'nother.*
4. Negation, rejection, denial: *no, not, don't, dirty.*
5. Location: *here, there, up, duck-water, sit-lap.*
6. Notice: *hi, see, look, here.*

Between 18 and 22 months, several additional semantic intentions tend to emerge.

7. Cessation: *stop.*
8. Possession, association: *my, mine, daddy-coat, mommy-nose.*
9. Question: *what's that?*
10. Action: *push, run, go, up, off.*
11. Attribution: *hot, dirty.*

Since Brown (1973, p. 170) has estimated that 76 percent of the meanings expressed by children at stage I employ the semantic intentions of nomination, recurrence, or nonexistence, the importance of these meanings and the typical words used to express them should be appreciated by language specialists.

Styles in Learning First Words

The content of children's first vocabularies is remarkably similar in that all children comment upon or demand something in their immediate environment. Yet even within the constraints of a fifty-word vocabulary, the exact words differ from child to child. Bloom, Lightbown, and Hood (1975) noted that of the four children they followed in a longitudinal study, two used many nouns while the other two used many pronouns. K. Nelson (1973b, 1975) has suggested that children have different styles of learning their initial vocabulary. One style of language learning, which K. Nelson (1973b, p. 22) called expressive (E), is concerned with self and other people. This style of language learning appears to focus on the function of language. Words such as *no, go, more, hi,* and *thank you* are learned because they are useful in relating with other people and getting them to do things. The single words reported by Bloom (1973) for her daughter illustrate the use of this expressive style. At 16 months, Bloom's daughter used the following words most frequently (listed in order of frequency and followed by possible semantic intention): *there* (location or existence); *up* (location or action); *more* (recurrence); *down* (location or action); *no* (nonexistence, negation, rejection, or denial); *gone* (nonexistence); and *baby* (existence or notice).

Referential (R) style is primarily concerned with the name of objects and of people. Examples from Bloom's earlier studies (1970) show that Gia's most frequent single words were primarily referential in nature and all had the possible semantic intention of existence or notice: *mommy, 'cine* (machine), *Gia, noise, baby,* and *book.*

Other evidence (Bowerman, 1973a) confirms this tendency toward a style of learning. Examples of the most frequent words used by Rina as she learned Finnish include the following: *right here* (location); *yes* (agreement); *car* (existence or notice); *doggie* (existence or notice); and *uncle* (existence or notice). These words show that Rina was developing a referential style of language.

Follow-up studies have shown continuing differences between the R and E children. Initially, K. Nelson (1973b) felt that these differences tended to disappear by about 30 months; however, there is now accumulating evidence that these early styles of language learning persist. Of greatest significance to the language specialist is the fact that there is more than one way to learn language and that the individual styles of learning are apparent from the earliest ages.

Attrition of First Words

The attrition rate of early words is rather high. Bloom (1973, p. 66) reported that at 14 months her daughter used twenty-five different words, but during any one week only ten to twelve were used with regularity. Other diary studies (Leopold, 1939, pp. 159–160) also have reported "mortality" for words during this same period. The fact that a child has been heard to use a word does *not* indicate that he will consistently continue to use that word. Actually, it is rather likely that the word may be discontinued only to emerge later with a refined or different meaning, or it may reappear in different form, such as *doggie* reappearing as *bow-wow* (Bloom, 1973, pp. 66–67).

The subject of this experiment was observed while playing alone. As she looked through a magazine, she commented to herself about what she saw: for example, "that toothbrush" or "that nut." Another time, as she played with two gorilla dolls, she scolded one with "Bad, bad," while telling the other doll "Good gorilla. Good. Good." Such language is not unusual for toddlers, but this subject is a gorilla named KoKo who has been taught American Sign Language. Her vocabulary has expanded in various conceptual domains, and parallels the development of human children according to her trainer, Dr. Francine Patterson (1979, p. 352).

An analogous loss in words comprehended has been reported by Huttenlocher (1974). Her study of the development of comprehension in three normal children indicated several instances of a loss of systematic response to words, indicating that words that were comprehended at, for example 10 months, may not be comprehended at 11 or 12 months. It is possible that as the child matures, some objects and activities lose their importance. Whatever the cause, it is important for the language specialist to understand that it is normal for children to show a loss in the number of words they comprehend and/or express during the early stage.

Holophrases

Traditionally, it had been postulated that single words represented one-word sentences or *holophrases*. It was felt that when a toddler used the word *water,* for example, the intention or meaning was not to name the item but to say "I want water." It was claimed (McNeill, 1970) that at this stage the child used the single word for predication (implying an underlying knowledge of syntax)—not simply to label an object. It was therefore assumed that the child had the concept of an entire sentence. Using the theory of an innate capacity or language acquisition device (LAD), it was theorized that the young child used only a single word because of the immaturity of infant memory and vocal apparatus. The fact that these single words had intonation contours suggested that the child possessed knowledge of the syntactic structure of interrogation or assertion. Proponents of the holophrastic position asserted that children had a knowledge of sentences before they used them.

This position was most seriously challenged by Bloom (1973). Her study of her daughter showed that during the one-word stage, Allison often used more than one word, but these words did not appear to express syntactic relationships. Impressive evidence of this was Allison's use of the "word" *widə*. She used this in utterances such as "Mama widə," and "widə pig." Initially, the investigators gave many meanings to this word, but after careful analysis *widə* was found to be an empty or meaningless word that functioned as a pivot, occurring either before or after actual words. This indicated that a child at this stage was capable of remembering and vocally producing more than one word at a time.

In addition, Allison at times produced two words that were uttered successively but that still did not have syntactic meaning. For example, she handed her father a peach, wanting it to be peeled, and said, "Daddy-peach," thus indicating that she knew enough about words to talk about more than one thing at a time; but analysis of intonation demonstrated that these were two separate words chained together. It was Bloom's conclusion that single-word utterances did not carry sentence meaning, and that children used one word at a time primarily because they did not yet know the linguistic code sufficiently well to combine words in syntactic patterns. Subsequent studies have cast doubt upon Bloom's claim that the intonations accompanying these one-word utterances lack linguistic structure. The theoretical dilemma continues with the suggestion that in order to properly consider the nature of a child's single-word utterances, the child's pragmatic system must also be considered (Dore, 1975).

Other researchers have also observed the use of empty or meaningless words in two-word combinations. Leonard (1976, p. 51) observed that one of his subjects, Phoebe, could produce a two-word utterance such as "that Fred" or an utterance with an empty word such as "Mommy gokig." However an analogous utterance like "Mommy-washing?" was chained and not expressed as a two-word utterance. Leonard hypothesized that initially a child can express a single concept like nomination ("that Fred") with a two-word construction but still lack the concept of relating words expressing agent and action, etc., in utterances like "Mommy wash." Leonard further observed the use of the same empty form "n-there" by two children. This form, rather like Allison's use of *widə* seemed to indicate notice of something and may therefore represent a precursor to two-word utterances of notice, despite the fact that the child may already express some other semantic intentions in two-word utterances.

A thorough review of all of the current studies of single-word utterances was provided by Greenfield and Smith (1976). They concluded that children use words in systematic combination with nonverbal elements of the communication environment. Essentially, it is this combination of a single word with gesture, intonation, and context that allows the child to be understood. There is essentially no support for McNeill's claim (1970) that a young child's single word represents the linguistic knowledge of an entire sentence.

LEARNING TO COMBINE WORDS: SEMANTIC RELATIONS

As the child enters the two-word stage, the same semantic intentions that were previously expressed with one word may expand to two words. For example the child who previously expressed existence with words such as *doggie, car, juice, this,* and *here,* and expressed nonexistence with words like *all-gone* and *no,* may now combine these words. Existence could be expressed in phrases such as "this doggie," "here car," or "this juice." Non-existence might be expressed with "all-gone juice," "all-gone doggie," or "no car." At this level, the child who expresses two words like the above may still need to chain words like *pot-meat, car-see,* or *baby-cook.* These chained utterances express awareness of things that go together before the child can express this awareness linguistically in semantic relations.

Once the child enters Brown's stage I grammar and is consistently producing multiword utterances, a commonly accepted method of charting language growth is by analysis of semantic relations, which are the relationships between pairs of words such as agent and action ("mommy hit"), action and object ("hit mommy") or possessor and possessed ("mommy ball") or even agent and object ("mommy ball"). The notion that the agent and object may be the same person, represented by the same word (in the above case, *mommy*) requires a knowledge of causality. This distinction forms a basis for the development of multiword utterances.

The term *semantic relation* was proposed by I. M. Schlesinger (1971), who noted that the semantic relation seemed to be the verbal representation of what the child perceived and related to; thus, the semantic relation goes a step beyond the referential meaning by accounting for the meaning expressed by the relation between the words. This term is commonly used by psycholinguists and is now being employed in various research projects (Freedman & Carpenter, 1976; Leonard, Bolders, & Miller, 1976).

The reality of semantic relations was first illustrated by Bloom (1970) and I. M. Schlesinger (1971), who proposed that the components of the utterances of children at stage I grammar were semantic concepts such as agent, action, object, and location, rather than the syntactic notions of subject and predicate. Both stressed the importance of the child's verbal intention, which was conveyed by the total context of the utterance.

This technique of including the context in the evaluation of each utterance was called *rich interpretation* by Brown (1973) and it so powerfully illustrated the weakness of the strict grammatic approaches of "telegraphic speech" and "pivot grammar" that these methods of analysis were not used again for several years. Bloom (1970, pp. 45–48) provided an example that has been quoted in so many texts that it is now called simply the "mommy sock example." This utterance illustrated the weakness of any approach that looked only at the actual words produced by the child:

1. "Mommy sock"—Child points to mother's sock
2. "Mommy sock"—Mother is putting child's sock on child

By looking at the context it was as apparent to the investigators, as it obviously was to the mother, that these utterances have dif-

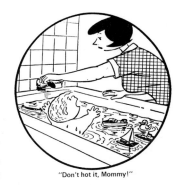

"Don't hot it, Mommy!"

Despite his substitution of an adjective for a verb, the context makes this child's meaning quite clear. (The Family Circus by Bil Keane, reprinted courtesy of Register and Tribune Syndicate.)

ferent semantic relations. The first expresses a possessor and possession relationship while the second expresses an agent and object relationship.

A list of approximately ten semantic relations is capable of suggesting most of the meanings children at stage I grammar express. These semantic relations and examples of words that have been reported as expressing them are:

1. Existence (nomination): *a, the, it, this, that, see* + noun (N).
2. Recurrence: *more, 'nother* + N.
3. Nonexistence: *no, no-more, all-gone* + N or verb (V).
4. Agent and action: "mommy fix," "mommy pull."
5. Action and object: "hit ball," "touch milk."
6. Agent and object: "mommy book," "Kathryn bear."
7. Action and locative: "put floor," "sit chair."
8. Entity and locative: "baby table," "sweater chair."
9. Possessor and possession: "mommy chair," "Kathryn sock."
10. Attribute and entity: "big ball," "party hat."

The relational categories of agent, object, action, location, etc., exist in most languages and provide one of the more productive means for analyzing the emerging speech of young children available at this time.

SCHEDULE OF DEVELOPMENT OF WORDS

Long before the current interest in psycholinguistics, psychologists were concerned with vocabulary size in relation to chronological age. The age of onset of speech is obviously affected by how a word is defined. Commonly, a "word" is any sound sequence that is produced spontaneously by the child, remains consistent, and has some relationship to the adult form of the word (Darley & Winitz, 1961; K. Nelson, 1973b). The inclusion of sound sequences as words was not based upon phonology nor upon the number of times the word occurred in certain samples. Comparison of diary studies (usually done by linguists studying their own children) with cross-sectional studies (where

Dorothea Agnes McCarthy

Working at the Institute of Child Welfare at the University of Minnesota as a research fellow from 1926 until 1928, Dorothea McCarthy participated in some of the most extensive cross-sectional research ever done in the development of child language. Her work, *Language Development of the Preschool Child*; her chapter, "Language Development" which appeared in the 1950 edition of the *Encyclopedia of Educational Research*; as well as her chapter *Language Development in Children*, which appeared in the L. Carmichael edition of the *Manual of Child Development* all were significant contributions to the study of child language. A revised and even more comprehensive review was published in the Mussen edition of *Carmichael's Manual of Child Psychology*. This chapter proved to be a "state of the art" description in child language for many years to follow.

McCarthy received her Ph.D. in psychology from the University of Minnesota in 1928 and remained there until she became a professor of psychology at Fordham University in New York City.

investigators interviewed children and their mothers) often shows wide differences in the number of words reported at various ages. K. Nelson (1973b) suggested that this may result because the mother and child initially form a closed communication circle and the mother is really the sole "expert" in what the child has said. Despite the differences evident between studies, there is a general consensus that children develop words around their first birthday.

The following schedule of development summarizes some of the vocabulary studies reported in the research literature. Norm-referenced vocabulary tests are discussed in Chapter 11, but the results of intensive studies of normal children are included here to show the wide variations observed among normal children. Children do not mature on a time schedule.

1. *Between 10 and 15 months.* Within the 6-month period around the child's first birthday, his first real words emerge. During this period, he acquires between three and ten words. (K. Nelson, 1973b; Slobin, 1967; M. E. Smith, 1926, 1941).

2. *Between 18 and 24 months.* As the child approaches his second birthday, it is expected that he will be using over fifty words and begining to combine words into multiword utterances (Lenneberg, 1966a; K. Nelson, 1973b). K. Nelson's study of eighteen children indicated that the mean age for acquisition of fifty words was 19 months, with a range of 15 to 24 months. The standard deviation in vocabulary size was ninety-five words. The lexicons of both Bowerman's (1973a) and Brown's (1973) three subjects ranged between 112 and 226 words when the children were 24 months old. Other vocabulary studies indicate that 2-year-olds have vocabularies ranging from 200 to 400 words (McCarthy, 1954; Slobin, 1967; M. E. Smith, 1926, 1941).

3. *Between 3 and 5 years.* By 3 years of age, a normal child may be expected to be using from 800 to over 1000 words. For the next year or so, the rate of growth in vocabulary tends to slow so that at 4 or even 5 years, the estimated vocabulary remains at several thousand words (Lenneberg, 1966, McCarthy, 1954; Slobin, 1967; M. E. Smith, 1926, 1941).

4. *Adults.* Studies of different languages around the world show that the size of adult vocabularies varies due chiefly to the differences in the advancement of science in that culture. When technical words are discounted, average adult speakers converse in everyday conversation using about 10,000 words expressing amazingly similar concepts (Carroll, 1964, p. 90). Actually, as few as 850 words might be sufficient to carry on a simple conversation, although an estimated 60,000 to 80,000 words are known and used by the average high school graduate (Carroll, 1964, p. 205).

outline

PRODUCTION

Increase in Utterance Complexity
Two-Word Constructions
Complexity and Word Order
Expansion Within Simple Sentences
Expansion to Complex Sentences
Mastery of Sentence Types
The Development of Grammatic Morphemes
Verb Modulation
Number Modulation
Person
Possessive
Prepositions
Articles
Pronouns
Development of Transformations
Negation
Interrogatives
Order of Acquisition of Linguistic Constructions
Grammatic Morphemes
Other Grammatic Structures

COMPREHENSION

Word Order
Interrogatives
Imperatives
Sentence Modalities

learning grammatic forms: syntactic development

8

THIS CHAPTER PROVIDES information that will be most useful to the language specialist who needs data regarding the developmental level of a child's grammatic knowledge for procedures of assessment and intervention. In order to make judgments about a child's stage of development in syntactic structure and to plan intervention strategies, the language-disorders specialist must know the sequence of development of grammatic structure in normal language. This chapter provides currently available data on the developmental sequence of grammatic structure. The emphasis is on *what* the stages are and not *how* they develop.

The chapter is divided into two major sections: production and comprehension. The section on the production of grammatic forms presents: (1) the general sequence of changes in sentence complexity; (2) the sequence of emergence of grammatic morphemes or functors such as the possessive, auxiliary, tense, and plurality, and (3) the sequence of emergence of syntactic transformations such as interrogatives and negatives. Additionally, the order of acquisition among these forms is given for those forms for which data are available.

The chapter is concerned with the development of formal linguistic structures, independent of their meaning. In studying the process of language development, it is difficult, if not impossible, to separate the development of semantic relations from that of grammatic relations, as the two are intertwined at every level. However, for the purposes of description and evaluation, it is fruitful to view the changes that occur in the grammatic aspects of language without reference to their semantic correspondents. This separation of the development of semantic relations from that of surface grammatic structures also has some intrinsic basis. Brown's studies (1973) of language acquisition place the development of *basic* semantic relations in stage I, and, except for some aspects of word order, the development of grammar—of what Brown calls *modulators* and *modalities*—occurs in stages II and III, respectively. In some respects, then, the developmental aspects covered in this chapter, except for early two-word constructions, relate to the structures developed from stage II on.

PRODUCTION   Increase in Utterance Complexity

At about 18 months of age, the typical child begins to use two-word utterances, and for several months thereafter the number of these utterances increases in an extraordinary fashion (Braine, 1963). This rapid increase, according to Braine, is illustrated by the cumulative number of different word combinations recorded in successive months in the developing language of one child: 14, 24, 54, 89, 350, 1400, and 2500 plus. Two-word combinations are more than two juxtaposed words; they also comprise the initial use of syntactic structure rules. The expansion from two-word utterances to fully formed sentences occurs in the short period of two years.

In listening to the language of the young child, the untrained observer will conclude that the child is using simple two-word combinations. This is not so: although the early constructions are comprised of only two words, they are by no means simple. Underlying these constructions are very complex semantic relations as well as some grammatic rules. One of the first rules of syntax that the child incorporates into his constructions, even at the level of two words, is that of word order. The order of words, which resembles the order in the adult language, is retained as utterances become more complex.

Two-Word Constructions

In describing the ways children "break into" the adult linguistic code, Bloom, Lightbown, and Hood (1975) identified two major entry types: pivotal and categorical.

One way children begin using adult constructions is by a pivotal strategy of the type described by Braine (1963). Braine suggested that the two-word combinations that children use are not comprised of words that are randomly juxtaposed. These words are selected on the basis of belonging to two types of word categories. One small class of words he called pivot (P) words; these occupy a fixed position (first or last) for each child and never occur in isolation. The second large and rapidly expanding class of words Braine referred to as open (O) class words; these are used with other open words, with pivot words, and in isolation to result in combinations such as pivot-open, open-pivot, and open-open. Words used by some children as pivots might be in the open category for other children and vice versa. A child's two-word constructions might take the following form:

P	O		O	P		O	O
↓	↓		↓	↓		↓	↓
big	boat		boat	all-gone		boy	sock

Subsequent research found Braine's analysis to be inadequate. In the first place, some of the restraints on class membership and combinations proposed by Braine were found not to apply to all children (Brown, 1973). Furthermore, not all children developed the type of grammar described by Braine, and therefore Slobin (1971a) concluded that such a grammar could not serve as a representation of a child's competence at the two-word stage.

The second method of entry into adult constructions (described in detail in Chapter 7) was labeled by Bloom, Lightbown, and Hood (1975) as categorical. This strategy, instead of exploring the surface structure of children's early utterances, describes the relationships between words. Bloom (1970) called these semantic relations; however, the semantic aspect does not describe the lexical meanings of the individual words but rather the meanings of the relationship between the words. Although two-word combinations are varied, their surface structure in no way reveals the complexity or breadth of the underlying structure.

Early two-word utterances of children, regardless of language, seem to be very similar. Bowerman (1978a, p. 141) compiled a list of the forms of these early surface constructions.*

1. *This/that/here/there/see/it + X* (to point out or name).
2. *More/'nother + X* (to express recurrence or additional exemplars).
3. *No/no more + X; X + all-gone/away* (to talk about nonexistence, disappearance, or rejection).
4. *Adam sit; Mommy push; bite finger* (to encode relations among agents, actions, and objects).
5. *Car garage; sweater chair; sit chair* (to encode relations between objects or events and locations).

*From Bowerman M: Semantic and syntactic development. In Schiefelbusch RL (Ed): *Bases of Language Intervention.* Baltimore: University Park Press, 1978.

6. *Dolly hat; my ball; Mommy nose* (to encode relations between objects or body parts and their "possessors").
7. *Big bed; hair wet* (to encode relations between entities and their attributes).

As is evident from these constructions, the early utterances of children are telegraphic; that is, they retain, for the most part, the information-carrying words (nouns, verbs, adjectives, and adverbs) and omit the functors (prepositions, articles, conjunctions, or auxiliary verbs). As the utterances become more complex, however, function words begin to appear.

Complexity and Word Order

Children begin using the rules of word order in early two-word utterances and continue the incorporation of these rules in complex sentences. Actually, word order is considered to be the basic device for indicating sentence structure in English. Brown (1973, p. 78) stated that in English declarative sentences, order distinguishes "subject from object, modifier from head, subject from locative, possessor from possessed, even when such structure signs as the possessive inflection, the copular verb, and the preposition are missing."

I. M. Schlesinger (1971) contended that the rules of order are learned before the rules of categorization, but Brown (1973) stated that there was not sufficient evidence to support this, since both rules of order and categorization were found in stage I of language development, and both were occasionally violated in that stage.

According to Bowerman (1978a), children learning English use consistent and usually appropriate word order when they begin to combine words. Brown (1973) labeled "Impressive" the consistency with which the surface order corresponds to inherent grammatic relations. In view of the fact that two orders are possible with two words, and six are possible with three words, the child's use of appropriate order in the language he is learning constitutes, according to Brown, a kind of discriminat-

You never know what will happen when word order is confused. (Reprinted courtesy of Field Newspaper Syndicate.)

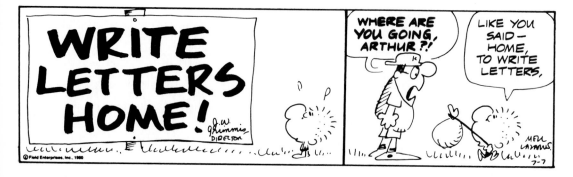

LEARNING GRAMMATIC FORMS: SYNTACTIC DEVELOPMENT

Dan I. Slobin

Dan Slobin's academic origins were in Cambridge, Massachusetts, where he was trained or influenced by psycholinguists such as George A. Miller and Robert Brown and linguists such as Noam Chomsky and Morris Halle. His doctoral dissertation, *Grammatical Transformations and Sentence Comprehension in Childhood and Adulthood*, was an important contribution to the early literature on methods of transformational grammar analyses. His subsequent contributions were made from studies done at the University of California in Berkeley. Slobin is best known for his reports on the acquisition of Russian as a native language and for his comparison of early grammatic development in several languages. He has studied child language and has been particularly interested in observing grammatic development through imitation. His research has led him to postulate universals of language development. Among his publications are *The Ontogenesis of Grammar* and *Studies of Child Language Development* (edited with C. A. Ferguson).

ing response—one that shows he is trying to communicate certain semantic relations.

Braine (1976) agreed that positional patterns for the purpose of expressing specific semantic relations (possessor *first,* object possessed second, etc.) are learned early. However, he found evidence that there may be a period of using a "groping pattern" before a particular position pattern is established. A groping pattern is a relatively flexible word order for expressing semantic content. When the possessor or agent in constructions such as possessor-possessed and agent-action were represented by *my* and *I,* respectively, Bowerman's (1978) daughter used fixed order, but when animate nouns represented the possessor or agent, she used variable order. The differences in the development of word order may be related to the speed of syntactic development, according to findings by Ramer (1976).

Slobin (1973, pp. 197–200) presented what he considers universal statements regarding the acquisition of sentence construction and word order. Some of these are as follows:

1. The standard order for functor morphemes in the input language is preserved in child speech. (This happens irrespective of language.)
2. Word order in child speech reflects word order in the input language.
3. Sentences deviating from standard word order will be interpreted (by children, *sic*) at early stages of development as if they were examples of standard (typical, *sic*) word order. (For example, passive voice order will be interpreted as active.)
4. Structures requiring permutation of elements will first appear in non-permuted form ("I can sit?" or "Where I can sit?" for "Where can I sit?")
5. There is a tendency to preserve the structure of the sentence as a closed entity, reflected in a development from *external* attachment to the sentence of various linguistic forms to their movement *within* the sentence ("No go," to "I no go," to "I can't go").

Expansion Within Simple Sentences

The early advance from two-word to three-word utterances involves filling in a three-term sequence with fragments that earlier occurred in a two-word utterance (Brown, 1973). This happens in two ways, according to Brown:

1. Serially linking more relations, with redundant terms omitted:

Agent	Action		Agent	Action		Agent	Action	Object
↓	↓		↓	↓		↓	↓	↓
John	drink	+	drink	milk	→	John	drink	milk

2. Unfolding simple relations so that one term becomes itself a relation—always either possession, attribution, or recurrence.

   Drink milk → Drink Daddy ('s) milk

Another method by which children increase sentence complexity is by the expansion of noun phrases or the addition of longer sequences of words that have the same privileges of occurrence as individual nouns in the child's speech ("That flower" becomes "That a blue flower" or "Put hat on" becomes "Put the red hat on" (Slobin, 1971).

Following this there is a gradual increase of specificity of each of the elements of the construction. For example, in a construction such as

$$\left\{ \begin{array}{l} \text{Noun} \\ \text{Pronoun} \end{array} \right\} \; + \; \text{Verb}$$

$$\begin{array}{cc} \downarrow & \quad\quad \downarrow \\ \text{Mama} & \quad\quad \text{go} \end{array}$$

the verb may be expanded to include (1) an intransitive verb and an adverb such as "mama go home" or (2) a transitive verb and a noun phrase with an adverb such as "take girl home." Noun phrases may be expanded by adding modifiers such as adjectives or by expanding the adverb to include a preposition such as "in house." Primitive transformations are added to basic constructions such as negation, "no mama go" or the question form, "where mama go?" Addition of determiners (*the, a*), auxiliaries (forms of *is*), and other morphemes are added gradually to complete the simple sentence.

Menyuk (1969) describes expansions by conjunctions of elements. For example, in a declarative statement the expansion may take the form of a topic comment:

"Fix it, Mommy's shoes."
"Read it, a paper."

Later, children expand utterances through juxtaposition and embedding of existing routines. For example, "like" and "take ride" combine into "I like take ride."

In demonstrating the elaborated forms of basic rules, Menyuk (1969) gives the following illustration:

"I see a house. It's made of wood."
    becomes
"I see a wooden house."
        or
"I see a house and another and another."
    becomes
"I see three houses."

Expansion to Complex Sentences

Complex and compound sentences involve joining two or more simple sentences, either by embedding or conjunction. Children begin to combine simple sentences into complex sentences between 2 and 3 years of age. According to Bloom et al. (1980), children accomplish this with considerable similarity in content but not in form. The first complex constructions are noun-phrase complements, in which a full sentence takes the place of the object of a verb as in "I wish you play with me" (Brown, 1973). Sentences are first conjoined by use of the conjunction *and.*

The connective forms used most frequently by children studied by Bloom et al. (1980) were *and, because, what, when* and *so;* the less frequently used connective forms were *and then, but, if, that,* and *where.* Both conjoined and embedded sentences appear before well-formed negative, interrogative, and passive sentences are used consistently (Menyuk, 1977).

D. Ingram (1975) reported a further change in complexity between the ages 3 and 5; children used utterances such as "Once there was a little boy and he went for a walk in the woods." At 5 years, this utterance resembled the following construction: "Once upon a time there was a little horse who lived on a farm." Ingram interpreted this as meaning that the younger children were not able to take two propositions and relate them to each other by embedding one within the other.

Mastery of Sentence Types

Limber (1973) compared the syntactic structure of a 3-year-old with that of a mature English speaker and concluded that the 3-year-old's utterances displayed the basic structural features of English, with some exceptions. Brown and Bellugi (1964) stated that by age 3, some children can produce all the major varieties of simple sentences in English up to a length of ten or eleven words. Past the age of 5 or 6 years, according to Dale (1976), the differences between child and adult grammar are not apparent from samples of free speech.

Palermo and Molfese (1972) do not agree with the concept

that the child's structure is complete by 3, 4, or 5 years of age. They reported data indicating that long after a child has passed his fifth birthday, he continues to make important syntactic advances. Menyuk (1963, 1964b) reported that children from ages 5 to 7 years failed to develop fully the auxiliary *have,* the participial complement, iteration, nominalization, pronominalization, and conjunctions with *if* and *so.* In a longitudinal study following children from kindergarten through ninth grade, Loban (1963, 1966) found that as children get older their speech performance improves, as indicated by (1) decreases in incomplete syntactic structures; (2) increases in the variety of structural patterns used, and (3) greater variations in the structures within sentences in terms of vocabulary, positions of phrases, nominalizations, etc. Muma (1975) stated that by 8 years of age, children have in essence acquired the grammar and reference of their linguistic community although they may not use it with facility. According to Muma, advanced and effective use of language involves identification of the correspondences between messages and situations. When a child's language reaches an advanced level of organization, it becomes difficult to describe his grammatic system (Bellugi-Klima, 1969).

The Development of Grammatic Morphemes

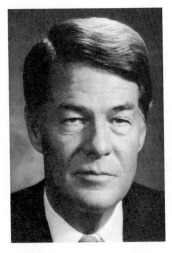

Brown (1973) considers the basic construction blocks of language to be nouns and verbs, and to a lesser degree, adjectives and adverbs. The group of words and inflections that are referred to as *functors* or semantic modulators (Brown, 1973) are words that are less essential to meaning than the words that carry relational meaning. The functors serve primarily to mark structure and secondarily to provide lexical meaning. Brown (1973) suggested that morphemes tune or modulate the meaning associated with content words. On the whole, the grammatic morphemes develop after the two-and three-word stage of language, which is in Brown's stage II.

Roger William Brown

Although he began his professional career as a social psychologist, Roger Brown's interest in language led him to be an innovator in the field of psycholinguistics. He received his Ph.D. from Michigan, and since then has been on the faculty at Harvard and the Massachusetts Institute of Technology. His first book in language, *Words and Things,* was a precursor to the studies in child language that he directed during the 1960s at Harvard. Together with his students and colleagues, he developed novel approaches to child language analysis. The group at Harvard was also one of the first research teams to utilize the then-emerging transformational methods in studying children's grammar. Brown's best known book in psycholinguistics is *A First Language,* in which he interprets the data obtained during a period of about 10 years. The children whom Brown studied so extensively—Adam, Eve, and Sarah—have become like friends to graduate students everywhere.

According to Brown (1973), the modulators have certain common characteristics:

1. They are phonetically minimal forms.
2. They receive light stress in sentences.
3. They belong to classes that have limited membership (as opposed to nouns, verbs, etc.).
4. They vary with the grammatic and phonetic properties of other words.
5. They develop slowly.
6. They exist in multiple linguistically contingent forms (as the plural allomorphs /s/, /z/, /ɪz/, which vary with the preceding phoneme.)

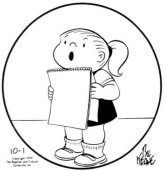

"Thirty days hath September. How many days does October hath?"

Is this what is called overgeneralization? (Reprinted courtesy of The Register and Tribune Syndicate, Inc.)

There are differences in the variety, scope, and regularity of the inflectional devices in or of different languages. Some languages express semantic relations primarily by word order, intonation, and functors, while other languages use inflectional affixes, accent shifts, etc. (Ferguson & Slobin, 1973).

Slobin (1973, pp. 192, 207) developed a set of universals of language development that specify the conditions under which some aspects of morphology are acquired before others:*

1. For any given semantic notion, grammatic realizations in the form of suffixes or postpositions will be acquired earlier than realizations in the form of prefixes or prepositions.
2. A child will begin to mark a semantic notion earlier if its morphological realization is more salient perceptually. [Perceptual saliency means that it is more observable auditorially because of stress, position, or other similar factors.]
3. When a child first controls a full form of a linguistic entity which can undergo contraction or deletion, contractions or deletions of such entities tend to be absent. [*I will* is articulated instead of *I'll* at the developmental stage where the auxiliary system is being learned.]
4. The following stages of linguistic marking of a semantic notion are typically observed: (1) no marking; (2) appropriate marking in limited cases; (3) overgeneralizing of marking, (4) full adult system [*drop* (past) becomes *dropped,* which becomes *dropted* or *dropped/drɑpɪd/,* which becomes *dropped*].
5. Errors in choice of functor are always within the given functor class and subcategory. [Children confuse prepositions with other prepositions, but not with conjunctions or other parts of speech.]
6. If there are homonymous forms, in an inflectional system those forms will tend not to be the earliest inflections acquired by the child; i.e. the child tends to select phonologi-

*Reprinted with permission from Ferguson CA & Slobin DI: *Studies of Child Language Development,* New York: Holt, Rinehart, & Winston, 1973.

cally unique forms, when available, as the first realization of inflections.

A child does not gain complete command of a functor all at once; each functor is acquired gradually and is used in some grammatic contexts before others. It appears that the child first learns the basic functions of an inflectional system before he uses the particular forms of the system in his speech (Slobin, 1973).

Verb Modulation

Present Progressive and Auxiliary. Brown (1973) stated that the verb is initially used in a generic unmarked form. At stage I, the verb is used in any of the following senses:

Imperative: "Get book."
Past: "Book drop."
Intention or prediction: "Mommy read."
Progressive, expressing temporary deviation: "Fish swim."

The present progressive tense is constructed by joining a form of the auxiliary *be* to a main verb having an *-ing* inflection. The auxiliary or helping verb varies with number. In developing language, children begin to use the inflection on the verb before using the auxiliary. This inflection emerges between Brown's stages I and III (Brown, Cazden, & Bellugi, 1973). During the period of acquisition of *-ing*, children distinguish process verbs (*sing, run, call,* etc.) that take *-ing* and the "state" verbs (*need, know, like,* etc.) that do not; rarely, if ever, do children add *-ing* to a state verb (Brown, Cazden, & Bellugi, 1973).

There is a group of semi-auxiliary verbs called *catenatives* (linkers), the most prominent of which are *gonna, wanna,* and *hafta.* These develop along with the progressives and the past and "are distributed in sentences as if they were, on some level, one thing" (Brown, Cazden, & Bellugi, 1973, p. 300).

The Copula. The verb *be* is also used as a main verb. When used as a main verb, *be* (as well as its present tense allomorphs, *am, is,* and *are*) is called a *copula.* Both the auxiliary and the copula emerge in stage II; however, the auxiliary use in obligatory contexts develops more slowly than copula use (Brown, 1973).

Brown found considerable variation in the acquisition of the allomorphs of the copula *be,* as well as in the use of these allomorphs with specific pronouns. The contracted form *it's* was used appropriately most of the time, whereas the copula in *what's* ("What that") and *who's* ("Who that") was omitted. Brown found data indicating that children did not analyze *it's* into component parts—the pronoun and the copula—but instead considered *it's* as the subject form of *it.* This was illustrated by a child's use of "It's will go" and "It's truck." Bellugi-Klima (1969) considered this behavior to exemplify incorrect segmentation on the part of the child.

Brown (1973) distinguished between the development of the contractible and uncontractible forms of the copula and auxiliary. In sentences in which it could not be contracted, the children in Brown's study almost never omitted the copula, but in sentences in which it could be contracted, the children frequently did omit it. He concluded that the uncontractible copula is acquired before the contractible one. In a subsequent study of the acquisition of morphemes, however, de Villiers and de Villiers (1973) found the contractible form of the copula is learned earlier than the uncontractible form.

Past Tense.   The English language contains both regular and irregular forms of past tense. The regular past is formed by adding *ed* to words and pronouncing the ending as /-d/, /-t/, or /ɪd/. The different pronunciations result from the ending of the stem verb: In verbs ending in a voiceless consonant, the *ed* is pronounced /-t/; in verbs ending in a voiced consonant, the *ed* is pronounced /-d/; and in verbs ending in /-t/ or /-d/, the *ed* is pronounced /-ɪd/. Verbs that have an irregular past are many; among those that are learned early are *came, fell, broke, sat,* and *went* (Brown, 1973).

In the acquisition of the past tense, the irregular past forms are always more frequent than the regular past (as they are in adult language). In learning the irregular forms, children use the irregular past (*came, fell, sat*) correctly and then go through a period of regularizing the irregular past (*comed, falled, sitted*) before totally mastering the irregular verbs (Slobin, 1971b). Exceptions to over-regularization are found in verbs whose past tense form ends in /d/ or/t/; these are called partially regular verbs and the final consonant of the past form seems to block over-regularization (*heard, told, hurt,* etc.; Slobin, 1971b). Bellugi (unpublished paper) stated that the speech of children during periods of overregularization appears to be impervious to attempts at correction.

The first efforts to modify the generic verb by using the past (either /-d, /-t/ or an irregular allomorph) are limited to the immediate past: "It dropped" or "It broke." The range of time gradually expands to include several hours on a full day (Brown, 1973). Cazden (1968) stated that the fact that the regular ending -*ed* is used initially in only a few words indicates that the words are learned as lexical items and by rote.

Number Modulation

The inflection for plural number exists in a regular and irregular form in English and is marked on the noun. The regular form is composed of allomorphs /-s/, /-z/, /ɪz/. The irregular forms are few but frequently used (*men, children, women*; Brown, 1973). The plural inflection was found by Brown to be entirely absent in stage I and often present by stage III.

Expression of plurality in English is more complicated than

Regularizing an irregular verb leads to trouble no matter which way you do it. (Reprinted courtesy of The Register and Tribune Syndicate, Inc.)

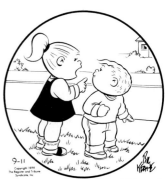

"We don't say 'I losed my dime.' We say 'I LOSTED it.'"

adding an inflection to the noun—the head noun and its determiners must agree ("The boy," "These boys"); the subject noun and the predicate nominal must also agree ("The boy is a male"; "The boys are males") as must the pronoun and its antecedent noun. The number and person of the noun determine the form of the verb (Brown, Cazden, & Bellugi, 1973).

According to G. A. Miller and Ervin (1964), the acquisition of the singular-plural contrast follows a simple pattern in most children. First there is noncontrast (between singular and plural), followed by acquisition of particular instances of contrast, followed several months later by generalization to many instances, and, finally, by differentiation of irregular forms. Miller & Ervin suggested that before the child begins to use the plural–singular contrast, he may assume that the use of a numeral preceding a noun is an adequate marker of plurality, as in "two book."

Pluralization rules seem to be observed within a phrase first, ("Some boys like apple"), then across a short sentence ("Some boys like apples"; Cazden, 1968), and finally across longer sentences ("Some boys like apples and bananas"; Menyuk, 1969).

The order of difficulty and, consequently, the development of the plural allomorphs seems to be as follows (Brown, 1973):

1. Those that correspond with the most general rules of phonology, i.e., the voiceless /s/ follows voiceless phonemes, as *jumps* /dʒʌmps/ and the voiced /z/ follows voiced phonemes, as *rubs* /rʌbz/.

2. Those that correspond with the general phonological rule when used as a plural for specific phonemes such as /l/, /m/, /n/ and /r/, although they are not always followed by voiced sibilant sounds, e.g., *pulse* /pʌls/.

3. The allomorph /ɪz/, which follows the sibilant sounds /s/, /z/, /ʃ/, /ʒ/, /tʃ/, /dʒ/ as in *washes* /waʃɪz/, *noses* /nouzɪz/, and *buses* /bʌsɪz/.

Person

The aspect of person that has been studied in developmental literature is third-person-singular present indicative. The inflection that expresses third person singular is prefixed to the verb but governed by the noun ("The cat jumps" or "The birds sing"). The regular morpheme is *-s* and it has three allomorphs, /-s/, /-z/, and /-ɪz/. The third-person-singular inflection is always redundant in English, since the person and number is communicated by the noun.

Brown (1973) found it difficult to operationally define the obligatory contexts for the third-person-singular inflection. For example, in the utterance "Mommy use it," is the inflection for the verb missing or is a modal, such as *can* missing? However, he reported the order of acquisition of this morpheme in the language of three children. In one child, it occurred in stage IV and in the other two children it occurred in stage V. The regular form ranked tenth in fourteen morphemes studied.

Possessive

In Brown's report (1973), the analysis of the possessive marker was treated as a noun inflection. Although children learn early when a particular object is associated or connected more often with one person than with others, the marking of the possessive morpheme appears much later in their speech (Bloom & Lahey, 1978). The form of the possessive is similar to that of the plural (/-s/, /-z/, /-ɪz/). He reported that the possessive inflection did not reach 90 percent until stage III or later, although it was clear in the children's conversation that they understood the concept of possession. This early form of expressing possession without inflection took the form of: "That Eve nose" or "That Mommy nose right there" (Brown, 1973). (Brown defined mastery as 90 percent correct usage in obligatory contexts, which are linguistic and nonlinguistic contexts in which a specific morpheme is required for an accurate grammatic utterance.)

Prepositions

Menyuk (1969) suggested that the early prepositions are nondistinguishable place markers, as in "Mommy sit uh table." The two identifiable prepositions that are used early in language development are *in* and *on.* Not only are they the first prepositions learned, but they are learned together (Brown, 1973). The children in Brown's study reached the 90-percent criterion in the use of the preposition *in* and *on* during stage II of development. Other early prepositions include *out, over, under,* and *away* (G. A. Miller & Ervin 1964).

In studying the comprehension and production of specific prepositions by children ages 3 to 5 years, Washington and Naremore (1978) found that comprehension of the prepositions preceded their production, and that evaluation by means of three-dimensional tasks yielded better responses than by two-dimensional ones. Prepositions whose meanings involve simple topological notions appeared easier than those involving dimensional spatial notions. The early learned prepositions were *inside, on, under,* and *around.* Those acquired later were *behind, between, beside, in front of,* and *over.* E. Clark (1971) conducted a study on comprehension and production of the temporal prepositions *before* and *after* and found that *before* was learned at an earlier age than *after.*

Articles

The indefinite articles most widely used by children in early language are *a* and *the.* In adult grammar, *a* is used for nonspecific reference and *the* is used for specific reference. Because the contexts for specific and nonspecific uses are numerous and complicated to identify, Brown (1973) combined the two articles in studying the acquisition of the article by children, using this combination; article acquisition ranged from stages III to IV, indicating variation among children in the acquisition of this functor.

Slobin (1971a) demonstrated the emergence of noun phrases by the addition of an article to a phrase; he obtained examples from Brown and Bellugi (1964) and Brown (1973). Earlier examples included "that factory," "that flower," and "put gas in." Later samples were "that a factory," "that a blue flower," and "put a gas in."

Pronouns

Some children express the early relations between persons and action through a *nominal* strategy, while other children express these relations through a *pronominal* strategy (Huxley, 1970). The nominal strategy, the use of nouns in relation to verbs, is expressed by the use of names in all positions, as "Mary home" or "See Mary cat," in which the speaker is Mary (Bellugi-Klima, 1969, Bellugi; 1971). Children who use the pronominal strategy substitute *I* for the name when the name occurs first in the sentence, but substitute *me* if the name is not first. Gradually the grammatic role of the pronoun supercedes the position and *I* is used in the subjective function and me in the objective function (Bellugi-Klima, 1969). Some children may replace previously learned subject forms (*I*) with the objective form (*me*) for a period of time before mastery (Huxley, 1970).

Huxley (1970) reported a general sequence of emergence of personal pronouns in two children: the pronoun *it* in the object case was learned first by both children; the pronoun *I* (subject), *it* (subject and object) and *you* (subject) were learned before *you* (object) or *we* (subject); *them* (object) was learned before *they* (subject); the plurals *them* (object) and *they* (subject) were learned before *we* (subject) and *us* (object). At all stages of development, the singular forms were used more frequently than plural ones.

In attempting to explain the sequence of emergence of the pronoun as well as some of the errors that occur during development, Waryas (1973) hypothesized that children make semantic distinctions first and case distinctions later. The child distinguished between pronouns that refer to the speaker and pronouns that refer to the listener, although he may confuse pronouns within the speaker or listener groups. The child may use *me* for *I* but not *you* for *I*. Gradually, the syntactic differentiation of subject and object takes place. Waryas observed that the order of emergence of pronouns in the syntactic differentiation follows that of the order in semantic development.

Ursula Bellugi-Klima

Ursula Bellugi-Klima was a graduate student at Harvard during the 1960s when Roger Brown began his studies of the acquisition of syntax in children. Together with him, she reported early studies of processes in the child's acquisition of syntax and the application of linguistic methods for studying child grammar. Bellugi-Klima's articles on the development of negation were of particular importance to psycholinguistic literature. Subsequent to her work at Harvard, she began linguistic analyses of the sign language of the deaf, which are now considered a classic contribution to the knowledge of the language of the deaf. Among her publications is *How Children Say No*.

Development of Transformations

Roger Brown (1973) wrote of mapping simple, declarative, sentences into modalities. The modalities leave the semantic relation and the modulations intact, and they involve a transformation of the sentence structure into the following forms: yes/no and constituent interrogatives, negatives, and imperatives. These transformations are developed in Brown's stage III.

Negation

The adult forms of negation include (1) the negative particle *not* and its contracted form *-n't* ("It isn't true"); (2) a small set of negative words including the negative pronouns *nobody* and *nothing* ("Nobody came"); (3) the negative determiner *no* ("No students passed"), and (4) the negative adverbs *never* and *nowhere* (Klima & Bellugi, 1973). At fifteen months, the child begins to use an intentional negative signal: shaking his head in response to some attempt to influence him (Spitz, 1957). Following this response is the word *no* used to resist commands and to answer yes/no questions (Brown, Cazden, & Bellugi, 1973). At the next stage, the negative is affixed more often at the beginning (Wode, 1977), but also at the end, of the nucleus of the utterance. This last stage is referred to as period 1 (Klima & Bellugi, 1973). Examples of period 1 sentences are:

"No sit there" (when "sit there" is the nucleus)
"No want stand head"
"No singing some"
"More . . . no"

The rules for the negation system of period 1 can be written as follows (Klima & Bellugi, 1973):

$$\left\{ \begin{matrix} (no) \\ (not) \end{matrix} \right\} + \text{nucleus} \quad or \quad \text{nucleus} + \text{no}$$

Slobin (1973) suggested that at early stages of development, the presence of a negative element in a sentence is accomplished by decreasing the complexity of the rest of the sentence. Bloom (1970) gave examples of the decreased complexity in

---

negative sentences uttered at the same period: "Kathryn have a socks on" and "Kathryn no shoe."

In Klima and Bellugi's period 2 (corresponding approximately to stages II and III of Brown), the negative is incorporated into the body of the nucleus utterance. The lexical representatives are *no* and *not* as in "He no like you" and "That not red, that blue;" and *can't* and *don't* as in "I can't find you" and "Don't hit me." Although auxiliary verbs appear in *don't* and *can't,* they appear at this stage only when accompanied by a negative. The affirmative modal auxiliaries have not appeared at this time. The negatives *can't* and *don't* are used as lexical items (Klima & Bellugi, 1973, p. 346). The rules for this period are

Sentence→noun phrase + (negative) + verb phrase

$$\text{where negative} \rightarrow \begin{Bmatrix} (\text{no}) \\ (\text{not}) \\ (\text{V neg}) \end{Bmatrix} \text{where V neg} \rightarrow \begin{Bmatrix} (\text{can't}) \\ (\text{don't}) \end{Bmatrix}$$

The speech of children in period 3 of Klima and Bellugi's analysis of the development of negation is characterized by inclusion of negative auxiliary verbs in addition to *don't* and *can't* as in "Paul didn't laugh" and "Donna won't let go." Since the auxiliary verbs appear in declarative sentences and questions, they can be considered as separate from the negative aspect of the sentence. McNeill (1970) stated that the negative sentences of Klima and Bellugi's third stage come from a grammatic system that has been fundamentally altered, and consequently the apparently few superficial changes don't reflect the extent of the change in the child's grammatic system.

Interrogatives

Asking questions takes two basic forms: those that require a *yes/no* response and those that require a response to *wh* words, such as *where, when,* and *why.* If declarative sentences are compared to their corresponding yes/no interrogatives, the transformations that take place in English interrogatives can be identified:

Mary can run.	Can Mary run?
He was playing.	Was he playing?
She had been crying.	Had she been crying?

From these examples, it can be seen that the auxiliary verb is transposed to the beginning of the interrogative sentence. If two auxiliaries are present, only the first is transposed. In the *wh* question, specific information is requested. An adaptation of Dale's (1976) examples illustrate the use of the *wh* form:

Mary will run.	(subject)	*Who* will run?
I will see *Mary.*	(object)	*Whom* will I see?
I am *running.*	(predicate)	*What* are you doing?

The big boy ran.	(determiner)	*Which* boy ran?
He went *home.*	(locative)	*Where* did he go?
She can go *now.*	(time)	*When* can she go?
Bill will travel *by car.*	(manner)	*How* will he travel?

Early versions of yes/no questions by children contain a declarative sentence or fragment with rising intonation at the end (Brown, Cazden, & Bellugi, 1973). Examples of this type of utterance were given by Klima and Bellugi (1973): "See hole?" "I ride train?" or "Ball go?" Klima and Bellugi consider the basic element the nucleus, which ordinarily consists of nouns and verbs with no indication of number and tense. They give a rule for this elementary form of interrogation:

$$\text{Sentence} \rightarrow \left\{ \begin{array}{l} \text{yes/no} \\ \text{question + nucleus} \end{array} \right\}$$

In period 1 of questioning, the most common use of *wh* forms are versions of "What's that?" "Where boy go?" and "What baby doing?" Klima and Bellugi suggested that this type of interrogative form is bound to specific words such as *go* and *do* and does not have the generality of the adult structure. Tyack and Ingram (1977) suggested that *what* and *where* questions are clearly tied to the child's immediate environment; the later-developed *when* is tied to time concepts and therefore appears later. Period 2 is characterized by the development of constituent questioning. The interrogative *what* appears in sentences that have a missing object, as for example; "What dollie have?" and "What book name?" The interrogatives *where* and *why* also are used in this manner, although intermittently. The third period of development finds the child's interrogatives similar to those of the adult. The yes/no questions may be formed by transposing the subject with verb forms, as in "Does the kitty stand up?" The *wh* question forms do *not* have the auxiliary verbs inverted or transposed with the subject noun phrase: "What he can ride in?" Brown (1968) traced the acquisition of transformational rules that relate *wh* question forms to the corresponding earlier-appearing affirmative statements. In the first stage, the children produced such utterances as "What John will read?" and "What John will do?" This is called preposing by Bloom and Lahey (1978). In a subsequent stage, the children transpose the subject and the verb auxiliary to form "What will John read?"

Brown, Cazden, and Bellugi (1973) concluded that children do not simply start to produce well-formed questions at a particular time; they first produce a form that requires only one major transformation, even when more than one is available. In yes/no questions, only transposition of subject and auxiliary is required, and it is performed; in *wh* questions, both transposition and a second transformation (preposing) are required, and children perform only the latter (McNeill, 1970).

Order of Acquisition of Linguistic Constructions

The preceding sections have described the gradual manner in which modulators and modalities emerge in children's language. Emergence *within* each of the forms occurs in a typical manner in children as does the sequence of emergence and mastery *between* forms.

Grammatic Morphemes

Three major studies have provided data on the order in which morphemes are acquired by children. Brown (1973) provided the rank order in which the children mastered fourteen grammatic morphemes. In a cross-sectional sampling of subjects at different language levels, de Villiers and de Villiers (1973a) presented the rank order of acquisition of these same fourteen morphemes. Bloom, Lifter, and Hafitz (1980) studied the emergence of verb inflections (*-ing, -s, -ed* and irregular endings) of four subjects through three successive developmental periods which coincided with Brown's MLU stages I, II, and III. The rank order of emergence reported by Brown (1973) and de Villiers and de Villiers (1973a) are presented in Table 8-1. Although there were differences in the rank order of acquisition between the results of Brown and de Villiers and de Villiers, the correlation was .87.

The acquisition order for verb inflections in the Brown and de Villiers study was *-ing,* irregular endings, *-ed,* and finally *-s.* In the Bloom, Lifter, and Hafitz study (1980), irregular endings ranked first. However, Brown and de Villiers and de Villiers were studying mastery of the forms, whereas Bloom et al. were investigating emergence. The difference in acquisition order may indicate a tendency toward word-by-word learning in the early stages of learning inflections (Bloom et al., 1980). Bloom et al. found that the three irregular verbs appeared at the same time in children's speech but that they were distributed differently; that is, one of the inflections was used with one verb population or type, another inflection was used with another verb population, etc. Apparently, they had learned the general rule for verb inflection, but the probability for using the endings differed with the type of verb.

Other Grammatic Structures

Slobin (1970, p. 16) provided the following order of emergence of linguistic means for expressing semantic notions: (1) intonation; (2) word order; (3) morphemes in words and sentences (e.g. inflections, questions, negatives); (4) positioning of morphemes inside of sentences; (5) permutation of morphemes;

Table 8–1
Rank Acquisition Order for Fourteen Morphemes*

Morpheme	Brown	de Villiers & de Villiers
Present progressive	1	4
In	2	1
On	3	2
Plural	4	3
Past irregular	5	5
Possessive	6	11
Uncontractible copula	7	10
Articles	8	8
Past regular	9	7
Third person regular	10	12
Third person irregular	11	6
Uncontractible auxiliary	12	14
Contactible copula	13	9
Contractible auxiliary	14	13

*As studied by Brown (1973) and de Villiers and de Villiers (1973a).

and (6) embedding. Cazden and Brown (1975) have concluded that the acquisition of syntax, unlike vocabulary or other communication skills, seems impervious to deliberate assistance.

COMPREHENSION

There are many problems inherent in studying the order of emergence of grammar in comprehension. The first is that it is unclear in studies of the development of comprehension whether the investigators are measuring the child's linguistic competence or performance.

Children do not begin to comprehend by decoding entire segments of speech. As is true of expression, children begin by understanding single words in a string of words and then gradually progressing to two and three words (Benedict, 1978). This occurs, according to Wetstone and Friedlander (1973), because children listen to what has meaning and is familiar. At the early stages, children respond more correctly to utterances having the form of children's speech than to well-formed commands (Shipley, Smith, & Gleitman, 1969), and they also respond to the referential or semantic aspects of individual words rather than to the syntactic forms or relationships. Sachs and Truswell (1978) found that children at the one-word stage of expression comprehended two-word instructions not cued by environmental factors; meanings were assigned by children to words combined in novel ways ("tickle shoe"), and the children responded by carrying out the appropriate action with the appropriate object. Considerable meaning is conveyed in reference words (note the effectiveness of a telegram), and apparently this type of response serves the children adequately at certain periods. Some achievement in language seems necessary before children begin responding to word order cues, modalities, and modulators.

Word Order

Research findings indicate that the English-speaking child's use of word-order cues to determine subject and object status is acquired late as compared to the presence of word-order performance in speech (Chapman & Miller, 1975). In fact, neither 1- nor 2-year-olds exhibit comprehension of word-order cues to semantic roles (Chapman & Kohn, 1978; de Villiers & de Villiers, 1973b; Wetstone & Friedlander, 1973). For example, Wetstone and Friedlander (1973) found similar responses to contrasting input such as "Where's the truck?" and "Truck the where is?" Word-order cues in comprehension are not mastered by children until about the third year or when the child has a MLU of about 4.0 (de Villiers & de Villiers, 1973b).

To study the effect of word-order cues, investigators have used reversible sentences, i.e., those that are similar except for the transposition of the subject and object ("The boy hits the girl" versus "The girl hits the boy"). Typical early responses to commands using reversible sentences have been summarized in Chapman and Kohn (1978) as follows: (1) the child acts as agent and thus acts on one or both objects; (2) the most probable event relation between the nouns is chosen, e.g., in "Mother washes the baby" and "Baby washes the mother," the mother is used as the agent; (3) the animate agent is chosen for action in preference to the inanimate one; (4) the smaller of two objects is used as the agent; (5) the position of an object relative to the child influences response; and (6) the noun first mentioned in the sentence is preferred as agent.

Interrogatives

There have been few studies of the developmental patterns of comprehension of questions and commands in language acquisition. This type of information is of general importance to persons interested in child language development, and is of specific importance to individuals working with language-disordered children, because much of the communication exchange in an intervention setting involves asking questions and requesting specific performance.

Early responses to question forms seem to appear prior to the emergence of speech. Crosby (1976) found that her subject, at the threshold of speech, was able to discriminate between yes/no and *wh* questions. The child either ignored or screened out information too difficult to process (32 percent of the yes/no questions and 44 percent of the *wh* questions).

The general order of acquisition of comprehension of the question form is fairly consistent from study to study. The rank order of the development of the interrogative forms is yes/no, where (intransitive), why, who (subject), how, where (transitive), what (object), and when (Carrow, 1968; H. H. Clark, 1970, 1973; Ervin-Tripp, 1970; Tyack & Ingram, 1977).

Tyack and Ingram (1977) found that the semantic features of a verb as well as its position in a sentence influences a child's response to interrogative forms. This means that the verb can dictate the correct response to an interrogative, even when the interrogative is not understood. Tyack and Ingram found that when a child heard *touch,* his attention was drawn to *what* was touched. The verb *ride,* on the other hand, placed the focus on *location.*

Menyuk (1977) reported that children first respond to identification questions as "What is that?" (with the person asking the question pointing) and then to action or entity questions as "What do you want?" Subsequently, children respond to questions that elicit action-word responses such as "What is Tommy doing?"

Imperatives

Shipley, Smith, and Gleitman (1969) found that children using holophrastic speech were significantly less attentive and responsive to commands that contained well-formed complex structures or nonsense material than to simple commands whose forms were only slightly more advanced than their own utterances. Well-formed commands were more effective than child forms in eliciting accurate responses from children whose speech was at the telegraphic level. Shipley et al. concluded that the effectiveness of well-formed commands increases with verbal maturity, implying stages of competence in comprehension developmentally preceding the ability to reflect them in speech.

Sentence Modalities

The primary approach to the study of the comprehension of sentence modalities or grammatic morphemes has been to present a child with pictures representing contrasting grammatic forms and to request that the child select the best fit for a stimulus containing one of the forms. Fraser, Bellugi, and Brown

Table 8–2
Developmental Order of Sentence Modalities*

Sentence Modalities	Fraser, Bellugi, & Brown[†]	Carrow[‡]	Miller & Yoder[‡]
Affirmative and negative	1	3-0 to 3-6	3-6
Subject and object in active voice (word-order cues)	2	3-0	
Present progressive and future tense	2	3-0 to 4-6	
Number, gender in third person, pronouns, nominative case	4	3-0 to 5-6	4-0
Masculine and feminine singular and neuter plural of third person, possessive pronoun	4	4-0	
Present progressive and past	5		5-0
Singular and plural marked by *is* or *are*	6	4-0	
Noun, singular and plural marked by inflection -*s*	7	4-0 to 5-0	4-6
Noun and noun + derivational, suffix -*er*		4-6	
Subject and object in possessive voice (word-order cues)	7	5-6 to 6-0	5-6
Indirect and direct object	9	4-6	
Possessive -'*s*			5-6

*As studied by Fraser et al. (1963), Carrow (1968), and Miller and Yoder (1972).
[†]Numbers represent order of acquisition.
[‡]Numbers represent age of acquistion.

(1963) used this procedure with twelve children and reported the results in terms of the rank order of difficulty of the items. Carrow (1968) studied 159 children and reported the results in terms of the age level at which 75 percent of the children passed each of the items. Miller and Yoder's procedures (1972) were similar to Carrow's. A summary of the order of development reported by these investigators, from which the order of acquisition of these items may be inferred, is found in Table 8-2. (The span in age reported by Carrow for specific items is a function of the stimulus; for example, in testing the affirmative/negative contrast, the age of 75 percent response differed when the stimulus was the affirmative than when it was negative.) Carrow (1968, p. 110) concluded that some grammatic contrasts appear to be more difficult than others. The children seemed to comprehend earlier "those categories which are fundamentally unmarked and specified, such as present tense and singular number, and to have more difficulty with grammatical contrasts which are derived and marked, such as past and future tense and plural number."

It appears that comprehension, like production, is gradual, and there seems to be a sequence in which children acquire the understanding of the specific grammatic means used to convey meaning. It is important for the language pathologist to be aware of the level of comprehension of the children for whom she is providing assistance, so that her expectations from the children are in line with their capabilities.

outline

THE TERMINOLOGY OF PRAGMATICS

FUNCTIONS OF LANGUAGE

Communicative Functions
Function 1: To Greet
Function 2: To Regulate
Function 3: To Exchange Information
Function 4: To Express Feelings
Function 5: To Use Language Imaginatively
Function 6: Metalinguistic Language
Noncommunicative Functions
Function 1: Concept Formation
Function 2: Self-Direction
Function 3: Magic

CONVERSATIONAL POSTULATES:
RULES OF DISCOURSE

Presupposition
Indirect Speech Acts and Polite Forms
Turn-Taking
Deixis
Deixis of Person/Object
Deixis of Place
Deixis of Time

THE CONTEXT OF LANGUAGE

DEVELOPMENT OF PRAGMATICS

learning when to use words: pragmatic development

9

A CHILD ACQUIRES LANGUAGE because the usefulness of communication becomes apparent even before he can say any words. Learning to communicate begins with the first social exchange between the infant and caretaker, and continues until the nuances and subtle rules governing polite forms, humor, and sarcasm are finally mastered late in the school years.

Although *pragmatics* was defined in Chapter 2, this chapter describes the terminology in greater detail. The function of language, the context of language, and the rules of conversation are discussed. As each function of language is described, an effort is made to summarize what is known about its course of development.

Pragmatics became the "fashion" of the middle and late 1970s, but, like so many fashion revolutions, this new interest represented less a bold step forward than a return to pre-Chomskian interest in language as a means of communication. In the pre-Chomskian era, pragmatics was mainly the province of philosophers like Pierce (1932), C. W. Morris (1946), and Austin (1962), who discussed the ways in which adults used language to communicate. They observed that in order for communication to take place, the speaker and listener were required to function as active partners in the ongoing process.

Pragmatic analysis must include information about both the speaker and the listener, as well as information about the relationship between the two and the environment in which they are speaking. Pragmatics has been rather frequently defined as the set of sociolinguistic rules that determine *Who* says *what* to *whom* in *which* circumstances.

Chapters 7 and 8 discussed the acquisition of words and grammatic processes with the focus on the child as the speaker who acquires this knowledge. This chapter stresses the speaker-listener dyad and the language context. The language specialist has particular need to appreciate how context influences language and to understand the multiple rules the child must master in order to carry on the simplest conversation. The child with a language disorder may fail to learn pragmatic rules as well as semantic and syntactic rules. This failure sometimes results in the "social ineptness" and inappropriate remarks that may characterize a language-disordered child even after he appears to have mastered other language systems.

THE TERMINOLOGY OF PRAGMATICS

Because several disciplines, including philosophy, linguistics, sociology, and sociolinguistics, have contributed to pragmatic theory, pragmatics now has a complex terminology. At times the same term may have a different connotation in child language than in adult language.

An important philosophical concept in the pragmatic analysis of language has been the notion that to speak is to act (Austin, 1962). Some types of utterances have profound effects on certain listeners and are events in themselves. These are clearly *performative* utterances (Dore, 1975). The judge who says "I sentence you to ten years in the penitentiary," the minister who says, "I pronounce you husband and wife," and the chairperson who says, "The meeting will now come to order" have all acted. A theory of speech acts has evolved based upon this recognition of speech as action. The term *speech act* is used to imply how the utterance functions (Rees, 1978; Searle, 1969). The focal point of the speech act theory is the *locutionary act,* which is the speech itself. In pragmatics, the speaker's reason for communicating is central to the analysis. This purpose is analyzed separately from the locutionary act and is called the *illocutionary act.* In some systems of analysis, this illocutionary act may be further divided based on whether the utterance is a simple statement ("Mary is my friend") or accomplishes some act, such as making a promise.

The purpose of an utterance may sometimes be explicitly stated. Analysis of the locutionary and illocutionary acts focuses on the speaker as does the analysis of the semantic and syntactic system. However, pragmatic analysis also includes the effect of the utterance on the listener, called a *perlocutionary* act. The effect any particular utterance has on a listener may be evaluated

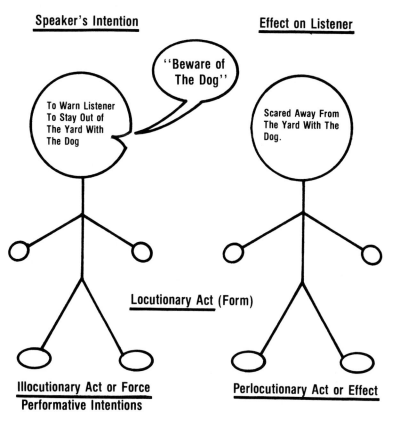

Speaker's Intention

Effect on Listener

"Beware of The Dog"

To Warn Listener To Stay Out of The Yard With The Dog

Scared Away From The Yard With The Dog.

Locutionary Act (Form)

Illocutionary Act or Force
Performative Intentions

Perlocutionary Act or Effect

Figure 9-1
Illustration of a speech act with the illocutionary force of warning the listener, and the perlocutionary effect of scaring the listener away.

in terms of the listener's action, thoughts, beliefs, etc. Sometimes this effect may actually be stated, using words such as *scare, inspire, enlighten, convince,* or *persuade* (Bates, 1976a; Dore, Gearhart, & Newman, 1978).

The terminology used to describe speech acts may be further illustrated by a simple example (Fig. 9-1). A speaker says to someone approaching his yard, "Beware of the dog." This statement is the locutionary act. The speaker's purpose is to warn the listener not to enter the yard; this purpose is referred to as the illocutionary act. The effect of the utterance on the listener is to scare him away from the yard; the perlocutionary act is made apparent by the listener's action—staying out of the yard.

Language exists because of the functions it serves. The functions of language may be divided into two main categories: communicative and noncommunicative (Rees, 1973a, 1978). Language that is directed to a listener and relies upon interpersonal reaction is called dialogue and has a communicative function. Other forms of language are called monologues and have noncommunicative functions.

FUNCTIONS OF LANGUAGE

Communicative Functions

A number of detailed lists of the communicative functions of language exist and have been reviewed by Rees (1978). The following communicative functions of language express a consensus of a number of researchers:

1. To greet and to express various social routines.
2. To regulate. This also includes language used to control, persuade, request, convince, nag, correct, criticize, threaten, demand, etc.
3. To exchange information. This also includes language used to question, inform, describe, assert, state, explain, answer, etc.
4. To express feelings. This also includes language used to express being happy, excited, sad, frightened, angry, mad, hurt, as well as to protest and to feel good.
5. Imaginative function. This includes langauge used in games and fantasy as well as figurative and artistic language.
6. Metalinguistic function. This includes the use of language to talk about language.

Function 1: To Greet

A few standard phrases have the primary function of establishing interpersonal contact. These social routines have their own set of rules and apparently their own unique developmental pattern. Utterances such as "Hello," "Goodbye," "I'll see you," "I'm sorry," "Congratulations," and "Merry Christmas" have social functions and are not always to be taken literally. Adults may say "I'm sorry" or "Excuse me" while continuing to push through a crowd; or they may say "Congratulations" to a rival.

Developmentally, it has been observed that some greetings are acquired very early. Social interactions occur even before the child associates adults with objects and seem to serve the

Charles W. Morris

Charles W. Morris is a philosopher whose outstanding contribution was his publication, *Foundations of the Theory of Signs,* which discussed the science of signs (semiotics) as including the investigation of syntax, semantics, and pragmatics. Specifically, Morris related pragmatics to the biosocial elements of communication. Almost fifty years ago, Morris stressed a truth that was forgotten for many years and was only recently rediscovered. He noted that pragmatic features were infrequently discussed in works on semantics and stressed that just as analysis of syntax must be supplemented by semantic information, so also must discussions of semantics be supplemented by pragmatics.

The writings of Morris owe much to C.S. Pierce (1839–1914), who was an influential philosopher and mathematician. Pierce's ideas had great impact on his colleagues but he wrote very sparingly. The works of philosophers like Pierce and Morris were neglected in linguistic study and were virtually unknown among clinicians, yet their ideas concerning communication are now considered current and relevant as demonstrated by the recent emphasis on the communication functions of language.

LEARNING WHEN TO USE WORDS: PRAGMATIC DEVELOPMENT

function of securing the adult's attention. Greenfield and Smith (1976) and K. Nelson (1978) observed the difference in styles of language learning with one group of children learning words of greeting such as *hi* and *bye-bye* very early, while others learned words having an obvious reference such as *cookie* or *doggie.* Halliday (1975) observed that some words that appear to have referential meaning, such as *cat,* could actually be considered a greeting when the intent of the communication is not to inform the adult "here is a cat" but rather to greet the cat.

An interesting insight into the way children learn social phrases has been furnished by Berko Gleason and Weintraub (1978). They studied the unique social routine of "trick or treat" because it occurred just once during the year. Some 150 children between 2 and 14 years old were observed with their parents on Halloween. The parents specifically taught the Halloween routine, which consisted of saying "trick or treat" when the door was opened, "thank you" when the children were given their treat, and "good-bye" as they left the house. The youngest children tended to say nothing, the 4- and 5-year-olds said only "trick or treat," the older children added "thank you," and those children over 10 years old correctly said the entire routine. The acquisition of social routines progresses in the opposite direction from the usual parental teaching of reference words. When teaching a social routine, adults first insist that the child learn the routine and only later, possibly years later, do the children come to realize the meaning of the individual words in the routine.

The acquisition of the social phrases *hi, bye-bye,* and *thanks* was studied in twenty-two children between the ages of 2 and 5 years (Blank-Greif & Berko Gleason, 1980). During these preschool years, *hi* and *bye-bye* were spontaneously produced 24 percent of the time while *thanks* was spontaneously produced only 7 percent of the time. One of the conclusions of this study was that parents must teach these routines; the usual method of teaching was the prompting of children to use the appropriate social phrase at the right time. When teaching words other than social phrases, adults focus on meaning; however, words like *hi* and *bye-bye* are events in themselves.

Function 2: To Regulate

The earliest vocalization of the infant is a cry, the function of which is universally interpreted by adults as a signal of distress and/or a need for attention. Once the infant comes to understand that the adult is the agent of comfort, these cries begin to constitute an attempt to regulate adult behavior. Another early emerging infant behavior is the exchange of gaze, which focuses adult attention on an object of interest to the infant. In the next developmental stage, the infant engages in pointing, showing, and giving objects to others. This behavior has been closely linked to the onset of words, and labeling emerges out of this pointing behavior (Bates, 1976a). It has been hypothesized that the frequency of this behavior can be correlated to the size of the earliest vocabulary (Bloom & Lahey, 1978).

Early preverbal communication often has a regulatory function, which has been described as consisting of sound plus gesture (Bates et al., 1977) and develops in three stages:

1. *Attention to objects* (The infant holds up an object and vocalizes.)
2. *Request for an object* (The infant reaches open-handed toward an object, and makes vocalizations.)
3. *Request for transfer of an object* (The infant holds out and gives an object and/or reaches for another object. These gestures are combined with vocalization.)

Much of a child's early speech is a request for attention, objects, or assistance. In his study of the illocutionary acts of 3-year-olds, Dore (1977) found that the largest single category was "requesting," which totaled 27 percent of all utterances. Likewise, much adult-to-child speech attempts to regulate the child through commands or requests for more suitable behavior.

Function 3: To Exchange Information

Adults appear to have strong motivation to inform small children about objects and events in their environment, and their speech appears well-designed to provide children with sufficient information with which to form referential categories. For example, as a child points, the parent might say, "See the bunny," "Look at the bunny's long ears," etc. Even the questions parents direct to young children are often instructive in nature ("What is the bunny doing? Is it hopping?") Such questions are not asked to elicit information but to provide it in a polite form.

The converse of this situation occurs when the child exchanges information with the adult. Initially, the toddler is unable to provide the adult with new information, instead commenting on what is obvious to the adult ("My truck," or "Me sit down.") As the child gets older, this type of remark occurs less frequently, possibly because it becomes apparent to the child that he cannot provide the adult with information, except in special situations, such as "tattling" on others. Information is exchanged when the child can both ask for and provide information by using *what* and *where* questions. By 18 to 24 months of age, the child begins to ask for the names of objects, their functions, and their locations. He can also provide that information when questioned.

Function 4: To Express Feelings

Initially, the child expresses all feelings nonverbally. From about age 2½ thru preschool years, caretakers use appropriate vocabulary to assist the child in expressing feelings verbally instead of nonverbally. Adults demonstrate that the child can say he is "hurt" or "mad" to express the condition for which he previously cried. In a novel situation such as a first ride on a merry-go-round, the adult may verbalize for the uncertain child what the adult thinks the child may be feeling ("This is exciting" or "You're having fun"). Adults routinely exaggerate their responses to situations, presumably to instruct and model the appropriate feelings for the child. H. H. Clark, (1973, p. 50) noted that when an adult plays with a child, the adult may comment with exaggerated emotion, "Look at all of these toys," "They are just great," or "Wow—this is a lot of fun, isn't it?" Since obviously the adult cannot be expected to find childish toys and activities this exciting, one reason for the exaggerated expression would be to teach the child how to verbalize appropriate emotions.

Function 5: To Use Language Imaginatively

Imaginative language has been closely associated with the symbolization process (Bruner, 1975). Only when children can function "as if" can they truly be credited with understanding the use of symbols. The normal preschooler displays a rich imagination and verbalizes this imaginative play: for example, "Let's pretend I'm a fireman and going to a fire." Between the ages of 2 and 5, imaginative social play with peers becomes increasingly frequent and complex (Garvey, 1977) as children engage in games of fantasy such as cowboys and Indians, cops and robbers, or teacher and students. Piaget (1955, p. 80) describes a 5-year-old boy who organizes a pretend game with his friends.

This youngster explains that they will pretend to be a balloon flying in the sky. He will be the basket, his friend will be the balloon, and another child will be the sand in the basket.

Another imaginative function of language is the use of metaphor. Very young children are, paradoxically, the ones who are most active in *apparent* metaphor production. These "figures of speech" contribute to the delightful and often amusing quality of conversation with preschoolers. "A middle-aged piece of cake"; "house hat" (to refer to a chimney; Gardner et al., 1978; "daddy's vacuum cleaner" (a lawn mower; Ferrier, 1978); and "horse with striped pajamas" (a zebra) appear to be figurative language. There is no evidence, however, that preschoolers appreciate that the use of "house hat," for example, is symbolic. Bowerman (1978b) has analyzed similar expressions, and she described common patterns such as the substitution of nouns for verbs and the confusion of semantically similar words. These expressions actually represent immaturity of the linguistic system. According to Gardner et al. (1978), true metaphoric competence does not emerge until adolescence, when children attain the level of formal logical operations.

Humor is another form of figurative language that develops late. During early school years, children derive great pleasure from games such as "knock-knock" and the telling of "shaggy dog stories." They also produce various noises that may sound foolish to adults. Gardner et al.(1978) found that by age 6 or 7, children begin to understand puns and riddles, but they must be at least several years older before they are able to grasp the point of a joke or retell a humorous story. Prior to that time, the child attends to the physical situation of a joke, for example, someone slipping, and thus the child may retell the joke describing only the situation he finds funny, while entirely omitting the verbal humor that is the point of the joke. In general, a child must have obtained the operational stage (after 11 years) before jokes are truly understood (Gardner et al., 1978).

Function 6: Metalinguistic Language

Metalinguistic language is used to talk about or to reflect upon language. The most common metalinguistic tasks for the average child are telling rhyming words and giving synonyms and antonyms. The task of rhyming involves the concept of "sounds like;" this ability to extract the phonological elements of words does not emerge until children are about kindergarten age (de Villiers & de Villiers, 1978b, p. 165). The ability to provide synonyms and antonyms requires a capacity to judge whether words or sentences express the same or different concepts. This involves thinking about language as an object, and most children have difficulty doing this until they are 5 or 6 years old (Foss & Hakes, 1978).

One of the more extensively studied forms of emerging meta-linguistic ability is the child's capacity to judge an utterance as grammatic or acceptable. (Most adults can quite easily judge whether utterances are acceptable or not.) One of the earliest attempts to elicit judgments about the acceptability of utterances from small children was by Brown and Bellugi (1964). They asked one of their subjects, Adam, at stage I grammar, "Which is right: 'Two shoes or two shoe' "? His answer, produced with explosive enthusiasm, was "Pop goes the weasel." This response illustrated the inherent difficulty of this task for toddlers. Subsequent attempts have been made with children at higher levels of grammar. One study (de Villiers & de Villiers, 1972) suggested that young children judge an utterance as acceptable if they can understand it, regardless of the deviations in word order or grammatic inflection. Four- and five-year-olds judged sentences as unacceptable if they did not feel the sentence was true or if they disagreed with the sentence. Thus, the utterance "The big rock was in the middle of the road" was judged ungrammatic because the children felt that it was bad to have a rock in the middle of the road. Adults, on the other hand, judge acceptability independent of their agreement with the sentence.

Noncommunicative Functions

Some language is not directed to a listener and has no essential communicative function, although it may be social; such language is known as *monologue*. A monologue is that form of speech that occurs when the speaker ignores the presence of another person and directs the speech to himself (Piaget, 1955). This uniquely personal and noncommunicative use of language has been outlined by Rees (1973a) and includes the following functions: (1) concept formation, (2) directive function, and (3) magical function.

Function 1: Concept Formation

The growth of vocabulary is intimately tied to cognitive development. Forming concepts is apparently useful behavior for the child, and the grouping or labeling of categories is a spontaneous activity. It has been theorized that assignment of a label assists in the child's cognitive growth. While there is no universally accepted theory of how a child learns words, the assignment of an object or activity to a particular category appears to reduce the cognitive load, allows the child to make increasing sense of his environment, and frees him for further interaction and learning. Observation of children indicates that they frequently label objects with no discernable purpose other than telling themselves what the thing is called. A child's early speech may constitute a symbolic verbal representation of what is seen and what is happening. His speech is tied to the here and now, so that words are linked first with his own perception or movement; only later do they *represent* that perception or movement.

Halliday (1975) noted that many of the first words that his subject, Nigel, learned had no communicative function. Instead, the new vocabulary had the sole purpose of observing or categorizing phenomena. Halliday speaks of this as the "learning function" of language, as opposed to the communication function of language. This dichotomy continued into the two-word stage when Nigel was 19 months old and clearly distinguished between utterances with regulatory functions, such as "more meat," and comments that categorized objects in his environment, such as "green car" or "two trains."

Among older children and adults, it has been observed (Carroll, 1964) that having a name or category for something facilitates perception. For instance, when a particular language lacks a word for a certain color the speakers of that language tend to ignore the difference between that color and other colors. Speakers of a language that had only the word *red* for a broad area of the color spectrum mixed red, pink, and orange indiscriminately, although they demonstrated that they could correctly distinguish the various types of red on perceptual testing (Bates et al., 1977). Such observations indicate the significance of language in concept formation.

In observing the conversation of the children he studied, Piaget (1955) noted that they often appeared unconcerned whether anyone heard them or answered them. All they wanted was for someone to be present. Piaget called this process of thinking aloud *egocentric* speech. He illustrated this speech by quoting one boy, P, who was drawing at the same table with his best friend, E (Piaget, 1955, pp. 30–31). P said to E, "But the trams that are hooked on behind don't have any flags." No answer. P to E, "They don't have any carriages hooked on." No answer. When E finally spoke, his comment was not related to the trams P was discussing. This type of verbalization led Piaget to classify children's speech as either egocentric or socialized. Piaget estimated that nearly half of the verbalizations of young children consisted of egocentric monologues. One reason for this, in Piaget's opinion, was that children do not know which thoughts should be spoken aloud, and so they speak as if thinking aloud.

Piaget's term *egocentric* has been widely quoted, and when used without explanation, it suggests that Piaget believed young children were "asocial." However, study of Piaget's later writings and analysis of the multitude of discussions of his work indicates that this interpretation is not true (Bates, 1975, p. 270). Simply because children did not require their listeners to indicate their attention does not imply that this speech does not have social goals. Actually, more recent studies indicate that preschool children engage in many fewer monologues than Piaget suggested.

Monologues with apparent "learning functions" may also be observed among adults, who, when faced with complex problems, may tend to verbalize their problem solving aloud. Such verbalization is not directed to anyone in particular; it not only does not require a response, but a response would probably be annoying to the speaker.

Function 2: Self-Direction

Russian psychologists such as Vygotsky (1962) and Luria (1961) have been influential in pointing out the regulatory functions of language. Both stressed the role of inner speech to regulate behavior. The emergence of this capacity is illustrated by the toddlers' tendency to echo their parents' prohibitions, often labeling forbidden objects or activities as *no-no's*. A mother recalled coming into the kitchen to find her 2-year-old dropping eggs to the floor as he said aloud, "No-no. Bad boy. Don't drop. No-no." This child had mastered the language appropriate to the situation, but had not yet internalized this language in such a way as to modify his behavior. Many parental injunctions remain with adults in the form of social mores such as "Don't talk with your mouth full," or "Don't put your elbows on the table."

Luria's experiments (1961) led him to outline three stages of development of self-direction. Between about 1½ and 3 years, verbal control resides with adults who direct the child's attention and issue commands. At that stage, commands can initiate but not truly inhibit actions. From age 3 to 5, verbal control must still be provided by adults, but the adult's command can really inhibit the child's actions. In the final stage, the child can regulate his own behavior. Although there have been problems with American replication of Luria's experimental work on verbal self-regulation, this theory continues to be influential. (Bloor, 1977).

Luria (1961) postulated that motor responses in children gradually come to be controlled by what he called a "second signalling" system of language. Once language is established, learning no longer needs to be trial and error, and language becomes capable of regulating both internal and external responses. Vygotsky (1962) felt that between 3 and 6 years of age, a child's speech to himself is so abbreviated that it is completely internalized, and thus constitutes what he called "inner speech."

Function 3: Magic

The linking of language and magic begins with the emergence of langauge and never entirely disappears. Young children have difficulty separating the word for a thing from the thing itself.

The inherent quality of names gives a word itself some of the aura of the actual article. One example of a link of words to magic occurs in infancy when the child may initially feel that *bye-bye* is a magic word because whenever it is said someone disappears.

In all cultures there are taboo words. A word is taboo when there are elaborate rules about its use. Some taboo words may only be spoken by certain people in the culture. Children as young as 2 to 3 years old recognize taboo words and warn other children not to say these words (Bates, 1976a). In some religions, the name of God may not be spoken, and euphemisms have been invented to use in its place. Some words, such as curses, became taboo because of religious strictures. In many cultures, the words connected with sex and/or elimination are taboo, and these are often replaced by colloquial euphemisms. In England, for example, the toilet may called a "cloak room," leading Americans to assume the speaker is referring to the room where coats are checked. Even the most sophisticated adults equate insulting language with actual abuse and react to such language with aggression—in some cases, physical aggression. Thus, the magical function of language remains part of the adult language system.

CONVERSATIONAL POSTULATES: RULES OF DISCOURSE

Discourse is at a higher level of organization than the speech act. A discourse may be a dialogue or a monologue. What is crucial is that discourse have a topical structure with successive utterances linked together on the basis of a common topic (Hurtig, 1977).

An effective conversation involves rules for turn-taking and learning such conventions as presupposition, indirect speech acts, and deixis. These conventions are called conversational postulates or rules of discourse. They concern the quality, relevance, and quantity of information contained in the discourse (D. Gordon & Lakoff, 1976), and constitute the assumptions that humans share about discourse. These postulates are generally and tacitly agreed-upon rules and include the following: (1) tell the truth; (2) offer new and relevant information; and (3) request only information you want (Bates, 1976a; Miller, 1978).

Presupposition

The conduct of conversation is probably the most complex as well as the most important target of the pragmatic approach to the study of language. To successfully conduct conversation the speaker must make a series of assumptions, which are called presuppositions. A presupposition is information that is not con-

Linguists have evidence that the place of women in our society is reflected in both the way women are expected to speak and the way they are spoken to. Even first graders can identify some patterns of speech that they regard as "talking like a lady" (Edelsky, 1977). The children agree that ladies are polite. Men use strong 'swear' words like "damn" and are perceived to be "mean"; but the children think that what they say is important. The speech of women is said to be characterized by use of particular adjectives, such as "adorable," "charming," "lovely," and "darling" (Lakoff, 1973). These adjectives not only suggest that the speaker is kind and sweet, but also that the topic of conversation is trivial. Another characteristic of women's speech is the tendency to overuse tag questions. Use of questions such as "John is here, isn't he?" instead of a direct statement or question, make women appear indecisive and unsure of themselves (Lakoff, 1973). The frequent use of tag questions and indirect requests (also in question form) tend to make women appear more polite than men, and guarantees that they will sound "like ladies."

tained in an utterance but must be known if the sentence is to be understood (Bates, 1976b; Greenfield & Zukow, 1978). Usually the information implied in the sentence must be assumed to be true. In the utterance, "Did you know John's sister?" it must be presumed true that (1) John exists, (2) John has a sister, and (3) that it would be possible for the addressee to have known the sister. None of this information is contained in the utterance.

When the speaker misses this presupposition, then additional information must be supplied in order for communication to take place. Somehow a joint referent must be negotiated: For instance, speaker A at a party says "Lois looks as if she's gaining too much weight to remain a champion tennis player." To which B might reply, "Who is Lois?" It would then be the task of A to decide what common information they shared so that the listener could tell Lois from all the other women at the party. The response might be something like "Lois is the blonde lady standing next to the tall man with the beard."

Interpretation of an utterance assumes previous knowledge of what to expect in various situations. Rees (1978) illustrated how the utterance "Would you like to eat here?" can be variously interpreted, depending upon the listener's understanding of the situation in which it was uttered. If the speaker and listener were driving into a town, the listener would suppose that the speaker wanted to stop and eat at a restaurant in that town. If they were both walking down the street, it would be assumed that the speaker meant the restaurant in view. If they were out on a picnic, it would be assumed that the speaker meant to spread the blanket and begin to eat immediately.

Very young children use presupposition to select the element of the communication situation that will be encoded (Halliday, 1975). When a child can say only a few words, the initial decision is what *not* to say. What can be assumed by the listener is therefore important. This requires at least a rudimentary ability to take the listener's point of view. By exploring the situation in which he is speaking, the child can encode the one most informative word (Greenfield & Smith, 1976). Consequently the very young child might choose not to say "want" but instead to say "cookie," trusting that in the circumstances the adult would understand that the child wanted a cookie.

Indirect Speech Acts and Polite Forms

Indirect speech acts and polite forms are considered to be in a special category of conversational postulates. The earliest polite forms consist of social phrases such as "please" and "thank you." When these phrases first emerge at 24 to 30 months, they are not understood by the children as polite forms. They are more often used to mark the end of an exchange. First requests are made very simply. Gradually, children learn to modify these requests to make them "more polite," by adding a reason, such as "cause I'm thirsty." If the request is not granted, the child next reduces the request through use of a diminutive like *little*. If reducing the "size" of the request is not successful, the child will then reduce his voice to a whisper, in an effort to be even more polite. The next stage of development of polite requests is to state a generic need such as "We want" or a direct need such as "I have to" (Bates, 1976a).

Children next learn that polite requests are frequently stated in the form of questions. The developmental nature of this is illustrated by the preschooler, who when answering the phone, is asked "Is your mother home?" and responds "Yes" and hangs up. Such a child does not understand that this question is in fact a polite request to call the mother to the phone. Indirect speech acts often use questions to make a request. Such questions as "Can you pass the salt?" do not inquire about the listener's physical strength, nor does "Do you have the time?" imply that the listener wants to know whether or not the other person has a watch.

This little boy has already mastered several aspects of polite request. His use of "borrow" however reflects his own creativity. (The Family Circus by Bil Keane, reprinted courtesy of Register and Tribune Syndicate.)

In indirect speech acts, the speaker is able to communicate more than is actually said by relying upon mutually shared background information. Sentences used as indirect requests share certain forms, which include verb forms such as *can, could,* and *would.*

Indirect requests could all be stated as direct commands. However, the principle motive for using an indirect request is politeness. In this way, compliance may be seen as a free action on the part of the listener (Searle, 1976).

Turn-Taking

The interaction of discourse has been compared to a game of catch (Fillmore, as cited in Bloom, Rocissano, & Hood, 1976). Each player comes to the game with a basket of balls and the

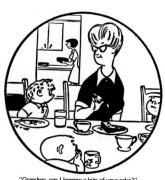

"Grandma, can I borrow a bite of your cake?"

knowledge that only one ball can be in the air at a time. This analogy suggests that conversation is a typical adult activity, yet turn-taking is apparent between mothers and their infants well before the infants begin to say words.

Developmentally, conversational turn-taking begins with preverbal exchanges between the infant and an adult. Only later is a formal lexicon and grammar added to this essentially social behavior. Freedle and Lewis (1977, p. 28) provide an illuminating example of social turn-taking from their research. This exchange takes place between an infant and her mother. During this exchange, the infant squeaks a rubber toy, kicks her feet, and then squeals, apparently in delight. At this, the mother turns toward her and smiles. Next, the infant vocalizes and reaches toward her mother, who then vocalizes while the infant watches and listens. The infant and then her mother vocalize and listen to each other for three more turns each. It is evident that even at this prelinguistic stage, this infant was aware that only one ball could be in the air at a time, figuratively speaking. Consequently the infant acted, the mother responded, and so on for several turns, until the activity was terminated.

Early discourse depends heavily on monitoring by the adult, who must provide proper input, based upon the child's capacity for output, as well as maintaining the topic at hand. Snow, in a 1976 lecture (Dore, 1979, p. 349), reported on two conversations with an 18-month-old child. In the first conversation, the child pointed out and named "band-aid" for an examiner. The examiner then attempted to elicit information as to whether the child had fallen and what part of the child's body the band-aid was on, but the child continued to repeat "band-aid." The next conversation was between the child and her mother. Since the mother knew how to ask questions of her child, she was able to find out the information the examiner had not been able to elicit.

By 36 months, children can respond to *what, where,* and *who* questions (Ervin-Tripp & Mitchell-Kernan, 1977) and this ability to reply to questions assists the adult in maintaining the conversation. By age 3, most children also demonstrate an understanding that the same topic is to be shared, and that they are able to add new information to the topic each time it is their turn to speak (Bloom, Rocissano, & Hood, 1976).

As children get older, it is expected, at least in conversation with adults, that the same "ball" be volleyed back and forth. Mothers teach this game to children by actually providing both sides of the conversation. For example, a mother might ask the general question, "How was school today?" and immediately follow it up with a more specific question, such as "Did you color a picture?" This might be followed by other specific questions, like "What was in your picture?" or "Did you bring your picture home?" In this way, the adult not only helps the child learn how to respond to general questions but also illustrates how a topic of conversation is maintained. (The number of turns that a young child can maintain on the same topic varies with the conversational partner.)

Although adults are helpful in teaching children about conversation, when more than two people are speaking, the young child is likely to be ignored and to experience considerable difficulty breaking into the conversation. In a study of 2-year-olds, as compared to 4-year-olds, Ervin-Tripp (1979) found that between 83 and 94 percent of the 2-year-olds' attempts to break into a conversation between adults and older children were unsuccessful.

Deixis

Deixis is a linguistic device that anchors an utterance to the communicative setting in which it occurs. The basic assumptions (presuppositions) are that during conversation the role of speaker and listener (deixis of person), their perspective of location (deixis of place), and their time frame continually shift. Deixis can only be understood as it relates to conversation.

Initial understanding of these presuppositions appears to grow out of the "give and take" games of infancy. In one such common game, an object is exchanged between adult and infant. At first the adult is always the agent, but later the infant learns to act as the agent and gives objects to the adult. Other games, such as peek-a-boo, also involve a change of role. It has been suggested (Bruner, 1975) that games like these, which children are already playing by 1 year of age, assist them in building the concept of changing roles. These concepts later contribute to the child's understanding of the changing perspectives of person, object, place, and time, which is essential to understanding deixis.

Deixis of Person/Object

In adult language, pronominalization is substitution of a pronoun for a noun. In both adult and child language the referent for a pronoun may be illustrated by either a gesture or by reference back to a person or object already mentioned. It is also understood that in a conversation the speaker always is *I* and the listener is always *you*.

As discussed in Chapter 7, very young children already have individual styles of language learning. Some studies, like that of Huxley (1970) describe the early emergence of the pronoun *it;* while other studies (Bellugi, 1971) suggest that in the first stage of language development children tend to refer to all objects and people, including themselves as speaker, by name. Bloom,

Lightbown, and Hood (1975) explored styles of learning nouns and pronouns and discovered a shift in the use of nouns and pronouns at an MLU of about 2.0. At that stage those children whose first vocabulary consisted mainly of nouns seemed to shift to pronouns, and vice versa. By the time the children reached an MLU of 2.5, most were able to use both nouns and pronouns, but they typically continued to use pronouns gesturally and there was poor evidence that they understood the alternate rules for the use of these shifting forms (Bloom & Lahey, 1978). The acquisition of pronouns requires not only an understanding of their structural complexity (see Chapter 8) but also an appreciation for the shifting of reference that characterizes discourse.

Adults intuitively appreciate the complexity of deixis of person and use nouns rather than pronouns when speaking to young children. Failure of person deixis was illustrated by Rees (1978), who described the confusion of a new husband who walked into the bathroom and found towels inscribed YOURS and MINE!

Deixis of Place

The referent for certain nouns, pronouns, and verbs alternates depending on the spatial orientation of the speaker in regard to the listener. Young children who have yet to learn to appreciate this shifting reference may have trouble understanding words like *nearby* or phrases like *next door*.

Pronouns such as *this/that* and *here/there* are frequently used to point out the location of particular objects or people. In adult language the forms *this* and *here* are understood to refer to the object or person closest to the speaker. In the speech of young children, the words emerge before the children have learned to understand this shifting of meaning. K. Nelson (1973b) found at least one deictic term each in the vocabularies of children who had mastered 30 words, and deictic terms often appeared in the first 10 words. These words, however, tended to be accompanied by gesture, which resolved any ambiguity. It was not until the MLU approached 4.0 that the deictic shift between *here* and *there* was observed (Bloom & Lahey, 1978).

In a series of studies, E. Clark (1977) also explored the child's emerging comprehension and expression of *here* and *there* during the ages of 2 to 5 years. Her subjects appeared to go through three stages. Initially, they used *here* and *there* as if both words had the same meaning. Next, the children established a point of reference that allowed them to make a partial contrast and by age 5, children mastered the contrast fully.

The contrast between paired verbs like *come/go* and *bring/take* is more complex. In another experiment, E. Clark (1977) gave children instructions, such as "Make the horse *come/go* to the circle." Children aged 3 to 5 years showed no consistent preference and used the terms interchangeably. Even 6-year-olds made a significant number of errors, although they seemed to realize that these words expressed variations in goal between speaker and listener. Clark concluded that by 3 to 4 years of age, children begin to appreciate speaker-based contrasts, but that they probably do not complete mastery of them until age 8 or 9.

Deixis of Time

Information about when an event occurs is relative to the time when the speaker chooses to speak of it: one can speak of an ongoing event, an event in the immediate or distant past, or in the future. This is done by marking the tense in the verb and by using words like *today, yesterday,* and *tomorrow.* A comment such as, "Let's have lunch together tomorrow" can only be interpreted by understanding that the speaker is referring to the day following the day on which he is speaking.

Another characteristic of words expressing time is their relationship to words of location. Linguists have long noted that in a number of languages, including English, the same limited set of adjectives *(long/short, far/near)* are used to describe both space and time. The relative nature of these references may be illustrated by the comment of an adult who is shopping for Christmas presents in September and who says that "Christmas is right around the corner." However, to a small child Christmas may still seem "far away" on December 23. Both place and time share the dynamic dimension of movement, and this too is reflected linguistically, as in the following examples: "Time *flew.*" "The plane *flew.*" "Friday *crept up* on us." "He *crept up* on us" (H. H. Clark, 1973).

At the present, there are more speculations than data on the order in which children learn the distinction between words expressing time. H. H. Clark (1973) feels that children learn to use words expressing space prior to using words to express time.

THE CONTEXT OF LANGUAGE

The recent emphasis on the pragmatic aspects of language stresses not only the function of language but also the context in which language occurs. The language context refers to the environment in which utterances are used as well as such listener variables as age, sex, and relation of listener to the speaker. Environmental variables also include the physical, cultural, and social setting in which speech occurs.

Chapter 5 illustrated how the speech of adults and even children changed when the listener was an infant or toddler. These predictable changes were called codes. The special code adopted by groups such as adolescents is dependent upon the listeners, and this code is used with peers but not with adults or persons in authority. Other examples of how speech changes to fit the listener include language used by lovers to each other, by the healthy to someone who is ill, and by employees to a person in power.

Speech is dependent not only upon the listeners but also upon the social context. Some topics are considered appropriate for parties; while others, like the weather, may be discussed with strangers in waiting rooms or elevators. Appreciation of the effect that the social context has on the topic of conversation emerges only gradually in the child and is related to socialization. Learning the rules for the use of language in different contexts constitutes a major task in the socialization of the child into the adult culture. The written, and unwritten, rules of etiquette for home, school, business, military, and social functions are all concerned with the specification of *who* should say *what* to *whom* in a series of differing contexts.

The context in which speech is uttered has an effect beyond regulating the speaker's code or even modifying the topic of conversation. Meaning in language is conveyed through the blending of the words with the social context (Bates, 1976a). The utterance "I love you" when said by a man to a woman on their first date is different than when said on their wedding day. These same words have a different meaning when a child says "I love you" to a parent, or when someone says this to a friend. In a different context, the same utterance may have a sarcastic meaning, in which the context overrides the literal meaning. No dictionary definition of the word *love* can convey all of these meanings.

The function and intended effect of utterances are also dependent on the environment in which the sentence is uttered. The function of the utterance "You must have some of this" varies depending upon circumstances in which it is used. When a hostess says to her guest "You must have some of this," it is a polite request or social phrase. The effect of this utterance on the listener may vary and it is perfectly appropriate for the listener to either accept or refuse the offered dish. When a mother says to her small child, "You must have some of this," the function of the utterance is to command, and the intended effect would be for the child to eat the designated food. Finally, if two guests were looking at a very unusual dish at a party and one said to the other, "You must have some of this!" the intent of this utterance might be sarcastic. The effect would probably be that both guests would laugh and neither would have any of the dish. No semantic or syntactic analysis can account for the range of meanings of social greetings, indirect requests, or sarcasm.

As children mature, they become less dependent on context. By age 3, they can talk about absent people and events. De Villiers and de Villiers (1978b) have suggested, rather whimsically, that that the ultimate achievement in freedom from context is

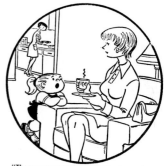

"Those are our very best cups. You have to be careful not to drop 'em."

*This little girl has learned to repeat a common caution. However, she has yet to learn the context in which the caution may be used appropriately. (*The Family Circus *by Bil Keane, reprinted courtesy of Register and Tribune Syndicate.)*

After an extended period in a preschool language development program, Robert had finally learned all the words in the little song that began his daily class. His rendition of this song was always praised by his teacher, his parents, and other family members, who were very proud of his accomplishment.

When he was taken to the airport to meet his father, Robert walked up to the nearest adult in the waiting room (a man busy with his calculator and his dictating machine) and proceeded to sing the entire song in a loud voice. The subsequent embarassment of his mother and the distress of the unknown man left Robert in tears.

Robert failed to understand the rules determining *who* should say *what* to *whom* under *what* circumstances.

the ability to lie. To lie convincingly, the speaker must be free from the true circumstances and present only the information best suited to convince the listener most effectively.

DEVELOPMENT OF PRAGMATICS

The use of language begins, as Leopold noted (1939), with the intention to communicate. Such intention may be clearly identified in children between birth and 8 to 10 months. Pointing plus vocalization constitute a common first step. Halliday (1975), in particular, has studied the functions of language in a child prior to the onset of words. His subject, Nigel, used four identifiable functions before he used words. These included (1) demanding ("give me"); (2) regulating ("do that"); (3) interacting ("I see you"); and (4) personal ("that's nice"). Nigel's language progressed through three identifiable phases. The first was preverbal. The next marked the transition to true verbal language at about 16 to 18 months. In this stage, Nigel learned to use grammar and also began to engage in verbal dialogue. As this phase progressed, Nigel learned to recite rhymes and social routines, tell stories, and provide information. The last phase is essentially the adult system, wherein the speaker controls devices for humor, sarcasm and indirect requests.

The following traces the development of pragmatics in child language.

1. *Between 2 and 10 months.* Eye contact and gaze exchange used to regulate joint attention on an activity—a prerequisite to learning reference. Eye contact, smiling, and attention indicate that the child takes notice of someone or something. Pointing plus vocalization suggests demand for someone or something.
2. *Between 10 and 16 months.* The regulatory function of language is strong at this stage. Gestures of giving, pointing, and showing draw attention to what is wanted. Nonverbal turn-taking in play lays the foundation for conversation. Early words are used to express instrumental ("I want"), regulatory ("Do what I tell you"), interactional ("hi"), and several other functions.

3. *Between 18 and 30 months.* In this time period, symbolic play, use of imaginative speech, beginning of discourse, answering questions, use of description, expressing some feeling, deictic use of pronouns, and ability to change topics are seen.
4. *Between 3 and 4 years.* Switches code when speaking to a baby. Recognizes taboo words. Increases ability to maintain conversation beyond several turns, especially if monitored by adult.
5. *Between 4 and 5 years.* Can give antonym, synonym, and rhyming words. Metalinguistic use of language emerges. Uses indirect requests.
6. *Grade-school age.* Uses at least three language codes. Can tell puns and stories. Follows most rules of discourse.
7. *High-school age.* Artistic use of language begins. Understands jokes, sarcasm, and social etiquette, but not necessarily debate and parliamentary rules.

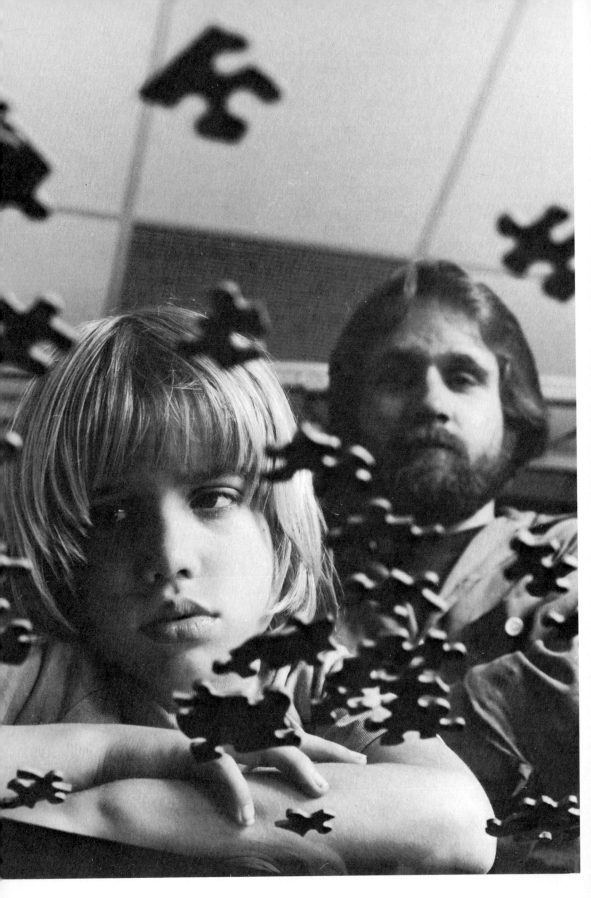

Photograph by Linda Stanford of the Media Production Center, University of Texas Health Science Center at Houston.

part three
disordered language

outline

PERSPECTIVES OF LANGUAGE DISORDERS IN THE INTEGRATIVE APPROACH

The Perspective of the Child
The Perspective of Disorder
The Perspective of Four Dimensions
The Perspective of Dimensional Interrelationship
The Perspective of Specification
The Perspective of Significance
Degree of Difference
Number of Dimensions Impaired
Rate of Change
Environmental and Intellectual Expectancies

DIMENSIONAL INTERRELATIONS IN THE INTEGRATIVE MODEL

Disorders of the Cognitive Dimension of Language
Disorders of Perception and Memory
Conceptual Disorders
Disorders of Representation and Symbolization
Disorders in the Dimension of Language Knowledge
Disorders of Grammar
Disorders of Semantics
Disorders of Pragmatics
Disorders of the Dimension of Language Performance
Disorders of Comprehension
Disorders of Language Production
Disorders of the Communication Environment Dimension

an integrative approach to language disorders 10

A REVIEW OF THE literature indicates that the term *language disorders* is neither clearly nor consistently defined. Although the term is used extensively, the professionals who use it often do not specify their criteria for and boundaries of disordered language; instead they use the term as if its meaning and scope were universally understood and accepted. However, the effectiveness of clinical management, theory, and research in language disorders is dependent upon the appropriate selection and classification of children according to a clear and valid definition of the problem. Such a definition cannot be evaluated from a theoretical basis only. It must be operationally valid; i.e., it must permit the identification of children with disordered language and account for the various manifestations of the problem.

This does not imply that there is only one way of answering the question, "What is a language disorder?" The complex nature of disorders of language does not lead to a single explanatory theory or model. However, it is possible for each language specialist to delineate and describe those processes, behaviors, and conditions that appear valid for her interpretation of language disorders, or to choose a model that has been thus delineated. This means that more than one theory or model of language disorders may be evolved. It also means that each language specialist must select the model or theory that appears to her to be most adequate for describing language disorders and must use it consistently.

The present chapter introduces an integrative model for describing and interpreting language disorders. Like the description of normal language used in the beginning chapters of this text, the integrative model for describing language disorders utilizes a concept of language based on four dimensions. The four-dimensional integrative model has been chosen because we believe it represents best the manifestation of the problems in disordered language.

The integrative approach to the description of disordered language has evolved from a consideration of six perspectives: (1) the perspective of the child; (2) the perspective of disorder; (3) the perspective of four dimensions; (4) the perspective of dimensional interrelationships; (5) the perspective of specification; and (6) the perspective of significance.

The first section of this chapter describes these six perspectives. Following this presentation, a second section provides a description of the interrelations among the dimensions of language with special reference to the effects of problems in one dimension upon components in other dimensions. Unless the complex nature and characteristics of language disorders are identified and clearly defined, the form of management will be ineffective and research results will be invalid. It is important to recognize that the dimensions are not equivalent in the sense that they describe the same type of process or level of category; nor are the components within each parameter parallel. The complexity of the language system in humans prohibits a "neat" organizational taxonomy. The simplicity and orderliness of the classification and organization must be sacrificed to obtain optimum validity, so that the system of classification represents the types of language disorders that are observed.

Individuals with extensive clinical experience with language disorders find that the application of a simple, one-dimensional, explanatory model of these disorders is inadequate for their understanding and management. What on paper appears to clarify the nature of language disorders only complicates understanding in practice and makes effective intervention difficult.

PERSPECTIVES OF LANGUAGE DISORDERS IN THE INTEGRATIVE APPROACH

The Perspective of the Child

Developments in psychololinguistics, sparked by Chomsky, led to an approach that emphasizes linguistic structure analysis in the assessment, intervention and definition of language disorders. The focus of concern in such an approach is primarily the language structure itself; language description is viewed as the main function of the language specialist.

The integrative approach proposed in the present text focuses on the *child* instead of on the language structure. This approach considers that language knowledge does not exist apart from other linguistic processes; language knowledge relates to and functions in an intrinsic cognitive system that learns and performs the language, and in an extrinsic environmental system that receives, responds to, and reinforces the language. A disorder of language in the integrative approach is viewed from the standpoint of the child and his intrinsic and extrinsic systems. Since the focus of concern is the child, in addition to a linguistic and cognitive description, the language specialists must determine how the language problem affects the child, his family and social relations, and his academic achievement. It seems that the early scholars stressed the role of the central nervous system in language but lacked the expertise to provide a linguistic description of language. Now, with the application of linguistic theory to psycholinguistic problems, there is a tendency to neglect the child as the learner of language and focus on the language behavior itself. The integrative theorist attempts to unite these two points of view. Emphasis on the child as the learner of language instead of on the language itself leads to a multidimensional view of language and particularly to a multidimensional view of language disorders.

The Perspective of Disorder

Within the past decade, methods for describing disorders of language have evolved from the methods used to study linguistic behavior in the normal population. The strategies that children use to learn language, the order in which acquisition takes place, and the principles underlying acquisition have been applied to the analysis and interpretation of disorders of language. In studying normal language, however, it is necessary only to observe language performance since it is assumed that all other aspects of the language-learning system are functioning adequately. In the language-disordered child, it is not sufficient to describe only the linguistic behavior of structure, and through it, semantics and use; the constituent skills involved in acquiring and using language are important to the definition of the disorder. Clinical observations have revealed that many disorders of language involve more than the language product—in fact, some language problems exhibit no outward differences from normal language performance. As a result, the normal language acquisition model may not be adequate for understanding the complex nature of language disorders. Furthermore, the evidence supporting the similarity in developmental sequences be-

The case of Milly illustrates a disorder of language in a girl with normal oral use of the linguistic code. Milly was 14 years old when she became a member of our car pool. I noticed immediately that she always asked for everything to be repeated. No matter who was speaking or what was said, she would respond with a high-pitched, "What did you say?" Her friends reported confidentially that she never knew what was going on at high school. She could not catch on to the conversation in small groups, did the wrong homework (although she had received As and Bs in the small private elementary school she had attended previously), and got upset in the cafeteria because the noise was too loud. I suggested that her mother take her for a hearing test.

The mother reported that Milly had been tested as a young child and was found to have auditory discrimination problems, vocabulary problems, and reading problems. However, she took Milly for an audiological evaluation, and her hearing was found to be normal. Subsequent tests found language production and comprehension to be at age level, but auditory discrimination, particularly in noise, to be significantly depressed. Her family made efforts to provide her with the help she needed, but her behavior gradually deteriorated. Her symptoms became so severe that she had to be taken out of school and placed with a tutor. Milly could not comprehend in her fast-moving noisy world. Although her oral language was normal, she in fact had a language disorder.

—Elizabeth Carrow-Woolfolk

tween disordered and normal language is not conclusive. Cross-sectional studies have indicated that certain aspects of the semantics and syntax of children with language disorders appear similar to those of the younger normal child. There have not been, however, comprehensive longitudinal studies of the language of the disordered across and within language parameters.

The limitations of a linguistic performance analysis have been pointed out by Bruner (1975), who stated that to write grammars at each of the levels of language development is not to explicate the nature of language acquisition. The complex set of perceptual, motor, conceptual, social, and linguistic skills that a child must acquire in order to master the language must be part of the study of language. The rules of grammar, according to Bruner, do not resemble, even closely, the psychological laws of language production and comprehension.

The integrative approach to language disorders sets the point of departure for the study of language disorders in the *disorders* themselves. The characteristics of disordered language, the order of its acquisition, the child's strategies for learning the language, and the condition of the child's language-learning system are the basis for understanding the disorders. This leads to the multidimensional approach to interpreting language disorders. Data on normal language acquisition are considered essential and are utilized, but only with the awareness of the differences between the learners of normal and disordered language.

The Perspective of Four Dimensions

The integrative approach views language disorders in much the same way it views language. (This view has been described in Part One of this text.) According to this approach, language is described in terms of both products and process, i.e. as a relationship between linguistic structure and meaning, which is learned by means of a cognitive system and performed through auditory-vocal processing systems in a social environment and for social purposes. The linguistic system, according to this multidimensional view (see Chapters 2–5), includes in the definition of language (1) the cognitive aspects that form the meaning of language; (2) the language-specific processing skills of perception and memory, together with the behavioral processes of comprehension and production; (3) the communication environment in which language is learned and used; and (4) the language content, use, and structure rules. The conceptual system, as it relates to structure, is an integral part of the language system, not a nonlanguage component.

The integrative definition of language disorders is much broader than the definitions provided by unidimensional approaches. The integrative approach considers that the selection of a single component of a dimension, such as oral language performance, as a criterion for identifying disordered language does not reflect accurately the nature and characteristics of such disorders—particularly if only oral language performance is used to infer the presence of other problems such as those of content and use. Although it is possible to classify samples of language on the basis of appearances according to problems in structure, use, and content, this classification may not accurately describe the language problem of the child, for problems in different dimensions can result in exactly the same oral language behavior. Failure to consider the multidimensional aspect of language may also cause the language specialist to overlook certain types of language disorders. For example, a child who has difficulty comprehending language in certain conditions (such as in a noisy environment) has a language disorder that may not be reflected in oral language performance. The varied manifestation of disorders in language has thus led to the multidimensional approach.

A distinction among language forms that is important to emphasize in language disorders is between structures (lexical, grammatic) that form *closed* categories and those that are *open*. The modulators are finite or closed within a specific language. Once they are acquired, they remain stable in the language of the child—as, for example, prepositions, plurality forms, and pronouns. There are other grammatic categories that are infinite and remain open; i.e., the number of members of the categories are so great that the learning process continues throughout adulthood. These are the categories that usually carry the semantic relations of language—the nouns, verbs, adjectives, etc.— and the category of word order with its related forms of conjunction and embedding. There may be as many different ways of expressing an idea as there are people trying to do it; the difference among these forms of expressions is in the open categories.

Children with language disorders may have problems with open or with closed categories. The child with moderate hearing impairment may learn the finite or closed categories but may have difficulty with open categories throughout his life. Because of this difficulty, the professional needs to make this kind of distinction in linguistic structure.

The Perspective of Dimensional Interrelationship

To understand language disorders from an integrative view, it is not sufficient to identify the various dimensions and features of language. It is also necessary to understand the relationship among them. Failure to understand the complexity of the relationships will produce oversimplification and misinterpretation of cause and effect among the dimensions of language and their components—in either a positive or a negative direction—and thereby produce misdiagnoses of language disorders.

The fact that language is described in stages and processes implies that there is a sequence of behavior that occurs both developmentally as well as in the performance of each communication event. Unless one chooses to consider each stage or process as being completely independent from every other one, the concept of relationship among stages, components, and dimensions of language must be accepted. These relationships can be ignored, with attention given only to the final product of language behavior, but the understanding and interpretation of the behavior, while appearing accurate, may in fact not be so.

A description of relationships among the various components and dimensions of language is similar to the description of the relationship between language and thought found in Chapter 3. These relationships may involve (1) a dependency effect, (2) a cumulative or complementary effect, (3) a reciprocal interaction effect, and (4) a relation-by-common-source effect. *Effect* means the manner in which some aspects of components are derived from others in development or maintenance.

One component of language may be dependent upon another in such a way that should the first fail to develop, the second will also:

$$C_1 \rightarrow C_2$$

The term dependence should not be interpreted as *cause*. Dependence means that one system requires input from another in order to build its structure (Bates et al., 1977). For example, the development of semantic features is dependent on, and derives from, the development of cognitive skills. Therefore, if there is a problem in cognition, one would expect a problem in semantics as well. (Not all problems in semantics are caused by cognitive disorders, however.)

Not only are the various language features dependent upon one another, the nature of the relationship in many instances is cumulative:

$$C_1 + C_2 \rightarrow C_3$$

For example, a problem in auditory acuity may affect auditory perception and the cumulative problem will affect auditory comprehension. The effects may also be complementary in degree; that is, the effect of one feature upon the other is such that, to the degree that one component is incomplete, inadequate, inefficient, etc., the component that is dependent on it is also incomplete, inadequate, and inefficient.

There may also be an effect of reciprocal interaction:

$$C_1 \rightleftarrows C_2$$

The interaction between two components involves their mutual benefit or their mutual constraint. The effect of interaction may depend on the timing of the interaction, that is, at what point in the development or execution of language they occur. For example, the interaction between concept formation and the linguistic code will have a different effect on a child of 2 who is learning language than on an adult.

The fourth effect arises from two factors being related in some fashion to a third, but not to each other:

$$C_2 \quad C_3$$
$$\nwarrow \quad \nearrow$$
$$C_1$$

For example, articulation and language comprehension may both relate to auditory memory but not necessarily to one another.

It is important to realize that the effects between components are never perfectly proportional nor completely predictable. The dependence, cumulative, and interactive effects exist between components that may in turn relate to the other components in different or similar ways. The adequacy of the other components may compensate for an inadequate relationship with the first. This indicates that the components cannot be considered as independent aspects of language, nor can any one of them, alone, be viewed as encompassing the totality of language.

The large number of skills, processes, and knowledge involved in language suggests that simple conclusions about any aspect of language are bound to be incorrect. Although one skill is dependent on a second, it does not follow that inadequacy in the second is caused by inadequacy in the first. It could be caused by any number of other inadequacies in other skills. For example, a moderate-to-severe auditory discrimination problem may affect auditory comprehension of language to some degree, but the extent of this effect will be determined by the adequacy of other skills and abilities related to comprehension, such as the ability to attend to spoken speech, and by the timing of the interaction between the auditory perception problem and auditory comprehension. It also does *not* follow that all auditory comprehension problems are a result of auditory discrimination problems. It would be erroneous, however, to conclude that because the relationship is not exclusive and not on a one-to-one basis that therefore the relationship does not exist.

The Perspective of Specification

A current position in the area of language disorders is that there is no need to classify disorders of language; instead, all individuals who have a problem in linguistic performance should be grouped together regardless of the nature or characteristics of the specific problem. The integrative position, however, is one of specification. This means that the nature and characteristics of a language disorder are important and should be delineated so that a more effective, valid, and informed program of research and clinical mangement can be carried out. The integrative approach considers the term language disorders similar to the term *sick*—a general problem is recognized but needs to be specified before appropriate solutions to the problem can be provided.

Specification leads to the recognition of the existence of systematic and predictable combinations of problems within the dimensions. These combinations of disorders produce identifiable and characteristic behaviors, which demand specific and characteristic management solutions. Combinations of problems that occur with frequency are grouped and provided with a label so that they may be studied as a unit. (The labels do not refer to etiology or cause; they describe a syndrome of behavior.) The groups that are most often identified and labeled are (1) language disorders of the emotionally disturbed; (2) language disorders of the mentally retarded; and (3) language disorders of the hearing impaired. Children in these groups have generalized and comprehensive problems in all four of the language dimensions; the language disorder is a *part* of their syndrome.

A fourth category groups children who have problems in specific components of three dimensions: language knowledge, language performance, and cognition. The characteristic difference between the fourth category and the first three is that in the fourth category the problems are selective rather than generalized, and they may occur in single components of a language dimension (e.g., syntax production) or in several dimensions. The result is a discrepancy among components within and between language dimensions. Where there is known injury to the language centers of the brain, these problems are called aphasic; where there is no demonstrable central nervous system involvement, they are labeled developmental or clinical language disorders. *Developmental or clinical language disorders* do not describe a single syndrome; there are different patterns of problems within and across various dimensions that are classified under this category.

Terminology confusion arises because some professionals do not distinguish among any of the above groups, simply considering members of all the groups language disordered, whereas other professionals use the term *language disorder* to refer to the fourth group only. Still other professionals classify in separate groups the *severely* retarded, hearing impaired, and emotionally disturbed but lump together moderate to mild problems in these areas under the category of language disorders.

For the purposes of this text, mild to moderate disorders associated with the categories of hearing loss, retardation, and emotional disturbance are grouped under those categories. Children whose language is quantitatively different from normal (mean or average) but whose differences or delays fall within the range of deviation considered normal, or those whose differences are in accord with delay in other developmental tasks, are not considered to be language disordered at all. In this text, the broad, unspecific term *language disorders* refers to any of the four categories described above; the term *clinical language disorder* is used to refer to the fourth category.

Group classification should not serve to categorize children nor label them, but to guide the study of language behaviors in all dimensions and of factors that often occur together. In this way, a better grasp of the behavioral dynamics of each child is obtained, and more effective management solutions are achieved. This is especially true in dealing with mild to moderate problems related to hearing loss, intellectual slowness, or emotional disturbance. The tendency might be to group them all under a loosely defined category of language-disordered children. Doing this would cloud the nature of the extensiveness of the problem and of the expectancies of success, and therefore make intervention less effective.

The Perspective of Significance

Because of the variability among children in the development of language, it is important to discuss the topic of significance as it pertains to delay or difference in language. Certainly, not all differences or delays are disorders of language, particularly since language development is judged in terms of stages through which all children pass—albeit at different ages. Differences in oral language performance need to be viewed in terms of the significance of the difference from what is expected behavior *for a particular child.* Some criteria upon which diagnoses of language disorder should be based are (1) the degree of difference; (2) the number of dimensions impaired; (3) the rate of change; and (4) intellectual and environmental expectancies. None of these criteria can be used independently from the others. They all play a role in diagnosis.

Degree of Difference

The issue of degree of difference is a critical one in the diagnosis of language disorders. It is not sufficient to determine that a child's speech is quantitatively different from what is expected. Some attempt at judging the extent of the difference should be made.

Although age reference is not as widely valued in the linguistic field as stage reference, the level of significance is ultimately determined by comparing performance among children in specific age groups. This can be done by judging from oral language performance data obtained either by naturalistic means or by testing language. The problem with the naturalistic data is that there have not been sufficient numbers of children whose language performance measures have been obtained. Therefore, the judgment of degree of difference seems to be made with greater validity by testing (Bloom & Lahey, 1978).

There is a problem, however, in using age scores instead of standard scores and percentiles. An age score can be misleading in terms of the child's level of language. A 4-year-old who is 2 years behind in language is functioning at 50 percent of what is expected for his age, whereas a 12-year-old who is 2 years behind functions at 82 percent of what is expected for his age. Although both are 2 years behind, the 4-year-old has a more severe problem. Standard and percentile scores, since they provide the relative position of the child on a scale that distributes the performance of other children on a specific language trait, are better means of describing the level of performance than age scores. The particular cut-off point for determining the point of significance cannot be given by the test. That point is determined locally, taking into account local levels of grammatic usage and standards. (The factor of environmental expectancies as they influence significance is described later.)

Number of Dimensions Impaired

In some instances, the number of dimensions impaired may lead to a diagnosis of "language disordered" even though none of the dimensions are significantly different from normal. If a child has a mild problem in hearing acuity, mild difficulty in auditory perception, some difficulty with vocabulary, a minimal number of semantic confusions, minor problems in comprehending under given circumstances, and a minimal number of misarticulations, the child would be considered language disordered, particularly if the intellectual ability of the child were normal or above. If the child has a minimal delay in semantic behavior only, his problem would not be classified as a disorder, but would be considered to be within the normal range of behavior. However, if one aspect of the language behavior differs

AN INTEGRATIVE APPROACH TO LANGUAGE DISORDERS

qualitatively from the expected—is truly deviant or discrepant—then only one dimension or one aspect of a dimension may be sufficient to consider the child language disordered, particularly if this difference interferes with life or learning.

Rate of Change

One very important aspect of a child's difference that helps in determining whether a child's problem is significant is the rate of his change in language behavior. Since the emphasis in language is upon stages, each child is expected to pass through the stages in a fairly consistent manner, although not necessarily at a particular age. It is important to measure the rate of change from stage A to stage B; i.e., does a child proceed through the stages in approximately the same time it takes a typical child? If a child is not talking at 3 years, it is more important to determine what he accomplishes in language between 3 years and 3 years, 6 months than to determine how different he is from other children. If his rate is slow, the gap between his performance and that of his peers will increase, and the chances of his needing assistance will also increase. If, however, his rate of improvement is substantial, the chances are that he will reach the level of performance of his peers, but at a slightly later age.

Environmental and Intellectual Expectancies

The final decision in the diagnosis of language disorders must be based on the expected language of a child within a specified environment at a specified level of intelligence. In other words, there is not an absolute cut-off level for determining disorders. If there were a single, absolute percentile rank or standard score for discriminating those who have from those who do not have disorders, some populations would have large numbers of children incorrectly classified. Populations having high linguistic performance criteria might have no child classified as language disordered, yet in fact, compared to the norms of that population, a number of children would be disordered. Conversely, populations having linguistic performance levels that consider numerous linguistic forms—ordinarily viewed as errors in other localities—as normal would have included among the disordered many children who are normal for that linguistic environment. It is important, therefore, that the level of significance for judging disordered language be determined locally.

The last factor to consider in determining significance is the intellectual ability of the child in whom the determination is to be made. If the child's language age is 2 years below his chronological age but within expected limits for his mental age, does he have a language disorder? If judged from the degree of difference of the linguistic output from what is expected for his mental age, he does not have such a disorder; if judged from the number of language dimensions probably involved, he does. It is not, however, a clinical language disorder as defined here; it is a language disorder associated with slow intellectual abilities, and intervention decisions based on expectations of change must take this into consideration. This is not to say that there is a perfect correlation between language and intelligence, nor that children with intellectual slowness should not receive language training. It does mean, however, that the language specialist should be ready to adjust her expectancies for change if such a child has difficulty in learning specific skills.

Therefore, the answers to the questions regarding the identification of language-disordered children (or the definition of language disorders) are based on judgments involving (1) the knowledge and understanding of external factors (social, ethnic) as well as internal ones (intelligence) that are related to language and how these factors operate in each individual child who has a disorder; and (2) data regarding the level of difference that is significant in all dimensions of language for each age and stage of development. Although the methods used to obtain these data on each child are in embryonic form, each language specialist must attempt to obtain information that will allow her to make decisions that are as accurate as possible given the existing state-of-the-art of assessment.

The definition of language disorder is a relative one. Language behaviors exist along a continuum from high to low performance. The responsibility of the language specialist is to decide, for each child, the point on the continuum to use for the determination of the child's problem. In order to do this with validity, analyses and descriptions should be made of the environmental, cognitive, and performance systems, as well as the linguistic one.

DIMENSIONAL INTERRELATIONS IN THE INTEGRATIVE MODEL

The four-dimensional description of language disorders presented in this section of the chapter is theoretical. Although extensive clinical experience supports the four dimensions and their components, scholarly research must provide validation. However, unless an attempt is made to confront this complex issue, *language disorder* will continue to be defined as "a disorder of language," a definition that serves neither the professional nor the child.

The description is not intended to be a basis for differential diagnosis, but simply a way of ordering the data so that a common ground may be established. Obviously, too, it may be difficult in specific instances to determine which of the components and categories may be impaired in an individual child. However, if there is a theoretical construct to which data can be added or deleted or changed, the knowledge of language disorders may be increased and the problems of the language-disordered child may be lessened.

Because the concern of this section is on the interrelationships of the dimensions, the developmental and performance sequences are important aspects of the description. For this reason, the order of presentation will follow, to some extent, the order in which these dimensions develop in the child; that is, (1) the cognitive; (2) the linguistic knowledge; and (3) the language performance dimensions. Since communication is both the beginning and the purpose of language, the communication environment could be presented at either end of the discussion; it is the final dimension discussed in this section.

Disorders of the Cognitive Dimension of Language

Disorders of Perception and Memory

Perception and memory play important roles in the development of concepts and in the relations between concepts and the linguistic code. During the developmental stages of language, perceptual disorders may limit the amount and accuracy of the visual or auditory input signals, and thereby interfere with the formation of concepts or with the linguistic signals that are stored in conjunction with the concepts. If the child's perception of the qualitative or functional characteristics of objects is inaccurate, if symbol and concept are therefore improperly matched, the semantic rules of language are affected. This, in turn, affects the accuracy of language comprehension and performance. Problems with specific kinds of perception (such as perception of space or perception of time) may be reflected in specific lexical items being affected (such as *near/far* or *up/down*, and *over/under* or *before/after*). The language of children with such a problem appears deviant because of the discrepancy between the level of the forms they use correctly and those they do not.

A problem in memory may limit the amount of information that can be processed by a child at a given time. The language input to the child is internally limited, which causes a delay in learning the code. If information is stored incorrectly—confused sequences of sounds or words, or inaccurate associations between words and their meaning—all aspects of language knowledge and performance reflect those inaccuracies. A child with this problem needs more experiences with language than a child with no memory constraint. Poor memory may cause a language delay.

Conceptual Disorders

Conceptual disorders have a significant effect on the development of all of the language dimensions. Concepts are the meanings of language, the ideas, thoughts, and relationships that are expressed by using the linguistic code. If a child is deficient in concepts, he is unable to provide adequate meaning to match the structure of language. Without meaning, words are not remembered, and, if they are, they are semantically empty. All aspects of the code reflect this problem—e.g., the substantive words, the morphemes, and word order. The code is simplified in the manner of a child younger than the one with a conceptual problem—in other words, the language appears delayed. Deficiencies in concepts are evident in the comprehension and production of spoken and written language. The problem of poor conceptualization is evident whether the input is of a visual or auditory nature or whether it is verbal or nonverbal.

The adults dealing with a child with a conceptual problem modify the type and amount of language input to the level of performance of the child (see Chapters 5 and 6). Consequently, the communication environment dimension of the child is different from that of the child without such a problem. Chapter 16 describes the child with a conceptual problem.

Disorders of Representation and Symbolization

As described in Chapter 3, before a child can learn to use language symbolically, he must be able to represent reality in some manner: through imitation, by pretending, or by some type of visual imagery. This representation forms the basis of symbolization in general and of the specific symbolization of the linguistic code.

A child who has difficulty in representation and symbolization may use words as signs, to indicate or point to an object or event, but will have difficulty in using words to represent meaning. Such a child learns to associate specific content with specific vocabulary but these associations are more likely concrete than abstract; there is a greater interest in things than ideas. The child has a generalized difficulty in generating novel utterances.

The concept development of children with symbolization problems appears better for nonverbal performance than for verbal functions. Other symbol systems, such as those of gesture, are correspondingly affected. Although the conceptual system is not directly impaired, the ability to develop concepts is affected, since words and symbols assist in the development of abstract and complex concepts. Deficiencies are observed in symbolic play and in the representations and imitations used to learn the pragmatic aspects of language.

Disorders in the Dimension of Language Knowledge

Disorders of the dimensions of language knowledge involve deficiencies in the knowledge of the *rules* of the linguistic code. They may be characterized by problems with the rules of grammar, semantics, or pragmatics. Disorders in language knowledge are always reflected in language performance but not all performance problems are the result of rule-based disorders.

Disorders of Grammar

A disorder of grammatic knowledge is one in which knowledge of the appropriate use of grammatic structures is impaired. Disorders of structures may take many forms, including omission of verb inflections, misplacement of negatives, unconventional word order, and incorrect use of morphemes. Some disorders of the knowledge of structure may be semantic problems—ones in which there is a mismatch between meaning and the manner in which the meaning is encoded in the grammatic structure of the language—but other disorders are due to the lack of knowledge of the rules of syntax.

A disorder of grammatic knowledge can be understood with greater clarity from the position of a second language learner; an individual who learns German as a second language must acquire the lexicon, the modulators, and the order in which these are used for expressing specific ideas. In the initial stages of second language learning, there are many words, prefixes, suffixes, and allomorphs the learner does not know; neither can he place the endings of words in correct positions because he does not know the rules for such placement. Consequently, the order of the words he uses will probably be quite different from that of the native speaker of German. In other words, he does not know the grammar.

A child who is learning language resembles the second language learner in some ways. There is one critical difference, however. The second language learner knows another grammar and its corresponding meanings or content. Consequently, when words and endings are omitted or word order is confused, the problem is clearly one involving the grammatic structures of the new language. The child acquiring language is learning the entire language system, and thus an analysis of the area of difficulty is more complicated.

There are some signals that may indicate that a child has a problem of grammatic knowledge, e.g., faulty recognition of his own errors when produced by someone else—the child cannot tell the correct grammar form from the incorrect one. If he does not know the rules of word order, he cannot recognize an un-grammatic sentence. If he can write, the same errors appear in writing as in speaking, and these errors are consistent. He demonstrates the same problems in the comprehension of the forms—in listening and reading—as in their expression. In other words, errors related to lack of knowledge of the rule system are more likely to be systematic than errors related to the performance system. There may be a discrepancy between levels of the child's concepts and his ability to code them. The child will use many lexical items to express an idea that could be expressed by grammatic means more effectively and efficiently.

The effects of problems of grammatic knowledge on oral language production is apparent—what is not known cannot be applied. The manner in which problems in grammatic knowledge influence comprehension is not so apparent. A listener uses his knowledge of syntax to structure the incoming message and to provide information that is missing. If the knowledge is not adequate, the decoding of the message will also be inadequate, and comprehension will be impaired.

Disorders of Semantics

The term semantics implies an association between words and grammatic structures and their meanings. When the semantics of an individual's language match the semantics of the individual's society and culture, the individual knows the semantics of the language.

The method by which the child learns the association between the form and the meaning of language is usually through the auditory system. The child hears the input, matches it to a situational context, and from there generalizes the rules of the linguistic input as well as those of the context; he thereby internalizes the language system for his own use. If, as the child hears running speech he has difficulty in segmentation—in isolating words and phonemes to match to content—he may develop a semantic problem.

The characteristics of a semantic problem help to differentiate it from other problems. A semantic disorder is not a conceptual problem; that is, the individual with a semantic disorder develops adequate concepts. The problem is one of inadequate rules of correspondence between the grammar and the meaning; the

A 5-year-old girl's responses to interrogative forms illustrates a poor match between forms and their meaning.

Q What do you eat for breakfast?
R Eggs and some toast.
Q When do you eat breakfast?
R Some eggs and toast.

Q When do you go to sleep?
R In my bed with a pillow.
Q With whom do you eat?
R With the hand.

wrong words or the wrong grammatic forms may be associated with specific meanings. Words may be overextended to take in incorrect referents, or the meanings of words may be incomplete in terms of the specific features associated with them. The problem is not one of using the wrong forms but one of not knowing the association of the forms with all the corresponding features of meaning.

A semantic problem is not a problem of comprehension—although it is reflected in comprehension. A semantic problem is more basic than the correct evocation of meaning from a stimulus. It is also not a problem of grammatic knowledge. The child with a semantic problem may know the grammar and use it in a grammatically correct form—he may not, however, use it appropriately for the meaning desired. Often, however, semantic problems are the cause of inaccurate grammatic forms. For example, a child who has not mapped the correct meanings for *in* and *on* will use them inappropriately in surface structure.

Examples of semantic problems are the misuse of words by overgeneralizing or substituting for words that have similar meanings; the use of *chair* for *stool* or the use of *delicious* for *delightful*. In the area of grammar, the individual with a semantic problem might, for example, confuse *she* and *he*. The concepts of masculinity and femininity may not be confused, but simply the ways of expressing them. A more complex grammatic confusion would be the use of *whether* for *if*. There may be a lack of association between the concept of plurality and the means for expressing it (not related to cultural or dialectal factors). The child may not know the relation between the plural morphemes and plurality; he may not comprehend the /s/ morpheme although he may use it automatically either in speaking or in writing—he may express the concept of plurality in other ways. Grammatic forms that use conjoining and embedding for expressing concepts are so complex that some children do not learn the associations of these forms with their meanings. If they wish to express a complex idea, they do so by using the simple forms that they know; the effect is that they seem to be "beating around the bush."

In the early stages of development of children with severe semantic problems, the content-form association has scarcely developed, and the children appear either retarded or autistic. When they hear language, they appear not to comprehend, but simply echo it—usually with correct articulation, inflection, and syntax—since for them the input is not associated with meaning. As the child begins to develop meaningful expression, he often passes through the stages of misarticulation and grammatic errors observed in the child with normal language development. In the later stages of development of expression, the child with a severe semantic problem may produce words and syntax cor-

An anecdote about Eric demonstrates a semantic problem. Eric was brought to the clinic when he was 4 years old because he had not started talking. At that time, he associated few words with meaning and was severely limited in comprehension. His speech was almost completely echolalic. After much hard work on his part and ours, he learned the rules of language and could use them, although not without subtle problems. One day when Eric had just finished the second grade at a small private school, he came to visit us. On the day of this visit, he went over to the coke machine and put in his money. He took hold of the handle and seemed uncertain as to the direction to move it. I said, "Down, Eric." He looked at me with a puzzled and pained expression. I said again, "Down, Eric, push down." He continued to look at me with uncertainty. Finally I demonstrated by moving my hand in a downward fashion. He imitated it and got his coke. This was only one residual among many, I'm sure, of his difficulty in matching words to meaning.

—*Elizabeth Carrow-Woolfolk*

rectly, but in inappropriate situations, as if the child has memorized the words but does not know exactly when to use them. A child might say, "Don't be silly," in response to a question he does not understand. These types of disorders are often referred to as receptive language disorders or receptive aphasia.

The language of children with mild to moderate semantic disorders may resemble the language of children with mild to moderate conceptual problems on the surface, particularly if the language alone is evaluated. The results of the evaluation would yield, among other things, low vocabulary scores, difficulty in expressing ideas, use of inappropriate and inaccurate words in speaking, confused word order, and incorrect comprehension of words and syntax. Important indicators of the child with a semantic problem are that (1) his conceptual development appears normal; (2) his errors are consistent; (3) he does not recognize the error in his own production of an utterance or if his utterance is imitated by others; and (4) the problem occurs in speech and comprehension *and* in reading and writing (Fig. 10-1).

Disorders of Pragmatics

For the purpose of describing the problems of children with language disorders, it is helpful to divide the topics that are grouped under the heading of pragmatics into two parts. One is discussed here and the other is discussed in the communication environment dimension section. Since this section of the chapter is concerned with language as object—the rules that govern the form, function, and use of language—the pragmatic topics that are reviewed here are those that pertain to the rules of language *use,* including *what to say, to whom, when,* and *where.* The rules that govern these situations are learned as are the other rules of language. They are abstracted from observation of the behaviors of others in the various situations where specific rules are required, or the rules are taught to the child by parents or teachers.

One important factor that influences the development of the rules is the frequency and extent of the situational opportunities for observation. If a child does not observe the use of appropriate language in appropriate situations, he will have nothing to abstract from. A second factor, related to the first, has to do with a child's perception. Unless a child observes and remembers the occurrences of language use, he will not have the elements from which to abstract the rules.

A third factor, one that seems to be particularly evident in clinical language disorders, is that of poor abstract ability. If a child does not observe and select the invariables and commonalities in situations, those aspects that make some situations alike and others different will not be abstracted, and the appropriate rules and consequent behaviors will not be adequate. In the case of poor abstraction, the resulting problems will be evident not only in the knowledge of pragmatic rules but in the knowledge of grammatic and semantic rules.

Frequently, the child with a pragmatic problem not only has difficulty knowing the rules of appropriate language use, but also has difficulty knowing the behaviors corresponding to this language; e.g., shaking hands when being introduced to someone or maintaining eye contact when speaking. Pragmatic disor-

Figure 10-1
Dimensional model illustrating the effects of a semantic problem on other language components. (Asterisks indicate components affected.)

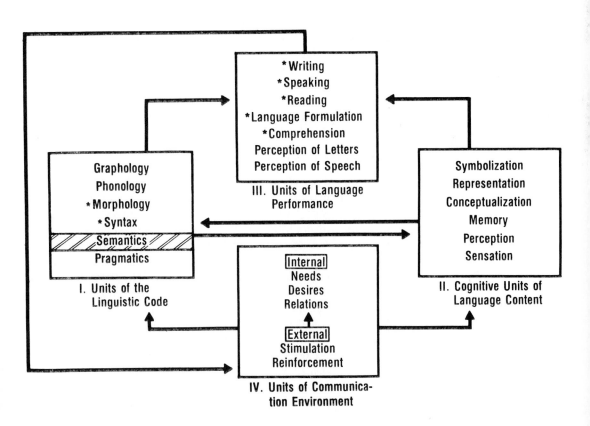

I. Units of the Linguistic Code

- Graphology
- Phonology
- *Morphology
- *Syntax
- Semantics
- Pragmatics

III. Units of Language Performance

- *Writing
- *Speaking
- *Reading
- *Language Formulation
- *Comprehension
- Perception of Letters
- Perception of Speech

II. Cognitive Units of Language Content

- Symbolization
- Representation
- Conceptualization
- Memory
- Perception
- Sensation

IV. Units of Communication Environment

Internal
- Needs
- Desires
- Relations

External
- Stimulation
- Reinforcement

ders often accompany other disorders in language, particularly disorders of semantics.

Disorders of the Dimension of Language Performance

Problems in language may involve disorders in the reception or expression of the language structure itself, even in the presence of adequate grammatic and semantic knowledge and conceptual development. Children who have linguistic performance problems may have developed adequate concepts and may have mapped these concepts to linguistic structure. They may, however, misunderstand the input and become confused as to its meaning in particular situations; i.e., the input fails to evoke the correct meaning. In the productive aspect of language, the child may not be able to match his output to what he wants to say. (In a way, it is like trying to hum a classical tune that can be heard in the "mind"—but what comes out does not match the auditory sound patterns that are rehearsed internally.) The result may be sentences with words out of sequence, with omissions of entire words or of morphological endings, or with words having syllables that are not in serial order.

The problems of performance present greater inconsistencies than those of knowledge of the rules of the code. Disorders of language formulation and execution may vary with the length of the utterance, with the particular productive mode (written or speech) being used for expression, and with the situation. Usually, the child recognizes the problem or errors, but has difficulty in correcting performance. These problems are disorders of the dimension of language performance.

Disorders of Comprehension

The process of comprehension, described in Chapter 4, includes speech perception and memory as stages through which the input passes on the way to being understood. Speech perception, with its integral short-term memory, relates directly to the performance aspects of language. It is therefore being considered in the present section as well as in the one on the cognitive dimension. The term *comprehension*, used in this context, does not refer to the *associations* between the auditory stimulus and meaning made in the early stages of language development. It refers instead to the process of decoding the incoming message by a native speaker of the language.

Just as learning language is more than acquiring linguistic structure, disordered language is more than a problem of the knowledge of the code. Language involves the ability to perceive and comprehend the ongoing stream of language that surrounds the child—the language of his teacher in the classroom and of his peers in the cafeteria and on the playground. Mishearing and misperceiving are also disorders of language, and a processing system that distorts the quality of perception of the linguistic input is part of the disorder.

Auditory perception is involved when the system does not perceive accurately under conditions of noise, or when the system cannot provide closure to auditory information that is distorted in any fashion, that is, when the listening conditions are not optimum or when the amount of information chunked into the input places a strain on the system. The individual with such a problem may ask for input to be repeated, may respond incorrectly, or may change the topic. At times, his responses will resemble those of a person with hearing loss. This type of problem will not ordinarily be reflected in oral language production, since under optimal conditions, the child can process language sufficiently well to learn the finite structures of grammar. In some instances, however, misperceived words will be stored incorrectly and therefore be expressed incorrectly.

Clinical experience has demonstrated that problems in memory, particularly memory of linguistic data, and language disorders do co-occur (see Chapters 3 and 4). The memory task has not been broken down with sufficient refinement, however, to describe the degree and type of relationship that may exist between memory and language. One type of memory problem may interfere with comprehension, particularly comprehension of complex, embedded sentences. The logical process of discovering the meanings in each part of a complex input requires that some parts be held in memory while others are being decoded. A child with auditory memory difficulty would have problems holding all the necessary elements for interpretation of a segment, and therefore have difficulty in extracting the meaning from the utterance. Such a problem may not directly affect the production of linguistic structures or semantics once these have been learned, although it may delay their development, and it most probably will affect the general communication function of the child. The solution, however, is not to attempt to improve the memory. This usually has no real effect on language functioning. The approach, instead, should be to teach compensatory behaviors to the child; i.e., to teach him ways to remember the types of information he needs to remember in life situations, ways that do not depend exclusively on the auditory system.

The clinical management of this type of disorder is not directed toward linguistic intervention techniques for improving auditory perception. The focus of the attention is not centered on the language as much as it is on the child and his environment. Helping the child to function in learning environments with an auditory system that makes communication difficult, and teach-

The case of Johnny illustrates a language disorder in which knowledge of the rules of language structure and their reflection in oral language is not only adequate but superior. When Johnny was 12 years old, his teachers wanted to place him in an accelerated English class because of his excellent grades and high performance in grammar and literature. Because Johnny had a history of problems in comprehending and using language, his mother sought the advice of a language specialist in the placement decision. Johnny had been slow in talking and had difficulty in learning to read. According to his mother, during development and up to the time of the evaluation, Johnny could not understand messages over the telephone; did not "pick up" the thread of conversations; totally confused names of people and places; did not complete thoughts in sentences; had difficulty in "word finding" and therefore in expressing ideas—both in speaking and in writing; and "scrambled" words. A language analysis indicated excellent knowledge of grammatic rules and superior semantic knowledge of words. However, auditory memory for unrelated words was significantly below his expected level. He had difficulty in repeating three- and four-syllable words. His problem was a problem of the performance of language in specific situations and with specific language tasks. Johnny's disorders were interfering with his communication.

Johnny was provided with specific suggestions for compensating for his problems in retaining non-meaningful auditory information and in retrieving stored information for production. With an increased understanding of the nature of his problem and of his learning strengths, he entered the accelerated class and succeeded.

ing people in his environment to understand the child's problem, are more important than teaching the child to discriminate phonemes. It is for this reason that a clinical approach to disordered language must include concern for the speech perceptual system.

Disorders of Language Production

Disorders of Formulation.   In language formulation problems, a child cannot match his output to what he wants to say, resulting in problems of word finding, omission of forms, changes in tense, and poor sequencing of syllables and words. The productive aspects of the language will reflect either auditory verbal imagery that is faulty, poor access to the mental lexicon, or the faulty transmissions of these images to output. A child with such a problem has difficulty evoking words from the auditory storage system to encode the meaning he wishes to express. He knows the words but they are not easily available to him to generate language with fluency and in sequence. Sentences are produced with words out of order; ("The witch saw outside a blackbird") and unfamiliar words are pronounced incorrectly (*jippy/jiffy, melonade/lemonade*). It is difficult for a child with this problem to generate complex linguistic structure for expressing an abstract idea or series of events such as conditionality or logical reasoning (even though the child's IQ and linguistic knowledge may be adequate for this purpose). The early stages of learning to read and spell, because of the role of the storage system in these activities, may also be involved; however, since reading and writing do not place the same kinds of fluency demands on formulation, the problems may not be readily apparent.

Auditory memory problems may be related to language formulation by causing difficulties in retaining and/or retrieving new and nonmeaningful information. A child hears new names in history class or new vocabulary words in English; for some children, the retention of this type of information is very difficult. They may recognize the words or sounds if uttered by someone else, but cannot retrieve the verbal material for accurate production. The search in the mental lexicon for appropriate words may result in selecting words with meanings or sounds similar to the desired word. A language problem of this type, if found in a person with brain injury, is termed aphasia. It is also found in children who have no history of injury to the brain. The source of the problem may be in the language processing system—if the system prevents the accurate reception, storage, and retrieval of auditory information. In the educational and social worlds of the child, the child may appear to be "spacey" because he does not pick up incidental information and is not tuned in to what is happening around him.

Disorders of Execution. Chapter 4 described the automatic aspects of speech production. In some children, the automatic productive system does not function adequately for error-free speech. The child knows what he wants to say—that is, his mapping of concepts to structure is adequate, as is his word recall and formulation—but in the act of producing the utterances, the integration between his formulative and automatic system breaks down. The result is inaccurate articulation and morphological use. Perhaps the complexity of chunking information by grammatic coding devices expressed in phonological terms causes the child to concentrate his efforts on the information-carrying aspects of the utterances—to the neglect of the inflectional, morphological, and phonological aspects. In other words, since the child's production span is limited, it can only handle a specific number of chunks of information, and those chunks carrying the least information are either omitted or distorted in some fashion. The child's automatic system does not function with sufficient fluidity to track the morphophonemic aspects of words as they are generated for utterance.

The disordered system functions this way in a somewhat consistent manner during the language-acquisition period, and thus specific omissions, substitutions, and distortions—those that are the most difficult to encode automatically—become a part of the child's linguistic utterance format. The grammatic errors in the output may take the form of "There is rabbit" or "Somebody pull his hair this morning." The phonological errors usually take the form of approximation of the desired production, or omissions. The omissions and distortions continue past the chronological age and MLU stage when they are acceptable. When the problem is in this aspect of the productive system, the child usually can recognize the errors if produced by someone else and may even recognize his own errors. It remains difficult for him to encode the utterance grammatically and phonologically in its accurate and complete form, particularly if it is long and grammatically complex.

As with the previous disorders, this type of problem may be present in aphasia. Some aspects of it are referred to as apraxia. It is not a muscular problem as one would find in cerebral palsy; it is a linguistic disorder. Children with motor dysfunction of the type produced by cerebral palsy may exhibit some symptoms of the type described above. There is a difference, however. The child with a motor problem will have consistent difficulty producing the sounds, whether the sounds are in long utterances or short ones and whether they are related to grammatic forms or not. Difficulty in cerebral palsy will also be evident in nonlinguistic, nonvolitional activities, such as in eating, involving the structures used in articulation.

As indicated in the previous sections, the severe aspects of apraxia are more easily differentiated than the mild to moderate problems. Because the morphology, as well as the phonology, is involved in apraxia, children with moderate forms of these problems are classified under the heading of language disordered.

Disorders of the Communication Environment Dimension

There are two aspects of problems related to the internal and external communication environments in which language is learned and used; the needs and motivations of the speaker to communicate and the environment (people and situations) that encourages and supports the communication. These two aspects are mutually dependent.

A child who has no need or desire to communicate may not begin to talk at the age when other children begin. His language is said to be delayed with respect to that of other children. In some instances, the child's needs are met by those in his environment, without them expecting or requiring an effort to communicate verbally on the part of the child. When the individuals in a child's environment change their expectancies, the child, in many cases, will begin to talk. It is important in such cases to identify the source of the problem and to distinguish it from problems associated with other factors. If a child begins language at an age later than other children, he may remain somewhat behind throughout most of the language-learning period. However, if his problem is due to lack of environmental stimulation, the amount of progress made within a span of time should be that which other normal children make within the same time period. The important issue, then, with children who are delayed because of environmental factors alone, is the adequacy of the rate of change and not the level of performance.

Other environmental factors that may delay language onset include inadequate language models in the home and insufficient language stimulation due to long absences of the caretaker during the critical ages for learning language. These environmental factors will not only delay the onset of language, they may also have a deleterious effect on the open systems of language, particularly vocabulary. It is the external environment that determines the language performance that is acceptable for each individual, as well as the range of variability within which "normal" lies within a specified population. The dialectal standards in Black English, and in various bilingual populations, determine the reference for disordered language within these subcultures.

When the relationship between the child and his environment is seriously disordered, as in childhood psychoses, the language behavior of the child will reflect the disorder. Language can be supported only if the child identifies with his world and wishes to communicate with it. (The types of language problems related to autism will be discussed in Chapter 18.)

outline

assessment of language and language disorders

11

THIS CHAPTER IS concerned with the assessment of children with suspected language disorders, especially as that assessment relates to the integrative approach to language. Previous chapters have indicated the complex interaction between the cognitive endowment of the child, his communicative environment, and his own unique style of acquiring the knowledge and use of the linguistic code. In this chapter, the evaluation of the various dimensions of language, including the use of differential assessment, naturalistic observation, and history-taking, will be discussed. Although students and pressured examiners always hope to find a brief, yet objective, evaluation protocol capable of providing a basis for assigning children to specific categories, this chapter demonstrates that complex, multidimensional behavior like language cannot be adequately evaluated with a unidimensional procedure.

Assessment is traditionally involved with several concerns. The first concern is the identification of a problem; the second is the determination of the significance or severity of the problem; the third is the description of the nature of the problem; and the fourth is the description of the person who has the problem. Determination of the existence of a problem and its severity requires comparison to normative data. Description of the nature of the problem and the child with the problem requires naturalistic observation of the child, interviews with parents or teachers, and probably the confirmation of observations

---

through the use of individually selected tests or checklists. Once a problem is identified, the focus should change from an emphasis on the problem to an emphasis on the child. It is the child who has the disorder—not the language.

This chapter begins with a discussion of the purposes of assessment. Next the various approaches to assessment as they have evolved through the years are reviewed; this review provides a basis for looking at some issues in assessment. Finally, the integrative approach to assessment is presented.

PURPOSES OF ASSESSMENT

The answers to several preliminary questions determine the type of assessment needed. These questions (Carrow, 1972b) include (1) Who requested the information? (2) What information is needed? and (3) How will the test results be used?

The source of referral helps to determine both the type of assessment needed and the type of report required. A child referred to determine the adequacy of his class placement prior to a formal hearing appealing his assignment has different assessment needs than the child referred by his classroom teacher because of inadequate communication skills. Not only would the assessment procedures differ but the discussion of results would differ. If the information is requested to plan intervention rather than for the purpose of defining or describing the child's problem, still other assessment procedures might be required. The classic example of the mismatch of factors is the complaint of the classroom teacher who told of referring a child for testing because he was not reading at grade level; after extensive testing she received a report saying that the child was reading two semesters below grade level. This assessment could have been made meaningful if the classroom teacher had clearly stated what she needed to know, and if the examiner had interpreted the evaluation results in response to the questions raised about the child.

Assessment protocols should not be determined solely on the basis of available and familiar tests but on the need for specific information to be used for a definite purpose. Sometimes the referring source may fail to provide this information. The first step in assessment therefore is to assist the individual making the referral to clearly state her concern. It is impossible to provide a clear, well reasoned answer to a vague question.

The type of information needed for the assessment is determined not only by the referral source but also by the philosophical approach of the examiner. An examiner who views language disorders primarily in terms of deviations from normal language structure, based on verbal output, will assess a disorder according to the quality and quantity of difference from normal. A language specialist who believes that language disorders are caused by identifiable medical, psychological, or social deficits will focus on the identification of these deficits during assessment. A language specialist who functions within an integrative framework defines the nature of a language disorder more broadly than this. In addition to describing the child's language, such a specialist seeks to describe the child who has the language disorder. One aspect of the description of the child is the identification of the "clinical classification" of the child. The reason for this is *not* to specify a cause for the language disorder; this classification influences the clinical management of the child's problem. Factors that are affected by clinical classification include decisions regarding the type of intervention, prognosis for eventual improvement, classroom placement, home management, and the need for further referrals and consultation. Besides describing the child's language and identifying his clinical classification, if any, the language specialist who works within an integrative framework will also explore the cognitive dimensions of language and the child's communicative environment. In the integrative approach, all of these are considered to be related, and consequently a disorder of any one may co-occur with a disorder in another, or one disorder may actually be present because another fundamental ability is defective.

The use that will be made of the assessment results is important in organizing the report. Some information may be gathered during the assessment that may not be relevant to the primary question asked of the examiner. The length, style, and specificity of the report should be structured in such a manner that communication is established between the examiner and the referring source.

If the referring source only wishes to identify the presence or absence of a language problem, then screening would be all that is required. If information is needed about the nature of a language problem, then differential assessment would be required.

Screening

An essential factor in any screening process is that the screening instrument have the capacity to differentiate, in the briefest possible time, normal individuals from those with suspected problems. In addition, it is important that the fewest possible normal individuals be referred for in-depth testing and the fewest abnormal individuals pass the screening. The concept of screening arose from the medical model where brief procedures, requiring only a minute or two of a paraprofessional's time, could correctly identify such problems as sickle cell anemia and diabetes. The identification of suspected language disorders is more complicated than this type of medical screening because language is a complex behavior that is dependent on context. The artificiality, formality, and stress inherent in most screening situations inhibits rather than facilitates language. In such a situation, a child might be silent for any number of reasons.

Despite these problems, there are a number of useful screening tests commercially available. Some of these tests, like the Birth to Three Developmental Scale (T. E. Bangs, 1979), were designed so that they could be administered by professionals other than speech and language pathologists. Some of the tests require less than 30 minutes to administer, such as the Bankson Language Screening Test (Bankson, 1977), and a few screening tests of articulation or syntax require only 2 to 3 minutes to administer. Except for tests like the *Denver Developmental Screening Test* (Frankenburg et al., 1967), which was standardized on over 2000 children, many of the instruments use relatively small norming populations, which is a cause for some concern.

Because of the complex nature of language, all language screening could benefit from the use of indirect evidence about the child. For children referred by schools, this information is available from teachers. Suggestions for an organized method of obtaining this information on a prescreening checklist have been presented by Lynch (1979). Other indirect evidence is also available from parents through the use of behavior checklists.

Differential Assessment

In the integrative approach, the term *differential assessment* is not used to refer to any specific test protocol. Instead, it means the testing and observation undertaken to describe the child suspected of having a language disorder and the nature of his disorder. This involves the exploration of the learning strengths and weaknesses of the child, the environmental factors that may affect language performance, and the use the child makes of language. In many cases, not all of this information will be provided by the same examiner, but it is the responsibility of the language specialist to interpret how the child's already diagnosed sensory capacities, intellectual abilities, and family situation, for example, may have contributed to his language problem and how they may affect his prognosis for improvement with intervention.

Differential assessment that emphasizes the child being tested rather than the child's ability under testing has the potential of revealing something about the child's style of learning. For example, evaluation of memory may indicate that the child can utilize visual imagery to improve his performance in auditory memory. Observation of the child in a natural situation may re-

ASSESSMENT OF LANGUAGE AND LANGUAGE DISORDERS

veal that the child is not spontaneously using this visual imagery in a functional way. This suggests that one goal in intervention might be to help the child to compensate for one weakness by utilizing an observed learning strength.

Following a period during which terms such as *objective, standardized,* and *accountable* were considered fundamental to assessment, an increasing number of warnings were sounded about the inadequacies of objective testing (Muma, 1973b, 1978; Siegel, 1975; Siegel & Broen, 1976). Descriptive assessment was recommended as a remedy for some of the problems inherent in standardized testing. Strong claims are still being made on both sides, and the language specialist who functions as an examiner of language may feel overcome with these "cautions" and impatient with the apparent need to keep changing assessment procedures.

APPROACHES TO ASSESSMENT

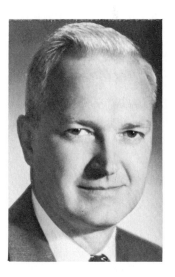

Early Descriptive Testing

In Myklebust's volume on differential diagnosis (1954), he presented protocols for taking and interpreting what he called a "differential history." The detailed case history he described explored not only the child's developmental milestones but also his verbal and nonverbal communicative behaviors as reported by his parents. After obtaining this history, the next step was the observation of the child during a period of free play. The behav-

Helmer R. Myklebust

The publication of *Auditory Disorders in Children* (1954) by Helmer R. Myklebust focused attention on "language disorder" as a symptom complex found in children with a variety of developmental problems. This book first organized and described the behavioral differences that are now so well known that it might appear that they were always recognized. This book also defined the techniques of differential diagnosis in language disorders.

Myklebust received his B.A. degree from Augustana College in 1933 and his M.A. in the education of the deaf from Gallaudet College in 1935. From 1935 until 1939 he was a teacher in the Tennessee School for the Deaf; he then became Director of Research and Child Study at the New Jersey School for the Deaf. Following this he obtained a second M.A., in psychology, from Temple University, and his Ed.D. from Rutgers University in 1945. From 1948 until 1969, Myklebust was a professor of Language Pathology and Psychology at Northwestern University. During that time he founded and was Director of the Institute for Language and Learning Disabilities at Northwestern University, where differential diagnosis and language therapy were carried out under his direction. Myklebust's professional interests and publications evolved from a focus on the deaf to a focus on auditory language disorders and finally to a focus on learning disabilities. His later publications, *Disorders of Written Language* and *Learning Disabilities* (with Doris Johnson), were followed by four volumes entitled *Progress in Learning Disabilities*. After leaving Northwestern University in 1969, he became professor of special education at Northern Illinois University, and then at the University of Illinois, Chicago Circle. In 1978 he returned to Northwestern University as a visiting scholar.

ioral characteristics of children with hearing loss, emotional disturbance, and mental retardation were compared and contrasted with the behaviors of children with clinical language disorder. Finally, certain objective tests were administered. Myklebust (1954, p. 240) considered a test a systematic procedure for comparing the behavior of people. The emphasis in Myklebust's technique of differential diagnosis was not on the administration of objective tests but on the skilled observation of behavior, both directly by the examiner and indirectly through the use of case histories.

During the period when Myklebust first described children with language disorders, McCarthy (1954) presented the definitive description of the language development of normal children. The techniques she reported had significant relationship to the assessment of the language of both normal and disordered children during the 1950s and beyond. In her analysis of children's language, McCarthy discussed total vocabulary size, parts of speech used, length of response, and sentence structures. The number of words used by children was ascertained in two ways: through the use of standardized tests and from naturalistic observation. Verbatim records were kept of the words produced by preschool children at play. Written records of these words were obtained from 30- to 45-minute periods of observation. Further analysis of the words used was carried out through use of the Type-Token Ratio (TTR). This ratio is obtained by dividing the number of *different* words used by the *total number* of words used. For many years the TTR was an important evaluation tool in the study of language. Next, the mean length of response was calculated, and the structures used in sentences were analyzed grammatically. In analyzing this data, McCarthy stressed that there were marked individual differences among normal children. She also considered the child's environment and the kinds of experiences that the child had had as significant to his language development.

Ascendancy of Standardized Tests

When accomplished by highly qualified examiners, naturalistic description, supported by several objective tests, provided sophisticated information concerning a child's language and overall development. However, not all examiners were equally qualified, and various psychological experiments were reported that demonstrated the effect of examiner bias on the results of the evaluation. The creditability of intelligence tests increased because it could be demonstrated that the standardized procedures incorporated in these tests removed much of the examiner bias. During the 1960s, the use and popularity of objective tests greatly increased.

With the increased use of tests such as the Wechsler Intelligence Scale for Children (WISC), which includes a verbal and a nonverbal scale, intratest differences within the same child could be observed. Psychologists stressed that the significance of the same IQ score differed between children if that score was generated in one child by equal verbal and nonverbal ability and in the second child by a high nonverbal score and a low verbal score. Differential profiles appeared to have the potential to describe the learning strengths and weaknesses of individual children. At this time, there was a lack of objective language tests; therefore, T. E. Bangs (1961) selected subtests from various standardized tests and arranged these subtests in clusters of behaviors in order to generate a profile of language-learning strengths and weaknesses. The scores of a child on each subtest were compared to the reported norms for that behavior. In addition, the differences between comprehension and expression of language, between visual and auditory memory, and between verbal and nonverbal skills could be compared as a basis for planning training. The child's level of functioning in each subtest was illustrated on a profile and compared to the norm for his chronological age.

A significant contribution to the objective analysis of language was the introduction of the Illinois Test of Psycholinguistic Ability (ITPA; Kirk, McCarthy, & Kirk, 1968). This test was based on Osgood's model of language (see Chapters 2 and 4), and it explored the relationship of various channels of learning. In addition to numerical scores, the ITPA also allowed the examiner to generate a profile of abilities that might have significance in planning intervention. The ITPA contained the more routine appraisal of comprehension, verbal expression, and memory, but it also contained several innovative subtests including a test of manual expression, morphological endings, and sound blending. Although the ITPA has been criticized for the bias reflected in some of the test items and in certain standardization procedures, this test was highly responsive to the expressed need of the profession at that time for an objective and standardized instrument for assessing language. Ironically, one weakness of this psycholinguistic test was its restricted approach to assessing verbal expression.

Carrow (1972b) presented a diagnostic approach to language disorders based on a taxonomy of language function. This taxonomy provided an integrated scheme for defining the basic process of language, the events that occur when any of these are disordered, and the assessment of these processes. This taxonomy identified levels of functioning. The lower levels were simpler and were learned earlier than the higher, more complex levels. In both the receptive and expressive systems, three levels of functioning were presented. This taxonomy identified these levels and the most important channels through which language and other data are received and expressed. Carrow suggested that any means, standardized or not, formal or informal, could be used to obtain information about the integrity of the language system.

The use of profiles to clarify the learning strengths and weaknesses of the language-disordered child was also discussed by Lynch (1978), who presented a series of differential assessment profiles of children with clinical language disorders and with language disorders associated with mental retardation, hearing loss, and emotional disturbance. These profiles provided a first step in identifying the nature of the language disorder, and also indicated the severity of the disorder of the individual child's performance as compared with the expected norm for that age. The profiles were generated on the basis of the administration of a series of objective tests.

As the advances in the study of normal language development were applied to language-disordered children by researchers like Menyuk and Lee, objective measures of various aspects of vocabulary and morphosyntactic development emerged. Examples of these objective measures include the Northwestern Syntax Screening Test (Lee, 1971), the Test of Auditory Comprehension of Language (Carrow, 1968, 1973a), the Carrow Elicited Language Inventory (Carrow, 1974a, 1974b), and the Assessment of Children's Language Comprehension (Foster, Giddan, & Stark, 1973). Other more general objective tests of language ability, such as the Preschool Language Scale (Zimmerman, Steiner, & Evatt, 1969) and the Utah Test of Language Development (Mecham, Jex, & Jones, 1967) also were published during the period between 1965 and 1975.

Return of Naturalistic Description

During the 1960s, Brown and his colleagues, among others, began their work on the analysis of childrens' language produced in a naturalistic setting—generally in the child's home. This and the subsequent psycholinguistic research into child language clearly illustrated the wealth of information that could be obtained from such analysis as opposed to the restricted information conveyed by a standardized test score. Language specialists involved with language disorders began to apply these techniques to their work. The Bloom and Lahey approach (1978) most clearly exemplifies a theory of assessment that focuses on linguistic description. Their assessment procedure is based primarily on the verbal output of the child, and little effort is made to evaluate behaviors other than expressive utterances. Their assessment goal is to identify the existence of differences from normal in one or more areas of language knowledge, such as semantics, syntax, or use. Bloom and Lahey viewed both the child's "specific abilities" (perceptual, conceptual, and feedback components) and his "clinical category" (hearing impairment, mental retardation, etc.) as outside of the domain that provides the framework for assessment and intervention.

A modification of this approach was applied to the assessment of language by J. Miller (1978, p. 271), who considered his approach developmental in that it attempted to identify language disorders using a developmental data base. This approach clearly focused on the definition and description of "linguistic behavior." In discussing the objectives of assessment, Miller stated that the structural and functional aspects of the language system should be assessed through the major processes of oral language use. However, he included the evaluation of comprehension as well as production in this process.

Muma (1978) presented a philosophy of descriptive analysis that included evaluation of the cognitive, linguistic, and communicative systems and processes. Muma (1978, p. 275) felt that developmental scales and other normative measures were of questionable value in assessment. This approach to testing was supported by L. McLean and McLean (1978, p. 137), who pointed out that a language sample can provide a much more complete picture of the child's language than any standardized instrument.

This brief review of the evolution of assessment of language and its disorders indicates how the earlier descriptive techniques tended to be replaced by objective, normative test instruments. More recently, after the use of normative tests was widely accepted and even mandated as a requirement for placement of children in certain programs, the trend in assessment is turning back to descriptive procedures. The integrative approach presented in this volume indicates that differential assessment must involve *both* types of analysis.

Structuring the Assessment

The literature on assessment has tended to focus on either standardized tests or naturalistic description. Proponents of standardized testing suggest that naturalistic description may produce only random, meaningless responses that could lead to incorrect diagnosis. Advocates of naturalistic description note that a child's score on a test may provide little significant information. When assessing many developmentally disabled children, what is needed is not a test score but examples of what the child *can do* despite his disability.

This apparent dichotomy in assessment philosophy may be resolved by distinguishing between structure and standardization. All meaningful assessment requires *structure,* which refers to the amount of control utilized in the testing situation. Structure may be either external or internal. *Standardization* refers to the establishment of a specified procedure for obtaining and analyzing information, in an effort to ensure objectivity, reliability, and validity. The specified procedure provides *external structure* for the examiner, which tends to be characterized by three conditions: (1) a formal assessment setting where the examiner may be told, for example, where to sit in relation to the child; (2) a protocol for obtaining responses from the child; and (3) criteria for judging the responses made by the child. Tests like the Illinois Test of Psycholinguistic Ability are called standardized because they provide structure that is external to the examiner. Any person who demonstrates the ability to accurately follow the instructions in the examiner's manual could administer and score such a test.

For a naturalistic description, which lacks external structure, it is assumed that competent examiners will provide *internal structure,* which includes knowledge of the normal ages and stages of development as well as familiarity with the research and clinical methods available for eliciting and analyzing the child's language. It further presumes that these methods will be individualized for each child. Good naturalistic description is therefore not without structure, but it does demand that each examiner provide internal structure.

Both standardized tests and naturalistic observations have limitations in terms of the value and applicability of the results. Naturalistic observations may be clinically impractical in terms of time and effort. Siegel and Broen (1976) indicated that even after extensive samples of spontaneous speech were obtained, there was no guarantee that all behaviors of interest would appear. On the other hand, methods employing external structure and yielding standardized scores may be limited in the types, variety, and spontaneity of the responses they elicit. Regardless of the method used, the examiner must bring structure to the assessment.

The Use and Misuse of Standardized Tests

Should the use of standardized tests be abolished? This is not a theoretical question since in some areas of the United States it is against the law to administer certain tests to some groups of children. Much of the criticism that has been directed toward tests and their value in assessment is a result of the manner in which tests have been misused. If a test clearly specifies that it has been normed on a population of middle-class children, the norms should not be applied to children at a low socioeconomic level. Because of the time and cost of standardization, it is frequently impractical to provide norms for every special population. One solution is to develop local norms for tests—a procedure that is relatively easy to accomplish.

In reliable administration, the use of standardized tests provides a good estimate of the level of significance of a problem. Standardized tests also indicate areas that need naturalistic observation. In other words, after tests have been administered in a standard manner, selected items can be explored in depth in a naturalistic setting. Consequently a second misuse of tests is using them exclusive of naturalistic observation, which can provide more extensive data on which to judge a particular aspect of functioning. As Leonard et al. (1978) noted, many features of language are not included in standardized tests; these features may be explored by modifying the procedures contained in both standardized tests and in research instruments. Leonard et al. provided suggestions for how this may be accomplished. Just because items occur in a test that has been standardized does not preclude the modification of the items to further explore a child's linguistic skill. If the child's performance improves with modification of the test item, this indicates what the child *can* do, and such information could contribute to planning the intervention program. Obviously, once the procedure has been modified, the norms may not be applied.

A third misuse of tests is drawing conclusions that the test data cannot support. Examiners may give two discrete tests and because a child has difficulty on both tests, the examiner may infer a cause-effect relationship. Co-occurence of two problems does not imply cause-effect even if one ability is dependent upon the other developmentally. The relationship must be explored in a variety of contexts, and by sequential modification of related variables, in order to determine a cause-effect relationship.

The fourth and final problem in the use of standardized tests is the misunderstanding of the concept of a norm. A norm is a statement of typical behavior. In developmental studies of children, it is used to refer to a base or reference against which to judge behavior. This base is usually in the form of an age level, but it can also take the form of stages of development. Both of these types of norms describe typical behavior. In some developmental tasks, such as motor skills, age level is the best reflector of acquisition; in other developmental tasks, e.g., language skills, stages of development seem to reflect most accurately the typical growth sequence.

Norms are obtained in different ways. Experienced observers obtain norms by documenting behaviors of children and analyzing the typical stages or age levels of these behaviors. For example, Brown (1973) studied the reports of the language development of three children and analyzed these in terms of the emergence of grammatic forms and semantic relations. The reported orders of emergence provide normative data that can be used as a reference for judging the language development of children. The drawback of Brown's data is not the method used for obtaining norms but the very small number of children upon which the normative data were based. In view of subsequent studies, the sequence of morpheme development has been challenged (see Chapter 8).

A measure of central tendency, such as a mean, is not valid unless there is also an index of the variation from the mean indicating the probability of an obtained mean being due to chance. Since there is typical variation in language acquisition by children, and since each of the children Brown used for developing the orders of acquisition varied from each other and from the mean, Brown's data should be used with informed caution. If it is used indiscriminately, children who have normal variations or who use a different learning style may be viewed as having a problem when they do not. Furthermore, because of the time and difficulty in obtaining norms of this type, these norms are available only for the language of children in the early stages of language development.

The Use and Misuse of Naturalistic Observation

Few language specialists disagree with the value of the naturalistic observation of language most commonly referred to as a language sample. This observation can provide valuable information about specific areas of linguistic development, the functional use of language, and the communicative relationship. A thorough language sample describes exactly what the child is doing. It allows the examiner to focus on the child's strengths and weaknesses and describes an individual child's style of learning. Despite its value in assessment, there are potential misuses of naturalistic observation.

A first misuse may occur in the size of the sample obtained for analysis. Research studies have relied on relatively large samples. For their cross-sectional study, the de Villiers (1973) obtained a mean of 360 utterances; Brown, Fraser, & Bellugi, (1964) obtained 700 utterances per child, and Bloom (1970) obtained 1500 utterances per child. Muma (1978) felt that 200 to 300 utterances should be obtained for clinical purposes and that these utterances should be collected under different circumstances. The commercially available systems of language sample analysis specify between 50 (Hanna, 1977; Lee, 1974) and 100 utterances (Lee, 1974; Tyack & Gottsleben, 1974). Crystal, Fletcher, and Garmon (1976) recommended a 30-minute language sample, which they indicated should yield between 100 and 200 utterances. Despite these recommendations, Bryne (1978, p. 121) reported that most clinicians obtained only a 3- to 10-minute language sample.

Another serious concern in the use of language samples is the context in which the language is elicited. The majority of research studies done since 1960 were audiotaped in the child's home as the child interacted with family members or with the investigator (Bloom, 1970; Bowerman, 1973a; Brown et al., 1964; Greenfield & Smith, 1976). Researchers who have studied the spontaneous language of disordered children have used a variety of settings and topics. Lackner (1968) gathered language samples of retarded children in a residential facility by audiotaping them as they got up in the morning and during their afternoon "rest" period. Morehead and Ingram (1973) taped a child and parent engaged in free play; Prutting, Gallagher, and Mulac (1975) had the mother, and subsequently a clinician, interact with the child in spontaneous dialogue; other studies had the parent and child interact at home (Freedman & Carpenter, 1976) or in the clinic (Leonard et al., 1976). Both the Applied Linguistic Analysis (Hannah, 1977) and the Language Assessment, Remediation, and Screening Procedure (LARSP) (Crystal et al., 1976) require the child to engage with the examiner in conversation and to interact with toys that may or may not be brought from home. The DSS and DST require the child to respond to toys and pictures, and to retell a story (Lee, 1974). Muma (1978) recommended that the child interact in three different situations: with a peer at school, with the parent at home, and with the clinician in the clinic.

Several studies have attempted to clarify the differences between obtaining a language sample in the child's home and in a professional setting. One study found that the sample obtained in the clinic was as representative of syntactic productivity as was the home sample (C. M. Scott & Taylor, 1978). However, the home sample contained more pronouns and twice as much questioning as the sample that was done in the clinic. Another study showed that syntax was the same regardless of where the sample was obtained, but that the MLU was longer when the sample was obtained at home (Kramer, James, & Saxman, 1979). These few studies suggest that language samples obtained in professional settings may tend to underestimate some aspects of the child's language ability.

Another potential misuse of the language sample occurs in the analysis of the sample. Although virtually all language specialists have courses in diagnostics, Muma (1979) reported that only twenty-one of the eighty-four training programs in speech

There were no textbooks on speech and language assessment until 1952, when the *Diagnostic Manual in Speech Correction* was compiled by Wendell Johnson (senior author) and F. Darley and D. Spriestersbach (co-authors).* This manual directed the attention of potential examiners beyond the speech defect to the person involved. The authors pointed out that a speech defect has no particular meaning apart from the person who has the defect. They noted that every individual reflects the interaction between his original endowment and the environment into which he has been thrust. In 1952, these criteria for good assessment practice were already time-tested, having first been articulated by Edward Lee Travis (one of the founders of the profession of speech pathology) almost twenty years previously.

*Wendell Johnson, Frederic Darley, D.C. Spriestersbach: *Diagnostic Manual in Speech Correction.* New York, Harper & Brothers, 1952.

pathology that he surveyed provided training for their students in eliciting and analyzing language samples.

THE INTEGRATIVE APPROACH

The goal of assessment in the integrative approach is to comprehensively evaluate the dimensions of language in order to describe areas of strength and weakness in each. This approach includes four tasks: (1) to identify rule-based deficits in the knowledge of the linguistic code; (2) to identify perceptual and conceptual processing problems in the cognitive dimension; (3) to identify possible inadequacies in the communication environment of the child; and (4) to identify factors that obstruct the performance of the receptive and expressive aspects of language. The integrative approach also seeks to relate these dimensions to each other. This approach endeavors to compare the cognitive with the linguistic; the semantic with the grammatic; the comprehension with the expression; and the knowledge with the performance of language. The ultimate goal is to understand how deficits in any of these dimensions affect the child's functioning in real life situations.

A practical example of the integrative effort to relate assessment to the child's major problem (which is very possibly the chief concern of the referring source) would be testing the following hypothesis during assessment:

1. Is this child's problem in understanding and following directions in school related to a memory or discrimination problem?
2. Is the child's failure to use specific grammatic structures in his conversation also evident in aural comprehension and/or in writing?
3. Is the child's failure to respond verbally the result of an inability to formulate language or is it due to inability to execute the rapid sequential movements inherent in speech articulation?
4. Is the child's problem with tense an expression of a further problem with temporal ordering? Is it also expressed in lexical aspects of expression?

5. Are the child's rule-based deficits in grammar responsible for his difficulty in learning to read or is this failure the result of generalized intellectual delay?

The results of assessment ought to be directly applicable to the problems the child exhibits. Information should not be gathered for its own sake or simply because it is part of a protocol with which the examiner is familiar.

Assessment is essentially a procedure of hypothesis testing. Based on the referral (the source and reason for referral), the examiner establishes her first hypothesis. The first standardized test or naturalistic observation should be chosen to verify or refute that hypothesis. A second hypothesis is then established and tested and so on until the nature of the child's problem can be described.

Use of Standardized Procedures

In the integrative approach, standardized procedures serve to identify the presence and extent of deviations in language behavior from an already established norm. When norms are used, these procedures should be chosen only for those children who can be appropriately compared to the population on which the test was normed. However, standardized test items may be adapted for use as a systematic method of observing a child's behavior, even though the norms are not used. For example, if on the Test of Auditory Comprehension of Language (Carrow, 1973), a child is unable to point to the word *ball,* he might be asked to repeat the word after the examiner and then attempt to point. Successful pointing following this modification would provide direction for planning intervention.

The Cognitive Dimension

In the normal child, cognitive abilities may be judged intact based upon the child's adequate language performance and ability to express concepts verbally. In the language-disordered child, however, this information may not be available directly from the analysis of semantic or syntactic abilities, and so must be tested directly.

The most sophisticated tests of auditory sensory and auditory perceptual processing systems are those performed by the audiologist. A major function of the tests administered by audiologists is to locate the site and the nature of lesions in the auditory processing areas of the central nervous system. Auditory perception tests developed for use by the language specialist cannot be utilized for this purpose; they can, however, describe how the auditory system functions when presented with specific types of information. For example, presentation of minimal pairs (words differing only in one phoneme) for discrimination can indicate the possible difficulty an individual has in recognizing words that sound very much the same. Comparison can be made between the ability to discriminate phonemic differences in quiet and in noise. This type of information can assist in the management aspects of language disorders.

Memory for auditory information is usually measured by repetition of words or digits. However, the use of unrelated words or digits may have little functional relationship to expressive language. Although expressive language problems and memory problems may co-occur, there may not be a cause-effect relationship between them in an individual child. However, memory problems may interfere with communication. Although most memory tests require a verbal response, there are some that do not (e.g., the Hiskey-Nebraska Test of Learning Ability). These request a child to point to pictures in a sequence, thus making it possible to measure memory in a child who has a severe speech and/or language problem. Other tests (e.g., Detroit Tests of Learning Aptitude) require the child to follow a series of increasingly complicated directions.

The recognition and discrimination of visual forms and features are basic to the development of some of the concepts that comprise the spatial meanings of language. Visual skills are also needed to transfer the skills of language comprehension and expression to the use of written symbols. As a rule, available tests (e.g., the ITPA and WISC) of visual perception require memory as well as perception. Other perceptual tests (e.g., the Bender Visual Motor Gestalt Test) require motor reproduction either by drawing or writing. If a child does poorly, it is difficult to determine if the problem is one of perceptual recognition, memory, or motor reproduction. The Carrow Auditory and Visual Abilities Test (Carrow-Woolfolk, 1981) distinguishes the functions of memory, discrimination, and motor reproduction. It is important to select tests that discriminate among these skills.

Concept development is the next level of cognitive ability that may be assessed. The most common means of obtaining information about the child's level of concept development is through language. Concepts are, by definition, internal structures of the mind, and as such are not available for direct observation or measurement. A gross idea of the level of conceptualization can be determined by observing a child's relation to his world and the objects and events that comprise it. If the child demonstrates that he knows the proper function of specific objects (e.g., a knife or a cup), in effect he has represented concepts. Myklebust (1954) recommended testing what he called "inner language" by observing how a child related to common toys and objects. If a child can group or categorize objects, basic concepts have been acquired.

Representation and symbolization abilities may be evaluated through a series of techniques, including the observation of play. Several observational techniques have been proposed to evaluate concept development. Chappell and Johnson (1976) presented children with common household objects and evaluated their response on different levels. The authors felt that the test pattern revealed the child's general developmental status. Westby (1980) presented a Symbolic Play Scale designed so that an observer could chart the level of play and compare it to verbal expression. Administration of such a scale allows a comparison of nonverbal cognitive skills and verbal language expression. The use of gesture combined with contextual clues also provides information on symbolization.

Piaget's observations of infant development during the sensorimotor period have been objectified and systematized in ordinal scales of development (Uzgiris & Hunt, 1975). There is evidence of a sequential order of development of concepts such as object permanence, means-end relationship, and causality. This test allows an examiner to assign a child to a particular level of development, but there are no age norms.

The most common means of obtaining information about the overall level of a child's concept and symbolic development is through language. Words, or word problems, are presented to the child and he responds by defining or pointing to pictures to represent the concept encoded by the word, or by explaining the solution to the word problem. For the child with an intact linguistic system, this method of assessing cognition is sufficient and is represented by most of the standard tests of intelligence. Several of these tests allow for differences between verbal and nonverbal concept development by having separate verbal and performance scales (WISC-R; Wechsler, 1974) or mental and motor scales (Bayley Scale of Infant Development; Bayley, 1968). Other tests of concept development are entirely nonverbal (Leiter International Performance Scale; Leiter, 1969) and are commonly administered to hearing-impaired or nonverbal individuals.

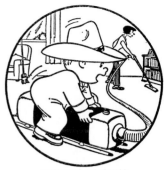

"GIDEE-UP! GIDEE-UP!"

A child's spontaneous play reflects his symbolic development. (The Family Circus by Bil Keane, reprinted courtesy of the Register and Tribune Syndicate, Inc.)

The Dimension of the Linguistic Code

Knowledge of the linguistic code is tested through performance; however, performance problems can exist without deficits in the knowledge of the code. Therefore, error analysis is fundamental to the interpretation of test results. A correct response suggests that the child possesses a functional knowledge of the rule under test, but an incorrect response may reflect any number of factors. For example, a child may fail to generate a structure because he does not know the rule; or he may know the rule but be unable to formulate an appropriate utterance containing that structure. This can be tested by reducing the length of the utterance containing the structure, by checking for the consistency of the error in naturalistic observation, or by exploring the child's ability to comprehend the structure. In addition, if a child knows a rule but can't express his knowledge, then he will very likely try to express the meaning in other ways. If the child does not understand the meaning of the rule, then the structure will be entirely omitted. There are a relatively large number of standardized tests that appraise performance of the various linguistic systems.

Semantics.   Vocabulary analysis is a primary means of evaluating the semantic system, and there are a number of ways in which vocabulary can be measured, including actual counts of words used, testing definitions of words, using picture recognition to identify word meanings, and word association tests. Users of vocabulary tests must seriously consider the relationship between vocabulary and general intelligence. This relationship allows the same charges of ethnic and cultural bias that have been leveled against intelligence tests to be made against many of the commercially available vocabulary tests. It is therefore vital that the language specialist verify that the test selected does not simply confirm the child's ethnic background, his intelligence, or his opportunity to attend school.

For some normal children, but especially for children suspected of having a language disorder, the ability to comprehend words is of special interest. Comprehension is often demonstrated by having the child point to the one picture, out of a possible four pictures, that best illustrates the word named by the examiner. A few tests of comprehension require the child to manipulate objects to demonstrate his comprehension of particular words. This leads to a more realistic situation but can also lead to ambiguity in evaluating the child's response. Deciding whether the child failed because he did not understand the word under test or whether he simply chose what he considered the most appropriate thing to do in that context requires considerable clinical judgment. A child who has had little previous experience with "school-type" situations may be baffled by why an adult is asking him to follow such commands.

Grammatic Forms.   Analysis of the syntactic level of a child's language involves studying the comprehension and expression of the various aspects of syntax construction, word order, and morpheme usage. The productive use of grammar may be analyzed through the use of specific tests or through the analysis of language samples. Menyuk (1969), Lee (1971), Carrow (1974a, 1974b), and others have all studied syntax through the use of elicited imitation. Comprehension of various linguistic structures have also been assessed by providing a linguistic signal to the child who then must select a picture corresponding to the signal or who must follow a command. Some of these situations involve the child manipulating objects to demonstrate comprehension of, for example, the difference between active and passive voice. The problem for the child might be to demonstrate, for example, "The boy is chased by the dog." Also, a number of commercially available systems for the analysis of language samples provide detailed instructions for evaluating grammatic structures, and some of the advantages and problems inherent to these systems are discussed later in this chapter (p. 249).

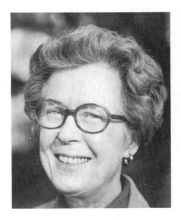

Pragmatic Use.   With the renewed emphasis on the communicative use of language, it is disappointing to realize how little assessment information is available in this area. However, already available knowledge of conversational rules allows the examiner to be aware, for example, that when an examiner and child enter the usual testing situation, the question and answer format, involving the pragmatic function of exchange of information, is used. Based upon analysis of questions in conversation (Rees, 1978), it is known that preschool children answer questions from adults based upon certain assumptions or conversational postulates. The child will respond if the following conditions occur: (1) The child comprehends the question; (2) The child knows the answer; (3) The child believes the speaker does *not* know the answer; and (4) The child believes the speaker *wants* to know the answer. In view of this, the examiner should be cautious in assuming that numbers 1 and 2 are the only possible reasons why a child did not respond.

Metalinguistic functions of language are also commonly measured on standardized tests. A task is metalinguistic when the child is required to view language as an object. Tasks involving the identification of individual phonemes and tasks asking the child to provide antonyms, synonyms, and rhyming words are all metalinguistic tasks. Examiners should be aware that failure on

---

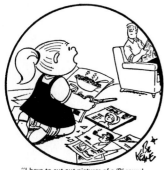

"I have to cut out pictures of a 'P' sound. Does PASKETTI begin with a 'P' or a 'B'?"

The reason for a child's error may have as much or more diagnostic significance than the existence of the error. (The Family Circus by Bil Keane, reprinted courtesy of the Register and Tribune Syndicate, Inc.)

such tasks may reflect an immaturity in development of the metalinguistic function of language rather than a perceptual or semantic deficit.

Despite the lack of commercially available tests of pragmatic function, several research methods have been adapted to measure the functional use children make of language (L. Miller, 1978; Prutting et al., 1978). These studies present systems for evaluating the function of speech produced by young children. The identification of possible pragmatic problems in older children was discussed by Damico and Oller (1980), who provided a checklist of behaviors that characterize the school-aged child with pragmatic problems. These include criteria such as nonspecific vocabulary, poor topic maintenance, and many requests for repetition without apparent improvement in understanding. These pragmatic criteria were successful in identifying language-disordered children.

The Dimension of the Communication Environment

Obviously, such internal states as "needs and desires" cannot be objectively measured. Needs are expressed by the efforts the infant makes to establish communication relationships. Initially, these are nonverbal efforts to exchange mutual gaze, to smile, to maintain eye contact, to grasp and offer objects, to point to objects, and to begin using words to describe the relationship of agents and actions to objects. These efforts of the child are stimulated by caretakers, other adults, and children who appear motivated to interact with the infant and to engage in the process of teaching language through the use of "motherese" (see Chapter 5).

The extent and variety of interaction may be judged by observation of the parent and child in naturalistic situations. In such cases, a language sample may be specifically analyzed for communication exchanges instead of for semantic or syntactic forms. Various methods of language analysis provide devices for noting direction of gaze and other nonverbal behaviors. In addition, case histories, parental diaries of daily activities, and behavioral checklists may provide supportive information concerning the amount and quality of interpersonal exchange. In obtaining this information, it is important that the examiner be sensitive to the effect the child has on parental behavior, so that these questions are not perceived by the parents as a means of establishing blame for their child's problem.

In the integrative approach, assessment procedure is always evolving in response to new information and in response to the needs of individual children. Examiners must be prepared to evaluate new tests and restudy old tests and classic techniques. A number of diagnostic textbooks are currently available that provide sound guidelines. These include texts by Emerick and Hatten (1974), Nation and Aram (1977), Bloom and Lahey (1978), Darley and Spriesterbach (1978), and Singh and Lynch (1978). In addition, there are books that describe and/or evaluate tests (McCabe, 1978; Darley, 1979). Professional journals like ASHA also routinely review newly published tests.

Use of Naturalistic Observation

Frequently voiced concerns about the use of language samples involves the amount of time required to obtain and analyze the sample, as well as hesitancy about reporting data from a "nonstandardized" technique. However, in view of the complexity of language and the significant constraints of context, language samples have emerged as a necessary part of differential assessment.

A *language sample* is defined here as the verbatim, written record of the exchange of spontaneous utterances between two people. Based on the studies previously discussed in this chapter (pp. 238–239), it appears that a language sample may be collected in a professional setting and that a sample size of approximately 100 utterances may be sufficient for most systems of analysis.

Language is fleeting and must be carefully recorded if the results are to be meaningfully analyzed. Ideally, a language sample should be tape recorded or video recorded with the examiner observing in the room in order to take notes on the context and nonverbal behaviors. If possible the sample should be transcribed on the day on which it was recorded. Unless articulation is to be studied, the transcription can be done in orthographic script rather than in phonetics. It is this written record, not the subsequent analysis, that is most important and that forms the *language sample.* This record should be preserved because it may be reanalyzed repeatedly. Researchers such as Brown and Bloom and their colleagues, for example, continue to analyze language samples obtained more than 10 to 15 years ago.

To date, the most detailed procedural methods for recording language samples have been provided by Ochs (1979) and by Bloom and Lahey (1978). In her detailed chapter on the transcription of language samples, Ochs recommended a form that allows for noting nonverbal and verbal behavior for *both* speakers involved in the situation. She also provided an array of notations for marking various behaviors.

From the time of the major developmental studies of the 1930s, it was accepted that the mean length of response was one of the most sensitive measures of a child's linguistic achievement. Brown popularized the use of the mean length of utterance (MLU), and this measure is now used as a basis for comparing children linguistically, in preference to other comparisons such as chronological age. This technique has been found to be an excellent index of language development up to an MLU of 4.0 (Brown, 1973). The closest relationship exists between MLU and grammatic development such as acquisition of grammatic morphemes. There is a less firm relationship between MLU and semantic development (Leonard, 1976). A recent study (Miller & Chapman, 1981) explored the relationship between MLU and age. Analysis of free speech samples supported the findings of early investigators and indicated a significant correlation between MLU and chronological age as well as between MLU and linguistic achievement. Rules for calculating the MLU in morphemes are provided in Appendix A.

Once the MLU has been determined, other methods of analysis may be used. For example:

- For an MLU below 1.00 (prestage I)
  1. Specify the lexicon
  2. Analyze semantic intentions
  3. Analyze pragmatic functions
- For an MLU below 2.5 (stages I and II)
  1. Specify the lexicon
  2. Analyze the semantic intentions and semantic relations and determine grammatic morphemes used
  3. Analyze pragmatic functions
- For an MLU over 2.5
  1. Analyze semantic relations
  2. Analyze sentence types and morphosyntactic structures
  3. Determine the function of the speech

For younger or immature children, the lexicon can be inventoried, and the listing of words may be compared with early vocabularies that have already been described (see Chapter 7). Analysis of vocabulary can assist in establishing the learning style of the child. More important than listing the words is the analysis of semantic intentions and semantic relations. The semantic intention implies the meaning the child intends to convey. This is determined by consideration of the context in which the word was used and cannot be correctly established by comparing the child's word or phrase with a printed list of semantic intentions or semantic relations. If, for example, the child said *car*, the semantic intention could only be ascertained by evaluating the context. If the mother had just said she did not know where the child had put his "special" blanket, and the child responded with the word *car*, the semantic intention would be location; if the child was impatiently waiting to peddle or "drive" his toy car, then the word *car* would function as object; if the child was pointing out the presence of a car then the semantic intention would be existence. Even with consideration of the context, there may still be confusion, so suggestions for establishing these intentions are provided in Appendix B.

Once the data regarding the vocabulary, morphosyntactic structures, and functional use have been analyzed, the language specialist can make initial judgments regarding the individual child's level of function by referring to the detailed discussion of development contained in Chapters 8 and 9. These chapters include the rate and sequence of development of these various units of linguistic code as well as the age range in which the behavior most often emerges.

The primary commercially available systems of analysis tend to emphasize sentence structure. They include Developmental Sentence Types and Developmental Sentence Scoring (Lee, 1974); the Language Sampling, Analysis, and Training Procedure (Tyack & Gottsleben, 1974); the LARSP (Crystal, Fletcher, & Garman, 1976); and the Applied Linguistic Analysis (Hannah, 1977). One of the most recent manuals on the analysis of free speech (J. Miller, 1981) discusses how research techniques may be adapted to elicit various language forms, and describes the analysis procedure for data obtained.

Two important considerations in analyzing a language sample are productivity and obligatory contexts. *Productivity* refers to the frequency with which a word or form occurs. This is an important consideration in judging whether a child has mastered a form. For example, if a child with an MLU of 1.9 described his fish as "in the water," how could the examiner ascertain if the child truly had the concept of *in* or whether he had simply learned the answer to "Where's the fish?" and was saying one long word, *in-the-water.* If *in* was used in other utterances, like "in the box," "in the house," and "in bed," then this form could be said to be used productively, and this would constitute good evidence that the concept underlying *in* had been mastered. The criteria for productivity varies. Morehead and Ingram (1973) accepted two occurrences, Greenfield and Smith (1976) accepted three occurrences, and the de Villiers (1973) accepted five. Bloom & Lahey (1978) expressed a more common criterion by suggesting that four occurrences indicated the productive use of a form.

Grammatical analysis also relies upon understanding of *obligatory contexts.* This applies especially to the use of commands and to responses to questions. The usual response to *wh* question is a word or phrase, not a complete sentence. In response to the question, "What are you doing?" the most usual response would be a single word such as "playing." In that example, the subject and predicate, "I am" is nonobligatory and its ommission should not be counted as a syntactic error.

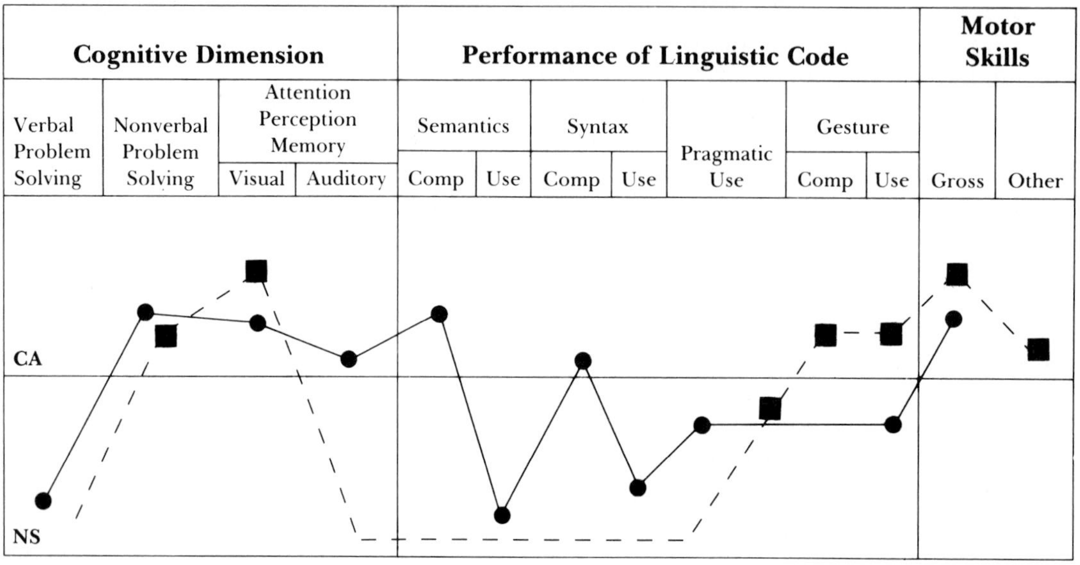

Figure 11-1
Differential assessment profile illustrating the performance characteristic of a child with a clinical language disorder (Pattern E*—solid line), and the performance of a child who has a language disorder associated with severe hearing impairment (dotted line). The line labeled CA represents performance on the test considered appropriate for the child's chronological age. NS indicates that the child was unable to respond to tests in that area. *See Chapter 13, p. 302. (Adapted from material in Lynch J: Evaluation of linguistic disorders in children. In Singh S, Lynch J (Eds): *Diagnostic Procedures in Hearing Speech and Language.* Baltimore: University Park Press, 1978, pp. 327–378.)

Once the data have been gathered and analyzed, the examiner must organize and interpret this information for the purpose of making decisions about the child and his problem. At this point, the examiner might return once more to the reason for the referral. It is important to relate the problems observed during assessment with the real-life problems the child is experiencing. If the examiner has proposed and adequately tested the various hypotheses suggested by the initial complaint, she will be in a position to account for the reason the child is experiencing the problems for which he was referred.

A profile that has proved useful for displaying assessment results is illustrated in Figure 11-1. The profile allows the results of any standardized test or naturalistic observations to be graphically compared to the level of performance expected for a child of a given age. The profile may be used to illustrate strengths and weaknesses in a single child, to analyze changes in a single child over time, or to illustrate the differences and similarities of two children.

The report that follows assessment should include a statement of the nature of the problem(s) as related to the problem for which the child was referred. Also, the nature of the child's problem(s), based upon evidence from standardized evaluation and supported and tested during naturalistic observation, should be reported. The severity of the problem(s) should be suggested based upon normative information. The interrelationship of the observed problem(s) in the various dimensions of language should be described. The particular learning

	Cognitive Dimension				Performance of Linguistic Code							Motor Skills	
Verbal Problem Solving	Nonverbal Problem Solving	Attention Perception Memory		Semantics		Syntax		Pragmatic Use	Gesture				
		Visual	Auditory	Comp	Use	Comp	Use		Comp	Use	Gross	Other	

ASSESSMENT OF LANGUAGE AND LANGUAGE DISORDERS

strengths and weaknesses of the individual child should be presented along with his clinical category, if any. Factors inherent in the clinical category may contribute to the maintenance of the child's problem. This leads directly to a discussion of intervention for the child.

The authors propose a series of obligations that language specialists functioning as examiners in the integrative approach should assume:

1. The language specialist should function as a professional who is responsible for making recommendations about a child—not just about one facet of the child's behavior. If assessment focuses exclusively on language performance, then the examiner functions only as a technician whose task it is to describe deviations in language expression so that those deviations can be "fixed."
2. The language specialist must be prepared to accept that most language problems are multidimensional and interrelated. They cannot be assessed on a unidimensional basis using a single assessment tool for all children.
3. The language specialist must be knowledgable about all dimensions of normal language acquisition, the expected deviations in language disorders, and the currently available assessment instruments for measuring these deviations.
4. The language specialist should be aware of the interrelationship of the different units of the dimensions of language. (A problem, such as immature articulation for example, may be apparent during preschool. Complete assessment may reveal that the child exhibits other perceptual, conceptual, or memory problems that will later cause him problems in written language and in subjects such as mathematics and geography.) The potential for future problems should be pointed out so that the family and other professionals do not progress from one problem to another to another—which all *appear* totally unrelated and unexpected.
5. The language specialist should serve as an advocate for the child in obtaining necessary referrals and proper intervention. In addition, the language specialist should assist the family in becoming informed advocates for their child.
6. The language specialist should participate in informing *both* the child and his family, as well as other professionals, about the child's problem.
7. Finally, a child cannot be described as language-disordered simply because he confuses several prepositions or fails to express past tense, for example. *A language disorder results in failed communication.* It is this failure in communication that must be investigated, and this failure is ultimately the criterion on which the designation *language disorder* is made.

outline

SELECTION OF CHILDREN FOR INTERVENTION

PROGRAMMING IN INTERVENTION

General Principles of Program Selection
Preplanned Programs

CONTENT SELECTION

Bases of Content Selection
    Developmental, Remedial, and Hierarchical
    Approaches
    Receptive Versus Expressive Approaches
    Process Versus Task Approaches
Content for Early Developmental Levels
    Cognitive Content
    Semantic Content
    Grammatic Content
    Pragmatic Content
Content for Intermediate and Advanced Language
Levels

INSTRUCTIONAL PROCEDURES

Procedures in Cognitive Training
Procedures in Teaching Semantic Relations
Procedures in Teaching Syntactic Structures
Nonspeech Language Procedures

GENERAL TEACHING STRATEGIES

STABILIZATION AND GENERALIZATION

INTERVENTION VERSUS MANAGEMENT

INTEGRATIVE APPROACH TO INTERVENTION

Applications of the Integrative Approach

THE LANGUAGE SPECIALIST AND INTERVENTION

intervention and management 12

BECAUSE CLINICAL PROCEDURES in language disorders are influenced to a great extent by current theories of language, the focus of clinical intervention shifts often, reflecting the changes in theoretical interest. The early therapeutic or remedial approaches to treating the language-disordered child were primarily drawn from structured methods of teaching language to the deaf and hard of hearing (McGinnis, 1963). Later, concern with the severely brain-damaged child—sometimes called the aphasic child or the child with central auditory problems—led to intervention procedures emphasizing perceptual, representational, and vocabulary functions (Barry, 1962; Myklebust, 1954; Strauss & Lehtinen, 1947). In an attempt to integrate the perceptual, representational, and linguistic structure aspects of language, Osgood and Miron (1963) and Wepman et al. (1960) devised models upon which approaches to remediation of language disorders could be based. The emphasis, which had been on language when techniques for teaching deaf children were used, began to shift to concern for improving perception, memory, and other cognitive aspects of language. However, when the influence of Chomsky's theories (1957, 1965) began to be felt in clinical areas, the emphasis turned again to language.

Chomsky's theories of syntax drew clinical attention to the nature of linguistic structure; language intervention models were developed that presented sequences of linguistic structure based on the transformational hierarchy of phrase structure described by Chomsky. The language-disordered child came to be differentiated from the non-disordered child in terms of linguistic structure differences only, and these differences became the focus of intervention. The interest in structure per se was short-lived; Bloom (1970) suggested that the grammatic structures reflected, and were based on, semantic content and that this content, the semantic relations of words, needed to be developed before structure. The language intervention models reflected this shift, and programs were developed to teach the semantic relations found in early language development such as agent-action and agent-object.

Subsequently, language theorists found that description of structure and semantics was insufficient to explain language and so expanded the concept of language to include its broader communicative functions, the pragmatic aspects. Following this shift of emphasis, clinical intervention programs were developed for teaching pragmatic rules of language to children. Simultaneous with the shift to pragmatics was a renewed interest in the cognitive aspects of language (Moore, 1973) with particular focus on the application of Piaget's theories of child development (Morehead & Morehead, 1979).

The instability of the definition of language has led to an instability in intervention practices with language-disordered children. The shifts in focus have caused confustion on the part of specialists involved with the application of theory to specific children in specific situations. The differences in the theories must be viewed as differences in focus; all of them validly explain some aspect of language and all of them need to be considered in intervention. Bever (1970) suggested that language be studied as a conceptual and communicative system that recruits various kinds of human behavior but that is not exhaustively manifested in any particular form of language behavior. If language is considered in this broader, integrative form, as in this text, the focus of concern is not on the application of a current theory but on the *child's* unique use of his learning and behavioral strategies and processes for acquiring the semantic, pragmatic, and linguistic structure rules of language within his own environment. Simplification of language theory and application provides a compactness that facilitates assessment and intervention, but does not necessarily offer validity in terms of assisting the language-disordered child.

The child, then, must be the focus of language intervention. The child is not separated into parts some of which perceive, others comprehend, and others use pragmatically correct utterances. The child functions as a total person, using his abilities and skills for learning and performing language. When emphasis is placed on one skill, the other skills, as well as the desired products, must be kept in perspective, and the clinical procedures must move back and forth among all the child's language behaviors so that there is gradual change in ability to communicate effectively.

This chapter considers some of the tasks of the child in learning to communicate, as well as some of the methods and procedures that the clinician may use in teaching the tasks to the child. Because of the necessity for organizing the data on intervention, the content, tasks, and procedures for intervention may be presented at times as if they comprise isolated, mutually exclusive approaches. This is not intended. The approach to intervention used in this text follows the broad eclectic approach to language and its disorders that has been described in previous chapters.

The selected issues in intervention discussed in this chapter are (1) selecting children for intervention; (2) developing a program for treating the language-disordered child; (3) developing program content; (4) devising instructional procedures for effective intervention; and (5) stabilizing and generalizing new behaviors and skills. Where applicable, the issues are viewed in terms of language theory. The purpose is not to teach specific procedures or systems, but to present general principles that can guide the clinician in an intervention program.

SELECTION OF CHILDREN FOR INTERVENTION

Selection of children for intervention is based on a number of factors: (1) the theory and definition of language espoused by the clinician; (2) the significance of the child's problem; (3) the appropriateness of the child's language to other developmental milestones of the child; (4) the appropriateness of the child's language to external factors; (5) the probability of success; and the need for the clinician to make judicious use of time and cost factors.

If the clinician holds the linguistic structure view, that is, the view that language disorders are defined only by differences from normal children in linguistic production (indicated by problems in form, content, and use) then a child with such a difference, regardless of the nature or degree of the difference, would be accepted for clinical assistance in language. The integrative approach, on the other hand, considers the type, degree, and significance of the difference to be critical in the selection of children for intervention, particularly as these relate to factors other than language. This position considers that intelligence and emotional well-being, as well as cultural and ethnic factors, influence the type and effectiveness of intervention. The integrative approach also views the differences that affect the communication behaviors of comprehension, listening, and perceiving to constitute language disorders, and therefore considers children with these problems also eligible for intervention.

The integrative approach to intervention considers the appropriateness of the child's language to aspects within and without the child to be a key factor in selecting children for language intervention. If the child's language is different from that of the average child but is within normal variations and is appropriate for his intellectual level or mental age as determined by nonverbal means, the child would not be considered a candidate for intervention. If the child's linguistic difference is appropriate to the language spoken by the adults in his culture or ethnic environment, he would not be considered language disordered and might or might not be a candidate for intervention. A linguistic difference should be considered indicative for intervention only if it differs *significantly* from normal or if it creates significant communication problems in the environment in which the child lives and learns.

The probability of success should also be considered in selecting children for intervention. A child may be treated for a difference in language, but if his emotional or personality dynamics are unbalanced, the success of treatment will be minimal. A child cannot be forced to change. At times, no amount of motivation and encouragement provided for a child can bring about an interest in or awareness of his own linguistic differences. There is no value to the child, to the clinician, nor to the community to involve such a child in language intervention without first seeking a solution to his other problems, which may prevent success.

PROGRAMMING IN INTERVENTION

Once a child is selected for language intervention, the task of the clinician is to prepare to select a plan for bringing about the desired linguistic changes.

General Principles of Program Selection

Regardless of the type of program that is ultimately used, there are certain components that all programs must have. Also there is one principle that should always guide selection: the program must be suited to the needs of the child.

The single most important aspect of direct intervention is the construction of an overall plan that delineates all aspects of the instructional and learning process. The basic components of such a plan should include (1) the overall goal of the program and a series of intermediate goals expressed in terms of behavioral objectives or targets; (2) selection of content to be taught; (3) specification of the content in terms of priority and hierarchy of tasks and procedures to reach the objectives; (4) specification of instructional and motivational strategies; (5) identification of measures for evaluation of progress; and (6) procedures for stabilization and generalization.

Graham (1976) proposed that the goal of intervention should be to provide a system of communication that is both effective and functional for the individual within his own environment. This means that the beginning and end of language therapy is communication. Communication implies the ability to understand the messages conveyed by others and the ability to encode messages so that they can be understood by others. If therapy does not lead to this ultimate goal, the program is not a language program.

Preplanned Programs

A major issue regarding programming is the use of programs planned by clinicians to meet specific individual needs of children versus the use of preplanned programs that incorporate the components listed above. The use of preplanned programs has advantages. The time, effort, and knowledge required to plan a thorough, systematic, and sequential program is considerable. A preplanned program offers the user a means of providing quality instruction to the child with a minimal amount of clinical time and effort. It is also probable that the developers of the program have more experience in program development than the typical clinician-teacher. However, all children have different areas of disability and different areas of need. Furthermore, children are easily "lock-stepped" into preplanned programs without regard for their unique learning styles (Carrow-Woolfolk, 1975). Preplanned intervention program should (1) be suited to the children's needs; (2) have a sound theoretical base; (3) be developed by experienced language specialists and successfully used by them; (4) be cost effective; (5) provide for measurement of change or learning; and (6) lend themselves to group treatment. No single program can be used for all language-disordered children. It may be that a child needs only parts of a program; this judgment must be made by the language specialist.

Siegel and Spradlin (1978) suggested that in order for a language specialist to select an appropriate preplanned program for a child, she must seek answers to two questions: (1) What is the definition of language that has been used in developing the program? and (2) What degree of flexibility is built into the program design? An answer to the first question, according to Siegel and Spradlin (1978, p. 366), answers other questions as well: "Does [the program] focus on syntax or semantics? Is it concerned with teaching the child how to manipulate the environment, or how to manipulate sentences? Is it appropriate for children who already have some vocal communication skills?" An answer to the second question assists the clinician in determining whether or not the program can be individualized to the needs of the child.

The less experienced the language specialist, the greater the need for a preplanned program—but also the greater the need for care in its use. It must be emphasized that, if a preplanned program is not used, the teacher-clinician must take the time to carefully structure a plan for *each* intervention. Ruder (1978) recognized the problems inherent in detailed planning and cautioned clinicians against substituting less-structured play therapy, in which the term *play* refers to *play-it-by-ear*. There is no substitute for careful planning.

CONTENT SELECTION

The problem of content selection for intervention programs in language is a complex one. There is considerable professional disagreement regarding the areas in which skills and abilities should be taught and the order of their presentation. There are some who believe that syntax should be the primary focus, while others are concerned with cognitive, semantic, and/or pragmatic skills as well. There is also disagreement about the order of presentation of content.

Bases of Content Selection

Once a child has been accepted for language intervention, the language specialist must decide on the content she will use in teaching language skills. There is no clear-cut method of choosing content to fit the child. The bases for the selection of content are varied, and no single approach is superior to the others in all situations.

Developmental, Remedial, and Hierarchical Approaches

The developmental approach to language intervention stresses the ordering of content (whether cognitive, semantic, or syntactic) on the basis of the order of development in normal children. Some proponents of the developmental sequence of teaching language skills are J. F. Miller and Yoder (1974) and Stremel and Waryas (1974). The basic tenets of the developmental approach, according to Graham (1976), are based on the assumption that the task is to teach the child an effective language system rather than to eradicate deficiencies in the system.

Opponents of the developmental approach question its use in teaching language content (Gray & Ryan, 1973; Guess, Sailor, & Baer, 1974). They believe that there is little evidence to indicate that the sequence of development in the language-disordered child is the same sequence that has been identified in the normal child. Also, the critics of the developmental approach note the great variability among normal children in language development, and they question the use of a single sequence of progression as the best fit for all children. Siegel and Spradlin (1978) suggested that a developmental sequence in language may be useful in guiding research on language development but not as a base for all therapeutic intervention for all children: "Across categories, language seems too complex to be captured by a developmental progression" (Siegel & Spradlin, 1978, p. 370).

Graham (1976) described what she called "nondevelopmental content procedures" as those that are independent of prerequisite cognitive skills and the sequence of linguistic skills. Other writers call this a remedial approach. In this procedure, cognitive or linguistic forms are selected for teaching on the basis of child deviance and need. If, for example, a child does not use the negative form, proponents of the remedial approach will initiate instruction by teaching the negative form in its final or mastery state. Guess, Sailor, and Baer (1978) considered the remedial approach to be one that accomplishes improvement in a child's communication most quickly.

The problem with the remedial approach is that of determining which, among many, linguistic deficiencies will accomplish improvement in communication most quickly. A second problem is that changing a specific, surface manifestation of a linguistic problem may not indeed be what a child needs. He may not have the concept of the structure that is disordered, and thus working on the "error" will not bring about the desired results.

A third manner of selecting content is the hierarchical approach, in which the content is ordered in sequences of complexity *or* in sequences of developmental dependency.

Increases in complexity may be provided in the stimulus series, in which each set of presentations is more complex than the previous one: e.g., a linguistic stimulus is increased in length or number of morphemes or in transformational complexity, or a stimulus for visual discrimination is made more complex by adding color and size to the discrimination of a single form. Increases in complexity may also be provided in the required response, which may involve pointing, selecting, matching, copying, reproducing, formulating, etc.

Use of the hierarchical ordering in sequences of developmental dependency is based on the assumption that, for example, concepts develop before semantics and semantics before syntax. Teaching is then structured to follow such an order; the final product (syntax) is not taught until there is evidence that prior functions have been developed. The criticism of this latter aspect of the hierarchical approach is that the ordering by dependency is theoretical and not always supported by research.

Receptive Versus Expressive Approaches

It has been a commonly held belief that comprehension should precede production in intervention; i.e., children should not be taught to express a form they cannot understand. The rationale for this belief came from language theories and research that found comprehension to develop prior to production. The rationale was strengthened by evidence in delayed or disordered comprehension (hearing loss or aphasia) in which production was correspondingly affected. These data seemed to support the thesis that comprehension precedes production, and, conversely, that production is dependent on comprehension and should follow it on a hierarchical ordering. This position has been challenged by Bloom (1974), who presents arguments and research suggesting that there is little evidence to support the prior development of comprehension (see Chapter 6).

Siegel and Spradlin (1978), in their review of this controversy, reported suggestions by cognitive writers that both language production and comprehension may be a reflection of underlying cognitive or linguistic competencies. Siegel and Spradlin also proposed that the notion of simultaneous development of comprehension and production may be supported by some of the literature. Regardless of which develops first, some researchers (Asher, 1972; Mann & Baer, 1971; Winitz & Reeds, 1972, 1975) suggested that comprehension training is an effective means of teaching expressive language. They believe that training based on receptive language can facilitate the improvement of verbal production; in fact, they consider comprehension training more effective than imitation. Ruder and Smith (1974) concluded from the review of research and from their own studies that both imitation and comprehension training are needed to achieve verbal production.

It seems that from the position of intervention a distinction needs to be made between the *process* of comprehension and the *product* of comprehension. In the early stages of learning language, a child's comprehension involves not only processing a speech stimulus and decoding it, but also providing the establishment of a link between the stimulus and its meaning. As the child listens to speech and observes the context in which speech is produced, the meaning of language is learned. Then, when a child is said to comprehend a word, what is meant is that he has learned its meaning. It is obviously possible to utter words or morphemes without understanding their meaning, and it' often occurs in development in echolalia or in aphasia. It is also possible to acquire meaning by producing words in contexts that are not completely understood. It is important for the clinician to realize what may occur if children are only taught to produce semantically empty linguistic structures; Functional language is more likely to result if the child comprehends a structure before he uses it.

Process Versus Task Approaches

Another consideration in content selection involves the effectiveness of intervening in the process as opposed to intervening in the task. *Task* means the actual behavioral activity of comprehending, speaking, reading, writing, following directions, etc. *Process* means those cognitive systems that are essential to learning and maintaining the tasks, such as discrimination, memory, and sequencing. Hence, the clinical question is: Should the focus of intervention be on the processes that undergird the tasks or on the tasks themselves?

Arguments supporting teaching the process before the task suggest that unless the child's processing systems are strengthened to support the task, there will be little or no improvement in the task itself. Furthermore, since children often present more than one manifestation of a language problem, (articulation, syntax, reading, spelling, etc.), intervention in the processes that support these tasks would provide a more efficient and effective means of ameliorating the problems.

Unfortunately, the carry-over from process to task does not

The nature of the language disorder should dictate the type of intervention used. In this case, although oral language was delayed, the intervention approach of choice was teaching language comprehension.

Stephen, who was 4 years, 8 months old, was referred to the hospital language clinic from another agency because after 6 months in an oral language development program, he had made little progress. At the time we saw him, he was using a few isolated words and had considerable echolalia. Comprehensive evaluation indicated a severe auditory comprehension problem, although it appeared to the casual observer that he could comprehend oral material. We demonstrated to the parents and some physicians that his comprehension was of single words only. Stephen was instructed as follows; "Give the cigarettes to your Dad." He did so. Then, "Don't give the cigarettes to your Dad." He gave them to his father again. Another command was given, "Put the ball on the table." He responded correctly. Then, "Put the ball under the table." He put the ball on the table again. Stephen was enrolled in an intensive program for teaching him to associate and understand words and meaning. Although language comprehension was taught, his oral language improved. After 1 year, Stephen's verbal responses were approximately 3 to 5 words in length and were of telegraphic nature; articles and auxiliary verbs were omitted. After 2 years, he was using inflectional endings in verbs, as well as articles, pronouns, and prepositions: "Dog bumped his head. Peanut stepped on the dog tail. Dog gonna cry." Had he continued in a program based on oral language analyses stressing oral language imitation, modeling, and expansion, he most probably would not have made this progress.

usually take place automatically. A child can increase his memory for digits but still not remember classroom instructions. There must be a tie-in from process to task; i.e., the process should be taught in the manner in which it influences the task. If the child's memory problem interferes with following instructions in the classroom, he should be assisted in improving *memory for instructions*. If a child's perceptual and memory processing abilities interfere with comprehension, he should be taught compensatory means of holding the input (reauditorizing, visualizing, etc.), so that he will have time to segment and structure the input for comprehension. The functional use of language behaviors, not the development of specific skills, should be the goal.

Content for Early Developmental Levels

Content selection for children who have not spoken or who are just beginning to use oral language structure differs from that for children who have mastered the basic elements of language but whose language exhibits usage that is not appropriate for their age or general language development. For young children, or for children with severe cognitive or behavior disorders, the instructional process must include the teaching of behaviors that will make it possible to provide language instruction. Such behaviors include attending, responding, and sitting. These behaviors need to serve as the content of training prior to actual instruction in language skills. Once the readiness for instruction has been developed, the clinician chooses the language content area in which to begin intervention: (1) cognition; (2) semantics; (3) syntax; or (4) pragmatics. Her decision will be

Tina Bangs

Tina Bangs, an innovator in the field of language disorders, started her professional career at the University of Washington where she received her Masters degree in 1941. Bangs completed her Ph.D. degree in 1958 while already involved in developing new concepts of intervention.

Although Bangs' contributions to language assessment are considerable, her greatest impact has been in the area of preschool programs. In 1964, she introduced a preacademic program into a public school setting, because she recognized the need to develop in children the oral language and perceptual skills that are basic for learning to read, write, spell, etc. By introducing this program, Bangs shifted emphasis from the handicapping conditions to the educational needs of the child. Her continued interest in early intervention was demonstrated by her publication of books and developmental scales for children in the birth to three age range. Her initiation of concern with disorders at these early months of life brought about family involvement in the management of the handicapped child.

Among Bangs' publications are *Language and Learning Disorders of the Pre-Academic Child* (1968) and *Birth to Three, Developmental Learning and the Handicapped Child.* In all her writings, Bangs has stressed the importance of cognitive functions in language development.

based to a large extent on her theory of language disorders. Some programs, such as that of T.E. Bangs (1979), provide a comprehensive curriculum with attention given to all areas of content.

Cognitive Content

The renewed concern for the role of cognition in language (see Chapters 3 and 6) has stimulated the development of language procedures and programs that begin at the cognitive level. These programs are based on the Piaget's premise (1954, 1955, 1970) that language development is based on the prior development of sensorimotor, conceptual, representational, and symbolic behaviors, and, therefore, intervention should take into account such cognitive factors. Implied in this approach is (1) the existence of a dependency relationship between sensory and cognitive deficiencies and language-learning behavior; and (2) the need to provide a cognitive undergirding to the adequate social use of language. Since the same cognitive problems may be common to a number of language-learning activities, remediation provided at the cognitive level may anticipate and prevent subsequent problems in reading and spelling as well as in oral language.

The need for children to be able to discriminate and categorize on the basis of perceptual attributes in order to develop concepts has been proposed by many (Bricker & Bricker, 1974; E. Clark, 1971, 1974; Piaget, 1969). If a child cannot discriminate among colors, learning color names would not be an appropriate goal in intervention. Morehead and Morehead (1979) stressed the need for symbolic and representational behavior to have developed as a prerequisite to language. Ruder and Smith (1974, p. 577) suggested that if Piaget's notions are used to explain language acquisition, the ideal training program "must be capable of adjusting to a given subjects' level of cognitive functioning." They proposed that the use of such a framework in intervention may facilitate the acquisition and maintenance of a structured linguistic system, because it assigns a primary emphasis to the cognitive system, and because it is concerned with the child's manipulation of his environment.

Semantic Content

In the semantic approach, specific lexical items occurring either in isolation or in semantic relation (agent-action) to other lexical items serve as the primary base for intervention. This procedure stresses teaching the association of symbols with concepts.

The semantic approach usually begins with single items that reflect concepts of recurrence, nomination, rejection, agent, etc.

Once single lexical forms are established, the children are taught two-word utterances that represent semantic relations of different kinds. Using the same two words in different environmental contexts allows a wide semantic application of minimal structure. For example, "throw ball" can be used to urge a child to throw a ball, to remark on the clinician throwing a ball, or to ask if a ball has been thrown. Primary adherents of this procedure are J. F. Miller and Yoder (1974), who, although they suggested the need for cognitive prerequisites, feel the main thrust of intervention should be the pairing of individual experiences with appropriate lexical markers. The selection of lexical markers for a specific child is based on (1) the child's own communicative needs; and (2) the developmental hierarchy of semantic relations. Although Miller and Yoder's procedures are not directed at cognitive factors, they do in fact assist in the development of concepts through verbal mediation. The attachment of words to objects, events, and relations helps to define and refine the concepts with which the words are associated, and these relationships can also develop and strengthen the symbolic behaviors of children. Other programs using the semantic approach are those by Stremel and Waryas (1974) and MacDonald and Blott (1974).

Grammatic Content

In the syntax approach to teaching language, word strings are chosen on the basis of grammatic relations: subject-verb-object, noun phrase + verb phrase, etc. Differences between semantic and grammatical approaches are described in Bowerman (1973b). The syntactic approach stresses the teaching of grammatic forms and patterns with little or no attention to meaning, e.g., teaching a sequence of syntactic strings based on transformational grammar theory. Elements are added to fit into a specific grammatic form or pattern regardless of the semantic relations of the words selected.

The sequence in teaching syntax is established by gradually expanding the complexity and length of noun phrases and verb phrases. Sequences of this type may take the following forms:

verb (V) + noun (N)	throw ball
adjective (A) + N	little girl
possessor (P) + N	Mary doll
N + V + N	girl throw ball
V + A + N	throw little ball
V + P + N	throw Mary ball

These sequences may increase in complexity and length to the level of six or more words per utterance, and may include negative and question transformations as well as embedded and conjoined components.

Pragmatic Content

Intervention that begins at the pragmatic level emphasizes the use of language in the child's environment. The premise is that children who are not communicating have not developed the social needs and responses to do so. Consequently, a desire for communication must be established before formal attention is given to any of the other dimensions of language. Early pragmatic skills develop prior to language symbols in the normal child (Bates, 1976b; Bates et al., 1977), and, thus, according to the proponents of this approach, pragmatic skills should be taught before semantics or syntax.

Some of the pragmatic skills that are thought to precede language, and which therefore are suggested as intervention content, are skills such as drawing attention to self, responding to social approaches, initiating social interaction, and use of social agents to obtain ends. Once language is established, these pragmatic skills are evident in behavior of labeling, repeating, answering, requesting action, requesting answer, calling, greeting, protesting, and practicing (Dore, 1974). Later pragmatic skills that involve language are those of conversational turn-taking, appropriateness of language to the situation, use of language to express feelings and obtain information, etc.

Content for Intermediate and Advanced Language Levels

Intervention for children whose language performance has developed past the stage of basic syntactic elements presents different problems than does intervention for children in early stages. Most of the children in the intermediate and advanced levels of development are those who have clinical language disorders. Such children have ordinarily mastered the basic semantic relations, have developed many of the semantic modulators, and, in some cases use elaborate sentences. The language disorder may be expressed (1) by omissions or substitutions of a specific class of modulators (e.g., the omission of all negative forms in utterances containing other complex structures); (2) by omissions, substitutions, or transpositions of complex forms of specific grammatic elements (e.g. failure to use the correct question form with an auxiliary); (3) by deviation from the rules of word order; and (4) by an inconsistent pattern of complexity, with some forms representing a higher level of development than others within the same utterance. In fact, the disorder is signaled by discrepancy (1) in the levels of complexity between grammatic structures within the same group of utterances; (2) between the complexities of semantic relations and the grammatic forms used to express them; (3) between the level of comprehension of specific grammatic forms and their expression; or (4) between general cognitive development and the level of linguistic performance.

The language of these children is not viewed as much in terms of stages of development as in terms of the similarity of their language to that of the adult norm. The errors or differences are determined by comparison, not to early developmental models, but rather to the fully developed system used by native speakers in their community.

The issue of error analysis and content selection in this group of children illustrates the basic difference between the behavioristic and the integrative approach. Behaviorists examine the surface structure of language, discover differences, and proceed to modify the surface structure to resemble that of the adult model. The integrative approach leads to the analysis of the differences or errors and attempts to identify factors that may be operating to cause or maintain them in the child.

In the integrative approach, the language specialist explores the level at which the error occurs. Suppose, for example, a child does not use the preposition *in* correctly in obligatory contexts although he demonstrates mastery of morphemes that appear at later developmental stages of language. His MLU, however, is of sufficient length to expect the preposition *in* to have developed. The language specialist needs to know if the child's problem is in one or more of the following categories:

- *Conceptual.* The child does not distinguish among significant features of reality and therefore does not apply the linguistic marker appropriately. Applied to the instance given above, this means that the child does not distinguish the concept "in-ness" from other relations in space; he cannot identify the similarities among relationships showing one object *in* another. The word *in,* therefore is not used, or not used appropriately.

- *Semantic.* The child distinguishes the contrastive features of reality but does not know grammatic markers that code the features. In the case of the preposition *in,* the child would have the concept of "in-ness" and be able to distinguish it from other space relations such as "out-ness" or "under-ness," but has not correctly matched the concept with the word *in.* He may thus omit or substitute for the word *in.*

- *Comprehension.* The child distinguishes the contrastive features of reality and has associated the appropriate grammatic marker with it; however, the spoken word *in* does not evoke the appropriate meaning. This condition refers to the lack of comprehension of the spoken word, although the individual does respond correctly to the word in other language contexts (as in reading). This situation can be reversed—reading comprehension can be disordered, while auditory comprehension is fine.

- *Formulation.* The child discriminates the reality contrastive features and the associated markers but confuses the reality features and markers having minimal difference and uses them inappropriately in the process of expression. This condition would occur if the child consistently says the wrong thing, e.g. *on* for *in,* but knows that he is saying it incorrectly.

- *Execution.* The child distinguishes features of reality and knows the basic grammatic features that carry the semantic information, but cannot encode and articulate the feature automatically when uttering a sentence of a specific length.

A consideration of these conditions would lead the language specialist to a meaningful plan for intervention, which is different from trying to "teach" the child to produce the preposition *in* in a variety of linguistic contexts. Unless the first or prior conditions have been mastered, according to the integrative approach it would be fruitless to try to increase the percentage of use of the preposition *in* in obligatory contexts. Thus, in the integrative approach, intervention techniques may not be the same for children whose linguistic symptoms are the same.

The language specialist who uses the integrative approach also explores the possibility that some of a particular child's performance errors are transitional ones, which normally occur as part of the process of learning, and occur, to some extent, in all speakers. Such errors are not rule-based, either in the normal or disordered populations (Richards, 1969).

Children's "errors" may also reflect faulty learning strategies, and unless these errors are examined and differentiated in terms of their nature and source, underlying inadequate strategies or inadequate linguistic knowledge may not be identified. Consequently, future problems in language may not be predicted and prevented. These inadequate strategies, faulty knowledge, and consequent errors arise from the language-disordered child's effort to expand the functional capacities of his language. To describe the level or stage of language acquisition of the language-disordered child may not be sufficient.

INSTRUCTIONAL PROCEDURES

There are many ways of teaching specific content to language-disordered children. The basic elements of teaching have to do with (1) the type of stimulus the teacher presents to the child; (2) the type of response that is expected from the child; (3) the response of the teacher to the child's response; and (4) the amount of structure used in the interaction between the clinician and child. The first two are *instructional procedures* and the latter are *teaching strategies.* Variations within each of these four elements are the basis of differences among methods of teaching. These variations arise from the nature of the task that is to be taught—whether it is an automatic skill to be performed, an association to be learned, or a discrimination to be made. If the elements involved in most procedures are viewed in relation to the instructional tasks in cognition, semantics, and syntax, the role they play in language training can be identified more clearly. Items (1) and (2) are discussed below; (3) and (4) will be discussed under the section entitled General Teaching Strategies (p. 273).

Procedures in Cognitive Training

Stimuli and responses used in teaching cognitive behaviors are those involved in perceptual discrimination, stimulus recognition and identification, concept classification, representation, association, and generalization. Some examples are given below to clarify the use of these techniques.

Example 1.   The objective is to have a child discriminate visually between two sizes, large and small. The stimuli used are two sets of pictures of the same object. In one set, the objects are large; in the other set, the objects are small. The child is to respond by matching the pictures of the small objects and the pictures of the large ones. Increased complexity can be added (1) by providing a series of stimuli from small to large and having the child respond by ordering them to represent the gradation; or (2) by providing as stimuli a series of similar-sized objects with one large one and having the child respond by selecting the different one. Generalization occurs when the child responds by pointing, selecting or matching different pictures and objects than the ones used previously. The procedure can be used with all types of visual perceptual qualities—shape, color, number, spatial organization—and auditory perceptual qualities—tone, pitch, loudness, speech sounds. The essence of discrimination training involves the child's ability to identify those aspects of stimuli that are invariant and basic to the percept and those that are different—to generalize the likenesses and discriminate the differences.

Example 2.   The objective is to help the child develop a concept, e.g., "fruit." The stimuli are pictures, some of fruit and some of other objects. The child's response is to group (or classify) the pictures of fruit together and the nonfruit pictures together. Cueing and prompting in the form of demonstration are acceptable. Classification according to function can be taught by having the child group "things to eat" and "things that go in a room."

Example 3.   The object is to aid the child in developing representation behavior. The stimuli are toys representing real furniture and people. They toy people have either a picture of the teacher's or child's face pasted on their heads. The teacher matches the behavior of the objects to her behavior, i.e., the teacher sits in a chair and places the toy teacher in a chair. The child reproduces the teacher's behaviors by using the toys representatively.

These are random examples. It is assumed that the child has learned the appropriate responses through a hierarchy of simple to complex tasks. Complexity in the stimulus and in the response should be gradually developed by the teacher.

Procedures in Teaching Semantic Relations

The stimuli and responses used in teaching semantic relations are those best suited to developing associations between reality events (objects, people, and the relations among them) and the words that represent the objects, persons, etc. This is a later stage of representational behavior than that described in Example 3 above. In this procedure, sequences of vocal sounds, instead of toys, represent concepts of events and objects, and word relations represent semantic relations. The basic method of teaching semantic relations is by pairing (J. F. Miller & Yoder, 1974), in which an association is established between words and events by repeatedly presenting them together (the stimulus). The associations are presented in a systematic fashion to provide for reciprocal growth of both language and experience. J. F. Miller and Yoder (1974) suggested that the child's experience

David E. Yoder and Jon Frederick Miller

In 1965, David Yoder received his doctorate at the University of Kansas, where he began his studies in disorders of language and particularly in the language problems of the mentally retarded. In 1968, Yoder assumed academic duties at the University of Wisconsin. Jon Miller received a Ph.D. degree in 1966 from the University of Wisconsin and joined the faculty there in the Department of Communication Disorders in 1969.

Yoder and Miller have worked on projects in language development and language disorders at the Child Development Mental Retardation Center. By combining the content of linguistics with psychological principles of teaching, Yoder and Miller developed methods for developing the syntax and semantics of children at early stages of language development. Their approach is developmental and stresses the teaching of oral language production. Yoder's publications include *Language Intervention with the Retarded* (1972; with J. E. McLean and R. L. Schiefelbusch). A recent publication by Miller is entitled *Assessing Language Production in Children: Experimental Procedures* (1981).

should serve as a basis for selecting the linguistic members of the pair. The goal is not just the development of semantic relations but of linguistic production: "Through pairing explicit environmental experiences with their linguistic referent, the child will note these relations and their markers and begin to express them" (Miller & Yoder, 1974, p. 520).

Initially, no verbal expression is expected from the child; he observes and listens. The second step is to have the child indicate comprehension by responding to the linguistic marker appropriately. The next step is imitation of the lexical marker. The pairing of the marker with the experience immediately follows. These functions are then generalized to new situations, with corresponding markers representing the same semantic relations, and then stabilized.

Murray (1972) proposed a procedure similar to those described above; however, she did not classify it as a comprehension or semantic procedure, but as a reciprocal exchange approach. This approach also develops semantic mapping and comprehension prior to production. For example, in teaching the plural morpheme, the experimenter utters both the singular and plural forms, together with corresponding environmental conditions. Following this, the instructor requests either singular or plural objects ("I want the truck," "I want the trucks"), and then allows the child to participate by requesting the desired object with appropriate number inflection. This reciprocal exchange procedure should be particularly effective since it transfers the responsibility of initiating the communication exchanges to the child; i.e., the child provides the stimulus that receives a response. Placing a child in a teacher role is one of the best learning experiences he can have; it teaches the functional use of language.

Procedures in Teaching Syntactic Structures

There are procedures directed toward the improvement of production without concern for the semantic or comprehension aspects of linguistic structure. The main purpose of these approaches is to have the surface structure resemble a specified target or adult model. The three procedures most frequently used are those of modeling, imitation and expansion. The term modeling was borrowed from Bandura (1971), who proposed that a child acquires new behavior by observing the actions of others. With respect to language learning, the term is interpreted to mean the language input of the parent to the child—the *model* that the child can imitate or comprehend (Brown & Bellugi, 1964).

Modeling in intervention presents well-formed utterances to the child without requesting a response. Although considerable modeling by the language specialist is usually provided, it is difficult to conceive of a program consisting entirely of modeling procedures since the rate of progress would probably be restricted.

In imitation, the language specialist presents a model (Gray & Ryan, 1973) and the child responds by imitating the model. The imitation may be complete or partial, and its acceptance depends upon the goal of the teacher. Gray and Ryan (1973) and Bereiter and Engelmann (1966) developed programs using imitation.

Expansions have been the most widely used of the three procedures under discussion (J. F. Miller & Yoder, 1974). Ruder and Smith (1974) define expansion as the imitation of a child's utterance, using a modification of the utterance in the direction of a target—the next level of training. For example, if the child says, "Mary throw," the clinician would respond, "Throw ball," or "Mary throw ball." J. F. Miller and Yoder (1974), stressed that expansions may be telegraphic in nature and need not be complete sentences. They suggested that the order of using the technique after a child has been taught one-word responses through imitation be as follows: (1) expansions; (2) imitation of expansions; and (3) modeling (J. F. Miller and Yoder, 1972). The modeling described by J. F. Miller and Yoder (1972) follows a child's utterance, but instead of a slight modification of the utterance to a developmentally more complex utterance as in expansion, the clinician's model does not necessarily contain a content word from the child's previous utterance. For example, if the child says, "Daddy push," the clinician responds, "that wheel barrow heavy" (J. F. Miller & Yoder, 1972, p. 202). Cazden (1965) reported the effect of verbal support on the improvement of verbal behavior. She found more rapid change in situations where the teacher consistently modeled new structures for children than in those where the teacher consistently expanded the children's utterances.

The use of imitation in teaching language structures can be used in patterned drills. Patterned drills establish specific syntactic patterns (e.g., subject-verb-object), specific morphemes (e.g., auxiliary *is*), or specific word order. The patterns are repeated with the same lexicon until they become automatic, and then new words are substituted for those in the original pattern. The problem with patterned drills is that they can lead to incorrect uses of the grammatic forms:

The boy is throwing the ball.
The boy is winning a race.
The boy is jumping a fence.
The boy is looking a game.

Prior to having a child learn to produce a given grammatic structure, it is possible to teach him to perceive the grammaticality of utterances by pairing the correct form with a picture depicting it, then contrasting the form that he uses with the correct one, and having him choose the one that "sounds" best. Here the stimuli are the two utterances provided by the teacher; the child responds by discrimination and selection of the one that is gramatically accurate:

The boy running.
The boy is running.

Nonspeech Language Procedures

There are children whose physical and/or intellectual condition makes it difficult for them to acquire speech with sufficient speed to meet their immediate needs for functional communication, or at all. These children are said to be at risk for communication by speech, or in some cases by the use of auditory-vocal symbols. Severe cerebral palsy may, for example, interfere with the use of the peripheral speech mechanism for communication; severe hearing loss makes the early development of the auditory-vocal symbols used in language difficult. Children with these and related problems need substitutions to use as antecedents to speech until speech develops or to augment speech (Schielfelbusch & Hollis, 1980). The stimuli and responses may need to be in nonspeech forms. The decision as to which of the means are selected depends, of course, on each child's particular abilities and needs. In the case of severe sensory impairment, it is possible for the child to learn the syntactic rules of the auditory-vocal code through finger spelling or to substitute manual signs for auditory-vocal symbols. These two processes, when used in total communication, may be used to substitute for speech or to augment it.

A child with a severe problem in articulation, where intelligibility is essentially zero, may learn to write or type as a means of communication. If the child is too young to write or type, he may be taught to use a system of gestures or signs. McDonald (1980; McDonald & Schultz, 1973) recommended the use of communication boards, which may employ line drawings of everyday objects, painted words, or even a syntactic system for use in communication. He stated that children should be allowed to express their needs and desires in any way that is possible to them.

Chapman and Miller (1980) suggested a number of factors that are important in making decisions regarding the use of nonspeech intervention: (1) the developmental status of the cognitive, language, and communicative behaviors of the child; (2)

the language and communication characteristics of the nonvocal or nonverbal system; (3) the demands made on the child in learning and using the system; and (4) the speech community and overall situation of the child's environment.

GENERAL TEACHING STRATEGIES

In the introduction to the section on Instructional Procedures (p. 267), four basic elements of teaching were introduced. The first two—the teacher's stimulus and the child's response—were described there. The third and fourth elements—the teacher's response to the child's response, and the amount of structure provided in the relationship between the teacher and child—form the basis for teaching strategies. This is the aspect of teaching that is sometimes referred to as behavioral management. Unfortunately, the term behavioral modification is frequently confused with the content used in programs, when in fact it is a separate process, parts of which can be used with any content or procedure.

Behavioral management involves the structuring of the teacher's responses to the child's response for the purpose of strengthening or reinforcing the child's correct responses, or strengthening the association between a specific stimulus and a specific response. Most teachers try to encourage a child to respond. However, the manner in which they do so is not always conducive to achieving the desired results. It is possible to identify events that are reinforcing to a specific child (candy, points, stars, etc.) and to pair these with verbal reinforcers so that in time the verbal reinforcers have the same effect as the original reinforcer. Studies also indicate that the use of specified reinforcement schedules, which provide for variation in the frequency of reinforcement, identification of specific behaviors to be taught, and recording changes in behavior, will provide a situation that improves teaching efficiency. The structured management of behavior demands the ongoing recording and charting of behavior, and this provides better evaluations of progress and ultimately greater accountability.

Behavioral management techniques are applied more effectively to some behaviors than others. The teaching of behavioral skills (e.g., the utterance of a syntactic form) is better suited to the behavioral management approach than is the teaching of comprehension or meaningful language. However, no matter what is taught, the events that precede and follow the child's response should be carefully chosen.

STABILIZATION AND GENERALIZATION

Perhaps the most neglected area of intervention is ensuring the stability of newly learned behaviors and the generalization of these behaviors to other similar events. The desire to move too rapidly in intervention, and to teach too much, often results in poorly learned language skills. Stabilization will occur only if opportunities are given for the child to use a newly learned skill often, in different linguistic and environmental contexts. Children do not tire of some kinds of repetition—clinicians do; children enjoy the success experiences that come from repeated accomplishments of a goal. Also, stabilization procedures provide opportunities for the development of pragmatic skills.

The clinician must prepare lessons that provide different linguistic and environmental settings for the child. Intervention cannot be confined to a single room and a single type of clinician–student relationship (e.g., the clinician sitting on one side of a table and the child on the other). The clinician must plan various situations within and outside of the therapy room to give the child the varied occasions he needs for practice of a newly learned skill. The more informal the situation, the more formal and structured the planning should be to ensure numerous opportunities for practice.

As the stabilization process begins, the child must take greater and greater responsibility for his own linguistic change. In fact, one of the most important goals of intervention is to teach a child to become his own teacher. To do this, a child must be made aware not only of his linguistic needs, but of the general and specific goals that both he and the clinician are trying to reach. The dynamics of beginning therapy involve not a clinician trying to change a child's behavior, but a clinician and a child together trying to bring about the change. At the level of stabilization, the child becomes the primary person involved in the behavioral change. He needs to learn to be aware of his language; he must know the target to be reached; he must recognize when he does and does not reach it; and he must be able to monitor his output continuously so as to identify instances when he succeeds and when he does not.

The clinician must also have a systematic plan for including a child's parents and teachers in the stabilization and generalization of the child's linguistic change. Most parents and teachers are willing to help, and they have greater opportunity to relate to the child in naturalistic settings. However, the clinician must teach the parents and teachers how to help without too much correction and nagging.

Stability in learning comes from a knowledgeable teacher, one who understands the task or subject to be taught, the method to be used, and the child who is learning. A knowledgeable language specialist understands that every child has a unique learning style, and that she must be flexible in her approach so as to reach the child by *his* best avenue of learning. A knowledgeable language specialist knows that a child cannot learn if he is passive. A child must be an active participant in the learning process—he must think, do, speak, and write in his own way and in his own words. As Piaget (1954, 1955, 1970) counseled, simple responses are not enough; the child must reorganize his thinking in order to develop new patterns of response.

INTERVENTION VERSUS MANAGEMENT

An important consideration in intervention is the breadth of interpretation of the term. Intervention refers to the teaching of specific linguistic skills in cases where these skills are inadequate. Management means the total planning of the child's language learning, including referrals for other services, classroom seating, class placement, and the teaching of compensatory behaviors, as well as intervention. The child will not always be in a one-to-one situation with a language clinician; his language learning will not be limited to sessions held twice a week. He must be taught to function within his sensory and cognitive capacities, and, thus, must be provided with an entire program that may or may not be similar to the total program of other children with language disorders. The important consideration is not the language disorder and what to do about it, but the *language-disordered child* and how to help him.

Intervention in this context should be approached with a view to assisting the child to function in everyday life, in speaking, listening, remembering, and understanding. A knowledge of specific areas of difficulty, e.g., perception in noise or auditory memory, might assist the clinician in planning or modifying the environment for the child's learning and in teaching the child his own best learning style. The specific therapeutic technique used should have direct bearing on the child's problem in learning in his world.

INTEGRATIVE APPROACH TO INTERVENTION

While it is relatively easy to discuss intervention in the abstract, it is difficult to apply the principles to individual situations. The focus of concern for each child is his cognitive, linguistic, performance, and environmental needs. The integrative approach attempts to identify these needs in each child and to develop plans for meeting each of them in an integrative manner.

Applications of the Integrative Approach

Whatever type of language problems a child might have, the primary goal of intervention is pragmatic: to ultimately lead to improved communication at home and at school, in speaking, listening, reading, and writing. Intervention should assist the child in developing a desire to communicate and provide him with means to do so. A secondary goal of intervention is to make communication meaningful. The child must use symbols that are understood by others in his environment and that convey messages that are factually accurate. The accuracy of the medium or form in which the message is conveyed is not as important as the accuracy of the message and its meaning. Therefore, as long as the child's attempts are transitional and gradually approach a goal, these attempts should be accepted, regardless of how crudely they approximate language. The goal of surface grammatic accuracy is less important than the expression of semantic relations, since expressions of semantic relations are more important to communication. Last in order of priorities is articulation accuracy.

The order of importance of the goals of intervention does not necessarily reflect the temporal order in which aspects of language should be taught. It is possible, as well as beneficial, to include a number of goals within a particular intervention sequence and even within a particular lesson. Furthermore, working directly on a less important goal may indirectly aid a more important one. For example, in the early stages of the language development of a severely language-disordered child, the language specialist can choose a vocabulary or lexical item to be taught for pragmatic reasons—e.g., vocabulary that the child can use right away at home, such as *drink*. The concept of "drinking" can be taught and expanded by pairing the word with many different experiences of drinking—drinking milk, drinking soda, drinking water, drinking from a glass, drinking from a cup, and drinking from a bottle. Having the child repeat or imitate the word that is being paired with these experiences reinforces the association between the word and its meaning, thereby helping the semantic aspect of language. Grammatic relations are taught

Both Alice (in the first quotation) and the king (in the second) are expressing the frustration they feel in attempting to communicate effectively in situations where there are few words because there is little *need* for them. The environment does not require them. Intervention in language must include recognition that the need precedes the use of a form.

It is a very inconvenient habit of kittens (Alice had once made the remark) that, whatever you say to them, they *always* purr. "If they would only purr for 'yes,' and mew for 'no,' or any rule of that sort," she had said, "so that one could keep up a conversation. But how *can* you talk with a person if they *always* say the same thing?"*

But the extraordinary thing was that he could not ask such questions. In order to ask them, he would have had to put them into the ant language through his antennae: and he now discovered, with a helpless feeling, that there were no words for half the things he wanted to say. There were no words for happiness, for freedom, or for liking, nor were there any words for their opposites. He felt like a dumb man trying to shout "Fire!" The nearest thing he could get to Right and Wrong, even, was Done or Not-Done.†

*From Lewis Carroll: *Through the Looking Glass*. New York: Random House, 1946, p. 162. Reprinted with permission.
†From T. H. White: *The Book of Merlyn*. Austin: University of Texas Press, 1977, p. 51. Reprinted with permission.
Copyright © 1977 by Shaftesbury Publishing Company.

by using the word to convey different modulators: negative, by saying "drink" and shaking your head to indicate "don't drink"; interrogative, by inflecting the word upward at the end and holding a glass toward the child; declarative, by pointing to people or pictures of people who are drinking and saying "drink." As the association between the word and its meaning is developed, comprehension of the word develops; this can be tested by saying the word and having the child execute the meaning or select a picture, from a number of pictures, depicting the meaning. Application should be immediate and planned. The home and school can assist in having the child produce the word, perhaps by allowing him to play teacher and by expecting him to respond when it is used by others.

This integration of dimensions and processes can also be carried out with older children. At this level, it is particularly useful to explore the possibility of cognitive or semantic reasons for structural problems. If a child, for example, does not use verb inflections, particularly the past and future forms, the child's concepts of temporal order should be studied. Some children do not refer to past or future events at all. Their entire communication refers to the present. In such cases, teaching the concept of events in time, sharing these events, and referring to them in a meaningful way is basic to the development of inflections. Other children may have the concept of time but may use lexical rather than grammatic means to express their semantic intentions; e.g., "Before I go to school in the morning, I eat hot cakes," is used to describe a past occurrence. Such children need to learn to match the meaning to the efficient grammatic means of coding it. In both cases, once the concept or marker is learned, the performance will follow.

But suppose a child knows the concept and the marker but has difficulty generating it when speaking. In that case, the language specialist must observe the condition under which such a problem occurs. Does the length of the utterance influence the child's ability to use the inflection appropriately? Is his difficulty related to internal factors, such as fatigue or anxiety? Once a baseline is determined at which a child can successfully incorporate the inflection in an utterance of a specific type or length, then these factors can be changed gradually, and the child can, with practice, learn to express the grammatic marker in different situations and under different emotional conditions.

Just as the language specialist needs to be constantly aware of the dimensions along a horizontal plane—the conceptual, linguistic, performance, and environmental factors—she also needs to plan for vertical choices within the units and dimensions, i.e., she must choose the specific level of the developmental sequences to use for intervention. As was described in Chapters 7 and 8, the various grammatic and semantic forms are learned in sequences. Even after a form is used accurately, it needs a 90 percent use in obligatory sentences before it can be said to be mastered. The decision regarding the sequence stage or level of mastery to reach before moving to another form is a difficult one. The child should be at about the same level of development in all his semantic and grammatic behavior. This means that the movement must shift constantly between the vertical stages and the horizontal sequences and processes. A child is not taken through an entire developmental sequence of pragmatic or cognitive skills before he begins semantics or syntax, nor is he taught complete mastery of negation before he learns verb inflection. The sequences and levels of each should be at about the same point of development, and so the emphasis in intervention will shift back and forth, depending on needs of the child at each stage.

Language disorders, viewed from the framework of four dimensions, are complex problems needing complex solutions. One of the most important aspects of the solution is the knowledge and understanding of these disorders by the language specialist. Informed decisions are good decisions, and informed intervention is good intervention.

THE LANGUAGE SPECIALIST AND INTERVENTION

The language specialist must realize that the dominant factors in her success in helping the language-disordered child are the child, herself, and the relationship between the two. On one hand is the learner, his processing system, his style of learning, his way of discovery, and his awareness of his own strengths and weaknesses. On the other hand is the teacher, her grasp and understanding of the dynamic system of language, her excitement and enthusiasm for providing assistance in language, her understanding of each student's unique combination of abilities and disabilities, and her flexibility in following the student's lead in finding solutions to his problems. When these two persons are brought together into a relationship to change a behavior or a

Because the language specialist is necessarily concerned with improvement of the child's language, she often forgets to appreciate his good qualities and to let him know he is accepted. This quotation from W. Timothy Gallway provides a caution to this attitude.

When we plant a rose seed in the earth, we notice that it is small, but we do not criticize it as rootless and stemless. We treat it as a seed, giving it the water and nourishment required of a seed. When it first shoots up out of the earth, we don't criticize the buds for not being open when they appear. We stand in wonder at the progress taking place and give the plant the care it needs at each stage of its development. The rose is a rose from the time it is a seed to the time it dies. Within it, at all times, it contains its whole potential. It seems to be constantly in the process of change; yet at each stage, at each moment, it is perfectly all right as it is.

*From Gallway W T: *The Inner Game of Tennis.* New York: Random House, 1974, p. 37. Reprinted with permission.

group of behaviors in one of them, the behaviors of both should change. Together, they should analyze problems and arrive at solutions, however limited the child's ability and however difficult the problems may be initially. Both must always keep in mind that the one criterion of success is improved communication.

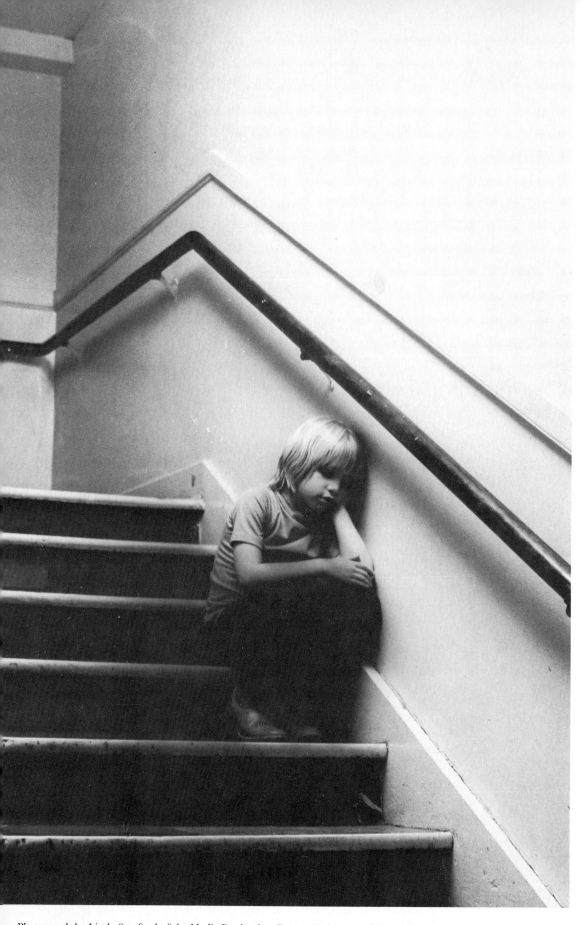

Photograph by Linda Stanford of the Media Production Center, University of Texas Health Science Center at Houston.

part four

range and variation of language disorders

outline

DEFINITION OF TERMS

Classification Criteria

EXPLANATORY THEORIES

An Auditory-Perceptual Defect
Defects of Temporal Ordering and
Rate Processing
Defects of Auditory Discrimination
Defects of Auditory Memory
A Symbolic Defect
An Attentional Defect

**THEORIES OF LINGUISTIC DELAY VERSUS
DEVIANCE**

Syntax
Semantics
Phonology

**CLINICAL LANGUAGE DISORDERS AND THE
COMMUNICATION ENVIRONMENT**

**INTEGRATIVE APPROACH TO CLINICAL
LANGUAGE DISORDERS**

ASSESSMENT

INTERVENTION

patterns of clinical language disorders

13

SOME CHILDREN WITH clinical language disorders appear to be developing normally except that they do not speak at all or speak very poorly. Since they have progressed well in other areas of development, their parents feel that they must be doing something wrong, or that their child is just "lazy" and "not trying to talk" or that their child has some "psychological" problem or "brain abnormality." The parents are given all sorts of advice: "Do nothing," "He will surely outgrow it," "Einstein was late to talk," "You must force him to talk," or "Don't give him anything to eat or drink unless he asks for it by name." Other children with clinical language disorders progress through the early stages of language development without attracting attention, yet as they get older it is noticed that their speech is excessively "vague" and filled with empty referents. They often misunderstand what is said to them and have an unfortunate way of saying inappropriate things and missing the point of humor or sarcasm.

This chapter will provide the language specialist with a description of what is known about clinical language disorders from a review of the literature and will present an integrative approach to clinical language disorders.

DEFINITION OF TERMS

Language disorders in children were first recognized and described by physicians (Gall, 1825; Vaisse, 1866; Wilde, 1853), who noted that there were children in schools for the deaf and the mentally retarded who were neither deaf nor mentally retarded but still could not speak. Their lack of oral language was compared to the loss of language in adult aphasics who had sustained brain injury. The term *aphasic* was applied to these children even though they, unlike adult aphasics, had never spoken and displayed no obvious signs of brain damage. However, the term *aphasia* continues to be used in some professional settings. Eisenson (1968, 1972) used developmental aphasia to mean a severe language disorder caused by central nervous system defect. The term *dysphasia* (deAjuriaguerra et al., 1976) is frequently used by European researchers and also by a few Americans (P. Weiner, 1969).

During the 1940s and 1950s, physicians and educators began to study the behavioral, visual-motor, and perceptual deficits of children with language and learning problems. The behavioral disorders in particular appeared comparable to those already described as occurring in adults with brain injury. Consequently, the terms *brain-injured child* and *minimal brain injury* (MBI) came into use both medically and educationally (Strauss & Kephart, 1955; Strauss & Lehtinen, 1947). The disturbing aspect of this terminology was that it proved difficult to establish a satisfactory relationship between the presence of positive neurological signs (such as abnormal reflexes) and EEG (brain wave) abnormalities and the severity of the observed symptoms. The use of terms such as *minimal brain injury* was criticized because it was felt that there could be nothing "minimal" about a condition that had such a serious consequence as failure to develop normal language.

Educators have countered the medical terminology with their own set of terms, with *language-learning disability* and *specific learning deficit* gaining the widest acceptance. The majority of American researchers, however, use terms such as *language disorder/deficit/delay* or *linguistically deviant/deficient*.

In this chapter, the term *clinical language disorder* is used for children who develop selective aspects of their native language in a slow, limited, or deviant manner. The selective nature of the impairment leads to a characteristic discrepancy in their performance on different tasks. *Clinical* was chosen rather than *developmental* because children with obvious developmental disorders such as intellectual retardation, hearing loss, and emotional disturbance are excluded from this classification.

Classification Criteria

Both the literature on language disorders and the integrative approach used in this text stress the importance of two classification criteria: exclusion and discrepancy. To classify a child as having a clinical language disorder, other handicapping condi-

The terminology conflict in the area of clinical language disorders was whimsically discussed and illustrated by E. Fry (1968) and Spreen (1976). They provided the following instructions for forming diagnostic labels in what was called a "Terminology Generator."

Choose any term from column I; combine it with one term from column II and one from column III and you have an accepted diagnostic label. Those terms appearing in a box in column II may sometimes be used alone.

I	II	III
primary	language	disorder
secondary	linguistic	disability
specific	learning	delay
minimal	cerebral	deficit
mild	brain	dysfunction
congenital	perceptual	impairment
developmental	visual-motor	pathology
chronic	neurologic	syndrome
childhood	educational	handicap
psychoneurological	aphasia	problem
functional	dysphasia	injury
	dyslexia	

All of these terms are still in use either in current diagnostic practice or in the literature.

tions must be excluded. Sensory deficits, particularly hearing loss, must first be ruled out, and then other serious developmental problems, such as mental retardation and emotional disturbance. The criteria of exclusion were explained by Myklebust in his manual of differential diagnosis (Myklebust, 1954) and were restated by Myklebust in 1971 (p. 1186): he indicated that the deficits are not a result of sensory, motor, intellectual, or emotional impairment, nor the lack of opportunity to learn. Zangwill (1978) reaffirmed that such children gave no "evidence of gross neurological or psychiatric disability." Menyuk and Looney (1972, p. 264) indicated that in children with language disorders, the "medical and psychological examinations of these children do not clearly indicate why this occurs." Despite the fact that many authors have presumed a subtle central nervous system (CNS) dysfunction, gross neurological disorders are excluded.

Children with clinical language disorders display an uneven pattern of abilities. As Myklebust (1971, p. 1186) has explained, "Children having this disability demonstrate a discrepancy between expected and actual achievement in one or more of the following functions: auditory perception, auditory memory, integration, comprehension, expression." The expected achievement is based upon the child's overall attainment of physical milestones (which tend to be within normal limits) and his ability to score within age level on selected nonverbal tests. Children with clinical language disorders do not initially arouse concern and even after the parents note the child's lack of verbal ability, they tend to reassure themselves because the children demonstrate in other ways their ability to solve problems.

EXPLANATORY THEORIES   Considerable research effort has been devoted to seeking the fundamental or underlying cause of the clinical language disorder. There are three significant explanatory theories; these theories propose that clinical language disorders result from one, or a combination, of the following: (1) an auditory-perceptual defect; (2) a symbolic defect; and/or (3) an attentional defect. In reviewing language-disorder theories, the language specialist should consider that some researchers believe that the language disorder is directly caused by, for example, the auditory perceptual defect. Other investigators consider that the defect under study may co-exist with the language disorder and that both the particular defect and the language disorder were ultimately caused by subtle central nervous system abnormality. Confusion regarding the relationship of observed defects to language performance has resulted in some unnecessary controversy in this area.

An Auditory-Perceptual Defect

It is theorized that listeners with normal perception use their semantic and syntactic knowledge of language to form internal expectancies of what the incoming auditory message will be. The expectancy is compared with the actual signal, and missing or distorted portions of the message are filled in as necessary. According to Lubert's (1981) review of the literature in this area, the neurophysiological data suggest that human beings have "feature detectors" that mediate the perception of speech sounds (see also Chapter 4).

Focus on the perceptual problems in children with language disorders began with Strauss and Lehtinen (1947), who felt that children with "brain injuries" demonstrated perceptual problems. A relationship between perceptual dysfunction and language disorder was proposed by Eisenson (1968, 1972). In his text on childhood aphasia, Eisenson (1972, p. 24) defined perception as "the process by which an individual organizes and interprets sensory data on the basis of past experience." His theory was based on the assumption that the language-disordered child's inability to process and produce language had its etiology in auditory-perceptual dysfunction (Eisenson & Ingram, 1972). This theory has stimulated considerable research into the abilities of children with clinical language disorders, particularly abilities in the areas of temporal ordering, auditory discrimination, and auditory memory.

Jon Eisenson

Jon Eisenson received the honors of the American Speech and Hearing Association in 1968 "for the body of published works in speech and language pathology which helped to forge a profession." Eisenson's publications include works on stuttering, speech disorders, speech correction, aphasia in adults, and aphasia in children. Eisenson's theory concerning the relationship of auditory-perceptual problems to aphasia in children significantly influenced the large body of research on the auditory and perceptual capacity of children with language disorders.

Eisenson received his B.S. degree from the College of the City of New York in 1928 and his Ph.D. from Columbia University in 1935. During World War II, he was a clinical psychologist for the War Department and supervised the language rehabilitation program for aphasics for the Surgeon General's office. In 1946 he joined the staff of Queens College in New York and remained there until 1962, when he became a professor of Speech and Hearing Sciences and Director of the Institute for Childhood Aphasia at the Stanford University School of Medicine. During this period, Eisenson was concerned with research in differential diagnosis and in the treatment of nonverbal children—especially those with perceptual impairment.

By the time he retired in 1973, Eisenson had been recognized as a Diplomate in Clinical Psychology by the American Psychological Association and a Fellow of the American Speech and Hearing Association. He served as president of the American Speech and Hearing Association in 1958.

Defects of Temporal Ordering and Rate Processing

A special deficit causing communication problems in language-disordered children is "malfunction of temporal ordering" (Lowe & Campbell, 1965). *Temporal ordering* refers to the proper ordering of syllables. An expressive error such as calling an "elephant" an "ephelant" is a mistake in temporal ordering. In learning language, the order of phonemes is crucial in distinguishing words. Monsees (1968) concurred that language-disordered children were impaired in their ability to report the temporal order of auditory stimuli presented to them. Aten and Davis (1968) also found that children with minimal cerebral dysfunction (as indicated by hard clinical signs such as abnormal EEG, seizures, and known head trauma) were deficient in sequential ordering of multisyllabic words.

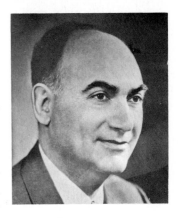

After reviewing this research, it appeared to Tallal and Piercy (1978) that these reported difficulties in perceiving the temporal order of auditory stimuli might actually represent a failure to discriminate the sound quality of stimuli when the stimuli are presented in rapid succession. In a series of studies (Tallal, 1975; Tallal & Piercy, 1973; Tallal & Stark, 1976), the ability of language-disordered children to process sounds was investigated. The subjects of Tallal and co-workers showed impairment in the ability to discriminate tones when the interval between the tones was short. The subjects displayed difficulty in discriminating speech sounds that incorporated rapidly changing acoustic spectra. The researchers concluded that the linguistic impairment of their subjects appeared to reflect a primary inability to analyze the rapid stream of acoustic information that characterized speech. This ability is essential for processing normal conversation. However, these children were able to understand single words presented in isolation (Tallal, 1975).

Defects of Auditory Discrimination

An individual must be able to differentiate important speech from nonspeech and from nonimportant speech. This ability is sometimes called *figure-ground* discrimination, and in the auditory realm this refers to the ability to attend selectively to a particular stimulus even though other auditory stimuli are present. This problem has obvious implications, especially for language-learning–disabled children in school. Keir (1977) tested 260 normal children and found that they could understand words even when the background noise was as loud as the words themselves. The language-learning–disabled children he tested could discriminate the same number of words only when the background noise was 10 to 15 dB *below* the level of the words. Keir then presented standard discrimination tests to the same groups of children. If the testing conditions were very quiet, the language-learning–disabled children did as well as normals, but once the background noise level increased they had serious difficulties. This led Keir to suggest that it may be poor figure-ground differentiation skills, not discrimination problems, that account for some language problems. Children with figure-ground problems are some of those about whom parents and teachers report, "this child can obviously hear but he only hears what he wants to," "he hears well enough but he won't listen," or "he just won't pay attention."

Defects of Auditory Memory

Based upon their review of the literature, Tallal and Piercy (1978, p. 77) indicated that there was a strong possibility that language-disordered children had additional defects in auditory memory. These children appeared especially vulnerable to demands placed upon auditory memory. Eisenson (1968) postulated that aphasic children may have defective storage systems for speech signals. Stark, Poppen, and May (1967) concluded that, based on their experiments, dysphasics have impaired auditory memory for sequences and tended to forget the first items in a sequence.

Keir (1977) explored auditory memory deficits in children with language-learning disabilities. He found a high percentage (63 percent versus 12 percent of normals) had significant short-term memory problems. The striking feature of his test results is the very sharp cut-off point between success and failure in these children. For example, they would repeat three digits quickly and confidently, but when an extra digit was added they would be unable to remember any of the digits. In his experience in following these children for a period of 6 to 8 years, this problem was most intractable to remediation. The best advice appears to be that parents and teachers should be aware of the child's memory span and accommodate their instructions to it.

Menyuk (1964a) also examined the ability of dysphasic children to recall and repeat sentences normally produced by children between the ages of 2 and 7 years. The language-disordered children made a considerable number of omissions and were not always able to successfully repeat sentences they produced spontaneously. When repeating sentences between three and five words in length, the structure rather than the length seemed most crucial.

Following an in-depth review of the literature concerning the various possible auditory defects, Rees (1973b) indicated that even if a primary perceptual difficulty was isolated in language-disordered children, there would still be little evidence to suggest that this defect was systematically related to language disability. She considered auditory perception a linguistic skill, and thought that imperception may co-occur with language disorders. Rees (1973b, p. 313) summarized her review by saying that "the inescapable conclusion is that the search for a single auditory skill, or even a set of auditory abilities, that is essential to language learning in all or most language disordered children seems futile." In another summary article, Tallal and Piercy (1978) reviewed the implications of their research and that of others. After re-exploring the arguments for and against the correlation of auditory and linguistic defects, their working hypothesis continued to be that "some cases of developmental dysphasia are the direct consequence of defective processing of rapidly changing acoustic information and an associated, possibly consequential, reduced memory span for auditory sequences."

The integrative model of language includes auditory perception and auditory memory as units of the cognitive and performance dimensions of language. Deficits in auditory perception or memory may delay the onset of language or impair its performance. The integrative approach suggests that these units may be impaired in some but not all children with clinical language disorders. The search for possible causes of all clinical language disorders tends to be hampered by the variability in the identification of the children used as subjects in various experiments. Some language-disordered children have hard clinical signs such as abnormal EEGs, head trauma, and/or seizure disorders, while others present none of these symptoms. Some language-disordered children are essentially nonverbal, while others verbalize rather freely, although their speech production is defective along a number of different parameters. Some comprehend language appropriately for their age, while others have severe comprehension defects. The failure to carefully describe the characteristics of all dimensions of language of the children serving as subjects in studies of clinical language disorders suggests that in some studies a rather diverse group of language-disordered children may have composed the experimental group. Therefore, it is not surprising that a specific symptom complex has not been identified as characteristic of the entire population.

A Symbolic Defect

The definition of language disorder by exclusion indicated that the intelligence level of children with clinical language disorders must be high enough to prove that they are not mentally retarded. However, a variety of experiments have suggested that language-disordered children have certain cognitive deficits compared to their normal peers.

In reviewing the research on the cognitive factors in language disorder, the relationship between thought and language (Chapter 4) is especially pertinent. The cognitive abilities that language researchers have most frequently hypothesized to correspond to language acquisition include sensorimotor skills such as the capacity for representational thought (Brown, 1973); the attainment of object permanence (Bloom 1973; Corrigan, 1978); and the recognition that other people serve as agents of actions (Bates, 1976a). Following a review of the literature discussing the relationship of cognitive stages and language production, Miller et al. (1980) concluded that cognitive development appeared to be correlated with development of both productive and receptive language (see Chapter 6).

Investigators have studied the performance of children with clinical language disorders on intelligence tests. Weiner (1969) studied the cognitive functioning of language-deficient children using the Wechsler Intelligence Scale for Children (WISC). Both the language-deficient children and their controls had performance IQs of 90 ($\pm$ 5 points). Weiner found that the experimental group displayed significant deficiencies on all tasks related to the auditory modality (not unexpectedly, since language-deficient children were included in the study on the basis of a verbal IQ 15 points below their performance IQ). Weiner observed that his language-deficient subjects functioned generally in a less integrated manner than the controls. Stark and Tallal (1981) administered the WISC or the Wechsler Preschool and Primary Scale of Intelligence (WPPSI) to all language-deficient children in their experiment. The children were first identified as language-deficient by speech-language clinicians, and only those with performance IQs of at least 85 (among other criteria) were placed in the experimental group. Although the purpose of this study was not to describe cognitive abilities, Stark and Tallal made several interesting observations. Of the 132 children originally identified as language-impaired by the speech-language clinicians, 50 had performance IQs below 85, and a few had performance IQs of 50 or less. It was suggested that these low scores were an artifact of the verbal directions inherent even on the performance items of the WISC and WPPSI. Consequently, 10 of these children were given the Nonverbal Hiskey-Nebraska Test of Learning Ability. They were still found to have IQs in the retarded range, and so they were excluded from Stark and Tallal's language-deficient category. Benton (1978) observed that even when such nonverbal tests as the Leiter International Performance Scale were used, there was a trend toward somewhat lower than expected levels of general intelligence in language-disordered children than in non–language-disordered children.

Inhelder (1976), a colleague of Piaget, explored the problem solving abilities of a group of children with language deficits. On nonverbal tests of operativity, one 5-year-old boy with diagnosed language deficiency was capable of solving problems in the same way as the most advanced children of his age group. In a test involving such verbal concepts as *some* and *all,* this dysphasic child demonstrated that he was capable of solving the problems despite his inadequate expressive vocabulary. In this study, Inhelder also explored whether dysphasic children developed figurative and imaginative symbolism as well as normal children. Her results indicated that development of the figurative aspects of thought was clearly impaired in her subjects.

Bartak and Rutter (1975, p. 193) felt that the dysphasic child lacked the imagination of the normal child. Johnston (1978) observed that language-disordered children tended to engage in less symbolic play. She suggested that they may have difficulty with visual imagery and associated conceptual development. Morehead and Ingram (1973) suggested that language-impaired children may have deficits in representational abilities, including symbolic play and imagery as well as language. Another study (Lovell, Hoyle, & Sidall, 1968) found that normal children spent

A child describes his own clinical language disorder in the following manner:*

I couldn't talk until I was five years old. I didn't learn to read until I was twelve. . . . My early school days were sad surprises for my parents. I could learn anything that didn't include words. Although I could hear I couldn't understand what people said. My teachers thought I wasn't paying attention. I tried but it didn't do any good. . . . My parents might have given up trying to reach me, but they didn't. . . . Neither my parents nor I believed I was stupid.

*Reprinted with permission from Zedler E: Social management. In Irwin J, Marge M (Eds): *Principles of Childhood Language Disability.* Englewood Cliffs: Prentice-Hall, 1972, pp. 383–384.

more time in symbolic play than did language-disordered children.

These studies evaluated the relationship of the various units of the cognitive dimension of language to the performance dimension. The integrative approach supports the observation that children with clinical language disorders are capable of demonstrating some normal cognitive skills despite deficits in other cognitive areas.

An Attentional Defect

Children with clinical language disorders may also display attentional defects, which may be exhibited as impulsive behaviors. Such children are commonly referred to as hyperactive. The classic description of this behavioral pattern includes distractability, lack of proper inhibition, overly intense responses, and perseverative or compulsive behaviors. Such children appear to be "always on the go" and display a low tolerance for frustration, to which they respond with emotional lability and a tendency toward temper tantrums.

For the wildly overactive child, the diagnosis is apparent. However, it has been stressed that ability to focus and maintain attention is really a "cognitive style" (Kinsbourne & Caplan, 1979), and acceptable styles vary from one culture to another. Chinese, for example, may deny children any opportunity to act out, while another culture would accept practically any degree of overactivity. Within the American culture, some homes are highly structured with rigid codes of behavior, whereas others allow children great freedom. In addition, the need for highly focused attention varies for all children from home to school. Consequently, the identification of attentional problems varies widely and, to some extent, is culture-specific.

Impulsiveness and lack of focus of attention not only vary according to the culture but also according to the situation. Almost everyone becomes overactive when faced with a monotonous task or a long wait. Some children in school or therapy may be "fidgety" because they face boring tasks—not because they are hyperactive.

The factors considered to cause these problems also differ according to cultures. Some cultures blame parents and family dynamics for all behavioral problems, other cultures blame the environment and toxins, while a few deny the possibility of the disorder even existing. Attentional problems have long been associated with children with language-learning problems (Strauss & Lehtinen, 1947; Strauss & Kephart, 1955). Efforts to establish a cause have indicated that these children may lack normal cerebral inhibition (Ong, 1968) or may have problems in selective attention and focused arousal (Sheer, 1976). Some researchers suggest that these patterns of behavior may be inherited (there is a distinct sex difference, with from 5 to 10 boys affected for every girl), or that they may represent brain damage (Eisenson, 1972), postnatal disease, food allergy (Crook, 1975; Safer & Allen, 1976), or a selective developmental lag in maturation of relevant areas of the brain (Kinsbourne & Caplan, 1979; Safer & Allen, 1976).

The treatment of choice for children with attentional problems that are severe enough to interfere with functioning continues to be with medication stimulants. It used to be thought that stimulants had a "paradoxical" effect on these children in that the stimulant "calmed" them. According to Kinsbourne and Caplan (1979), this is not true; the medication prolongs concentration and heightens attention in these children just as it would in any normal person. The use of this medication engenders many strong feelings, with some critics (Walker, 1974) expressing concern that the medications may have dangerous side effects. Yet other professionals report treating large numbers of cases with no ill effects. Regardless of treatment, this behavior tends to lessen spontaneously by 13 to 15 years of age, although in a few cases it may persist into adulthood (Kinsbourne & Caplan, 1979; Safer & Allen, 1976).

In the integrative model, attentional defects are considered apart from any of the dimensions of language. Their effect on language development is to reduce the child's potential for all learning and to interfere with child–adult and child-peer relationships in the dimension of the communication environment. No study has substantiated a causal relationship between attentional problems and language disorders.

THEORIES OF LINGUISTIC DELAY VERSUS DEVIANCE

Following the great advances in linguistics during the past twenty years, it appeared that linguistic analysis might be powerful enough to resolve the enigma of clinical language disorders. The pivotal concern around which many studies revolved was the question of whether language disorder represents a *delay* in the acquisition of the knowledge and use of the code or whether the language-disordered child has some fundamental *deviation* in his knowledge of the linguistic code. These studies provided the first careful linguistic analysis of language disorders, and consequently the methods and results used are of importance to the language specialist. Following trends in linguistics, the majority of the studies focused first on analysis of syntax, and more recently on semantic and phonological components of the linguistic code.

Syntax

Menyuk (1964a) was the first researcher to use the techniques of generative grammar to analyze the syntax of both linguistically deviant and normal children. She found that the deviant group used fewer transformations and produced more restricted and ungrammatic forms. It was her contention that these children displayed not delayed language, but deviant language that was qualitatively different from the language of normal children. In a follow-up study in 1969, Menyuk noted that language-disordered children produced various characteristic utterances, which seemed to indicate that they were operating with a different hypothesis about language. She noted deviant question forms such as "Where hang it?" and other deviant utterances such as "No ride feet" ("I ride without using feet"), "He'm put" ("He's putting") and "Big the dog" ("The dog is big"). In 1972, Menyuk and Looney again investigated language-disordered children and controls. They found that the language-disordered children had significant problems with syntactic structure. When asked to imitate sentences, they failed because of complicated structure, not because of the length of the sentences. Their omissions occurred selectively, and they omitted verbal auxiliary and the modal (*will, can, could, might,* etc.) most frequently. This study supported the hypothesis that the language system is somehow deviant in language-disordered children.

Menyuk's earlier studies were followed almost immediately by investigations by Lee (1966), who suggested that language-disordered children failed to make some of the linguistic generalizations upon which syntactic development rested. Although this observation supported the concept of deviant language, Lee modified this position in her 1974 book when she used the term "clinical children" and avoided the use of either *language delay* or *language disorder.* Lee's rather intensive study (1974) of the language of these children paid particular attention to verb elaboration, which is one of the most complicated features in English. She found that language-disordered children had particular difficulty with the copula, which they tended to simplify to the single word *be.* She observed a tendency for language-disordered children to use fewer and simpler grammatic rules. Lee's work is generally considered to support the deviant hypothesis.

Eisenson and Ingram (1972) stated that the difference between disordered and normal language was a quantitative one and constituted a delay. The aphasic child is slow to develop the rules for grammatic use and, rather than needing only about 50 words to begin to use phrases (as a normal child does), the disordered child must have at least 200 words. In Eisenson and Ingram's opinion, the quantitative nature of the problem supported the strength of language universals that were observed even in this population.

Morehead and Ingram (1973) made the important observation that most of the studies done in the 1960s matched subjects on the basis of their chronological age. In their own study, subjects were matched according to their level of language development as determined by the mean length of utterance. With this correction, it was found that while normal children passed very quickly through the two-word stage, disordered children remained at that stage for a long period. Disordered children not only were abnormally slow in learning first words, but the rate of further language acquisition was three times slower than the rate for normals. In particular, language-disordered children seem to use noun and verb combinations very late, tending instead to use more verbs and particles, such as "sitting down" or "fall down." Morehead and Ingram interpreted this to mean that the language of language-disordered children was delayed, not deviant. Further support for the delay hypothesis was provided by Johnston and Schery (1976), who observed that languaged-disordered children acquired grammatic morphemes in the same order as normal children. However, it took them much longer than normal children to reach a 90 percent criterion for correct use of the morphemes.

Semantics

The semantic development of the language-disordered child also appears to be characteristically delayed. Morehead and Ingram (1973) noted delayed acquisition of words. Eisenson (1972) found that some children may remain essentially nonverbal until age 4 or 5. Other investigators (Johnston & Schery, 1976; Leonard, Bolders, & Miller, 1976) found that their subjects were also late in learning to say words. After the language-delayed child begins to use words, he tends to remain less fluent than other children. Lee (1974, p. 83), noted that the children in her clinical sample tended to remain silent unless "prompted" or "prodded" to speak. In their case study, Crystal et al. (1976) reported that the 3-year-old language-disordered child they studied produced 80 percent of his utterances in response to direct questions. This impression of reduced verbalization was supported by Morehead and Ingram (1973), who noted that the mean number of utterances produced by normals in their study was 175.5, but it was only 148.7 for the language disordered.

Phonology

Possibly because of the tradition in speech pathology that articulation problems are a separate defect and should be studied apart from clinical language disorder, the articulatory defects of language-disordered children have received relatively little attention. However, following several studies (Menyuk, 1964a; Menyuk & Looney, 1972) of children with so-called functional articulation problems, a positive relationship between syntax and phonology was established. This was of particular interest because so many children with clinical language disorders have articulatory defects. DeAjuriaguerra et al. (1965) noted that 40 percent of the language-disordered children they studied had articulation problems. Eisenson (1972, p. 189) felt that virtually all children with developmental aphasia were speech-impaired, and Menyuk (1978b) concurred that most language-disordered children appeared to have difficulty with the phonological aspects of language. Again, the question of delay versus deviance appeared to influence the studies. D. Ingram (1976) felt that language-disordered children used phonological processes that were *not* typical of normal children. However, following a detailed analysis of the articulation of a single child, Grunwell (1980) concluded that the phonological development of this language-disordered child had been "arrested" at the very earliest stage of development. It was her contention that language disorders were expressed in the phonological system as well as in the other linguistic systems.

The literature on normal phonological development indicates that normal children show certain predictable tendencies, including consonant assimilation (gɔg for frog) and consonant re-

Paula Menyuk

Paula Menyuk's doctoral dissertation, submitted to the University of Boston in 1961, was one of the first descriptive studies of syntactic structures in the language of children. It heralded the beginning of the many studies based upon Chomsky's 1957 theories that were to be accomplished by linguistically sophisticated educators and clinicians. Menyuk was also a pioneer in describing the differences between the grammatic abilities of normal and language-disordered children. She hypothesized that the linguistic systems of language-disordered children were deviant, not simply delayed. Her application of distinctive feature theory to the acquisition of phonology in children was also a pioneer effort.

A native of New York City, Menyuk did her undergraduate work at New York University and spent several years as a teacher of speech and English in the New York City schools. She was then employed as a speech pathologist at the Massachusetts General Hospital in Boston. She subsequently obtained her Ed.D. at Boston University in 1961. She was awarded Fellowship in the American Speech and Hearing Association in 1967. Menyuk holds a research appointment in speech communication and psycholinguistics at the Massachusetts Institute of Technology and is professor of Psycholinguistics at Boston University.

duplication (baba for bottle). Leonard, Miller, and Brown (1980) studied eight language-disordered children and found certain common assimilation and reduplication errors that helped to illustrate the articulatory problems of these children. The authors concluded that assimilation and reduplication were used by language-disordered children in the same manner that they were used by normal children at very young ages. The difference was that the language-disordered children used these processes for prolonged periods. To further explore the question of the relationship between the phonological system and other linguistic systems, R. G. Schwartz et al. (1980) studied normal and language-disordered children matched for language age at an MLU of 1.14. They concluded that the processes used by the language-disordered were not different from those employed by normal children on a comparable language level.

An important effort to distinguish between delayed and deviant language was made by Leonard (1972), who reviewed the major studies and compared the results to his own data. His conclusions lent support to Menyuk's (1964) contention that the speech of deviant language users was not directly comparable to the speech of younger children. Despite these various studies focusing on the acquisition of syntax, semantics, and phonology by language-disordered children, there is still no consensus regarding the issue of delay versus deviance. This is possibly because of several problems with this type of analysis. Children may be chosen for study on the basis of their observed language delay, and so, obviously, when their language is measured, it will be found to be delayed. In some cases, this delay may reflect a generalized developmental problem rather than clinical language disorder. A second problem is that subjects may be evaluated on a single aspect of language without determining if other aspects of language are adequate or even above average. A delay in one aspect of language does not guarantee a generalized delay. If only a single component of language is delayed then *deviance* may actually be a better term than *delay* to characterize this discrepancy between one language behavior and another within the same child. Finally, and most importantly, a simplification of the language code is the expected result of a problem in any specific language area. A child with a clinical language disorder simplifies his language in the same manner as a child who is learning language. This simplified language will appear like that of the young child, but there will be differences in the reasons and the extent of simplification. As described in Chapter 8, the order of difficulty of forms is based on the cognitive difficulty of the meaning, the structural difficulty, the semantic complexity, and the frequency of occurrence of the forms in the environment. Language performance in the disordered child may *appear* to be like that of a younger child, but may in fact be different because of a cognitive, structural, semantic, or environmental problem. In this sense, then, the performance is not delayed but rather deviant or atypical.

CLINICAL LANGUAGE DISORDERS AND THE COMMUNICATION ENVIRONMENT

An obvious problem for the child with language impairment is that others will not be able to understand him. Before evaluating how disordered children respond to this circumstance, it is interesting to note how normal adults react when they are not understood. Longhurst and Siegel (1973) found that when normal adults could not be understood (due to mechanical distortion of their voice as a part of the experiment), they gave longer descriptions, restricted the diversity of their vocabularies, and talked more slowly. The investigators noted that the speakers' only reward for this behavior was that they could be understood.

This exploration was then extended to normal children. Gallagher (1977) taped an hour of conversation with children whose language was at Brown's stage I, II, or III. Twenty times during that hour the investigator indicated that she did not understand what the children were saying. The most common response of these normal children was to revise their utterance. In a subsequent experiment (Gallagher & Darnton, 1978), children with language disorders whose language level was also at Brown's stage I, II, or III were studied. In both experiments, there were three possible responses. The children could repeat what they had said, they could revise what they had said, or they could refuse to respond again. Over 75 percent of the time, both the normal and language-disordered children revised what they had said, but the language-disordered children tended to reduce the complexity of the structure when they revised and as a result, often deleted major sentence components. Their revisions were unsophisticated and qualitatively different from the revisions of the normal children at the same stage of language development. [Adults studied by Longhurst and Siegel (1973) gave *longer* descriptions].

The ways in which a silent or difficult-to-understand child may modify the responses of family members and ultimately affect his communication environment is of considerable relevance. To explore this aspect of communication, language-disordered children between 2 years, 8 months and 5 years, 6 months of age were matched with normal children of the same age, representing five social classes ranging from lower class to upper class (Wulbert et al., 1975). Mother–child interaction was studied using an interview technique. Some significant differences were found between the language-disordered and normal children in certain categories. One difference was in the manner of discipline. Mothers of normal children tended to reason with their children, which was often sufficient to change their behavior. Mothers of language-disordered children were quick to shout, threaten, and spank. The most significant difference was in the extent of maternal involvement with the children. Unlike the mothers of normal children, who played and interacted with their children, mothers of language-disordered children showed little interaction with their children. The study indicated that children affected parental behavior, and the mothers reported that the language-disordered children discouraged efforts to play with them, read to them, etc.

Cramblit and Siegel (1977) studied the speech addressed to a 4-year-old boy with a language disorder by his parents and a baby sitter and compared it to speech addressed to the boy's normal 4-year-old cousin. The results indicated that all speech directed to the language-disordered child was simplified. The adults used more single-word utterances and simpler constructions when speaking to the language-impaired boy than to his cousin. The authors concluded that there was reason to believe that adults other than those in the study would behave in the same fashion. The adults reacted to cues offered by the child, suggesting that the language stimulation the language-disordered child receives is directly influenced by his verbal proficiency. Thus, the child with a clinical language disorder may have a different verbal environment than the normal child.

INTEGRATIVE APPROACH TO CLINICAL LANGUAGE DISORDERS

It is apparent that no specific symptom complex has yet been identified as characteristic of the entire group of children with clinical language disorders. On the contrary, there is increasing evidence that *clinical language disorder* is a nonspecific term referring to a still undetermined number of *patterns* of language disorders, each of which appears to be characterized by differing degrees of impairment of certain units of the four dimensions of language discussed in this volume. An integrative model of language allows for this diversity.

In the earlier definition of terms, it was shown that the classification of clinical language disorder is made on the basis of exclusion and discrepancy. This discrepancy, which is characteristic of clinical language disorder, may be further illustrated by reviewing several illustrative patterns of clinical language disorders. The purpose of this presentation is not to add to the already overwhelming nomenclature in the field by suggesting that children be actually labeled as pattern A or pattern D or that there are only four or five possible patterns. Rather, the examples are provided to illustrate the effect of dysfunction in certain units of the dimensions of language. The continued use of the term *clinical language disorder* is appropriate. What needs to be done with greater care is to specify the strengths and weaknesses of each child. The variety of symptoms in clinical language disorders has been noted and described in terms of patterns by others (Aram & Nation, 1975; Crystal et al., 1976). More recently Stark and Tallal (1981) concluded that, despite their care in selecting subjects with language deficits, their experimental group was still not homogeneous. They felt that the children they chose displayed different patterns of deficits, especially in sensory, perceptual, and motor abilities. This trend toward the description of patterns of clinical language disorders has potential for clarifying this disability.

Pattern A

Some children with clinical language disorders may have a severe defect in auditory perception. This particular pattern of language disorder is shown in Figure 13-1. As the figure illus-

Figure 13-1
A model of one pattern of a clinical language disorder showing particular impairment in perceptual ability. Other deficits that may be predicted to occur in other dimensions as a result of this impairment are indicated by asterisks.

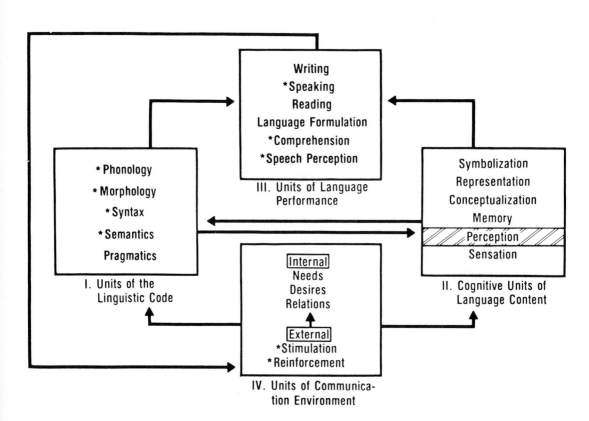

trates, the impairment in perception (one of the cognitive units of language) may be expected to affect various other units of language and contribute to the language performance problems observed during testing.

> From the earliest months of life, Abel did not perceive speech sounds accurately enough or quickly enough to make the proper association between the auditory stimuli and the concepts he developed. He obviously heard sounds. He also had developed many age-appropriate concepts about the permanence of objects, their function, and the relationship of objects to people. Abel seemed anxious to communicate, yet he failed to begin saying words, and his ability to understand what others said to him was impaired. His perceptual dysfunction was reflected in a semantic problem (knowledge of the linguistic code), which in turn affected his performance of both the comprehension and expression of language. Once Abel began to learn the code, his problems in mastering the open class of words persisted long after he had learned the closed class of function words and morphosyntactic structures. Although all facets of the linguistic code were delayed, the semantic problem was most significant. As he grew older, Abel had particular difficulty when he was expected to learn in noisy environments or against competing noise.

Pattern B

A rather specific deficit in one dimension of language may influence both oral and written language.

> Barbie had a deficit in auditory memory. She was able to match the auditory signal to concepts adequately, but in order to do so it was necessary for her to hear the word many more times than a normal child would require. Barbie was somewhat delayed in the onset of speech, but her problem attracted little attention, despite her "atypical" use of language forms. When she entered school, she experienced problems in learning to read. She had trouble recalling new vocabulary words and this was reflected in her expressive language. Barbie also had trouble following directions, and her assignments were often incorrectly done because she could not remember the entire direction. Barbie's memory deficit caused problems in language performance, such as reading, which places stress on the memory system.

Pattern C

The relationship of symbolic functioning to language performance is fundamental. Some children with clinical language disorders exhibit symbolic deficits, which may be expressed through problems in grasping certain abstract and shifting relationships.

As a toddler, Carl lacked the "pretend" function of language. He rarely participated in "make-believe" games, and he never pretended, for example, that he was mowing the grass or shaving like daddy. Carl learned to say his first words at the expected time, but as he grew older he had particular difficulty in learning and using abstract words—such as words expressing time and space—correctly. His prepositions were often in error, giving his speech a "foreign" quality. Carl is the type of child who might be expected to stop a teacher to ask where "around the corner" was located; Carl had great trouble in understanding that in order to follow directions the listener must appreciate that the direction was specific to the speaker's location at the time the statement was made. Carl was late to learn how to tell time and his tense markers were often in error. He remained confused and upset by the fact that by *tomorrow* the time he referred to as *today* would be called *yesterday*. As he progressed in school, Carl exhibited continuing problems with mathematics and geography.

Pattern D

As the integrative model of language indicates, concepts must be matched with the linguistic code. Failure to do this leads to significant problems in both comprehension and production of language.

As a preschooler, Dora showed evidence of purposeful use of objects, and she appeared to be trying to communicate her ideas. However, she produced little spontaneous speech beyond echoing and social greetings. Dora's ability to comprehend was limited to a few substantive words. Since she could repeat, it was apparent that her perception and memory were intact. Her semantic problem appeared to be related to a failure to match concepts with the linguistic code. Her automatic perceptual-motor system and meaning system were poorly integrated.

Pattern E

Still another group of children has specific problems with the formulation of language. They are unable to encode their ideas into the appropriate lexical and syntactic units.

Ernie's concept formation, memory, and comprehension of language appeared adequate-to-superior for his age. Still, Ernie was slow to speak. Once he began to talk, he combined his few single words imaginatively with gestures and context to convey sophisticated semantic intentions. While still producing only a few words, such as *daddy, go, car,* and *ball,* Ernie was able to convey to the clinician the news that his father had taken him to see a baseball game. With cooperative questioning, he could even demonstrate the home run that won the game. As his vocabulary increased, Ernie's speech continued to be slow and groping. He often seemed to be searching for the right word and failing that, made mistakes such as calling a "birthday cake" a "getting married cake."

To diagnose a child as having a clinical language disorder indicates that the child has failed to comprehend and/or express language appropriately for his chronological and mental age; that the child's language problem is not an expected component of one of the developmental disabilities; and that the problem is characterized by a discrepancy in and among the various dimensions of language.

Although many symptoms of language disorder are common (because the linguistic code can only be modified along certain specific parameters); the children who have the disorders differ widely. Understanding the differences among children appears to be directly associated with the success of intervention. Children with clinical language disorders may be expected to display both delays in the acquisition of the linguistic code and deviance in certain selected aspects of the expression of that code (see Fig. 11-1).

ASSESSMENT

For all children with suspected clinical language disorders, the importance of ruling out sensory hearing loss is apparent, yet sometimes this may be difficult to accomplish. In one of the earlier studies of language disorders, Ewing (1930) observed that six of the ten language-disordered children in his study had a high-frequency hearing loss. Mark and Hardy (1958) reported on language-disordered children who displayed what they described as "orienting reflex disturbances;" i.e., they failed to respond to newly introduced sounds that would elicit orienting responses in normal children. These observations indicated that, in the past at least, the audiometric evaluation of the language-disordered child was difficult. With current audiometric techniques, the kind of sensory losses documented in the past should be identified on initial diagnosis. However, the language specialist should be alert to the child who is particularly difficult to test audiometrically. Cromer (1978) felt that inconsistent response to sound may be either a contributory cause or an effect of language disorder.

After ruling out the possibility of hearing loss, the language specialist may focus on different test protocols, depending upon the pattern of the child's language disorder. In the assessment of children like Abel (Pattern A), it would be of particular importance to evaluate various aspects of nonspeech perception; whenever children demonstrate obvious impairment in comprehension, the development of nonverbal concepts needs to be carefully explored to rule out mental retardation.

In the assessment of children like Barbie (Pattern B), standardized tests of speech perception and verbal memory help clarify the limits of their ability. Naturalistic assessment revealed the sources of some of Barbie's atypical expressions. She produced utterances like "She cooking something" or "Smokes is here," indicating several morphosyntactic errors characteristic of delayed development. Yet another utterance in her picture description, "The woman running after the dog," utilized a complex prepositional phrase, despite the omission of the auxilliary. Analysis of Barbie's errors suggests delayed development of language, but analysis of her strengths from the same language sample illustrates that the delay may be specific to certain structures and may represent deviance in the development of the code.

Another assessment principle is illustrated by a child called Fred. Fred was considered immature by his parents, so he was screened prior to his enrollment in school. He fell below the mean on the language screening test, and a language specialist was consulted. When the language scores were compared to other scores, it was apparent that Fred was below the mean but still within the range of normal in all areas of performance and did not display a clinical language disorder. "Normal" includes children like Fred who are below the mean as well as children above the mean.

Another child, Greg, demonstrated what has been called *oral* or *verbal apraxia* (Chappel, 1973; Eisenson, 1972). Such children often demonstrate severe articulatory defects, even though they have no auditory imperception, no lack of ideas, and show an intact knowledge of all linguistic systems. Greg fell below the mean in expressive language. Unlike Fred, Greg scored above age level in every area except verbal production. However, he was persistently silent as a preschooler, and at school age still produced only a few single-word utterances. Testing revealed difficulty in combining and sequencing phonemes and inconsistent substitutions on the phonological level. In addition, he had difficulty in executing movements of the speech musculature on command even though he could perform the same task (such as licking his lips) spontaneously.

Once a clinical language disorder is confirmed, the classification of the units of language that show greatest impairment has significance for intervention. Analysis of verbal performance alone is not sufficient evidence on which to base assessment conclusions nor to plan effective intervention.

INTERVENTION

There is little question that significant clinical language disorders are not reversible without intervention. (Chapter 12 provides general principles for choosing curriculum.) Following the popularity of the tests such as the Illinois Test of Psycholinguistic Ability, the assumption was made by many language specialists that when a specific deficit was observed, that defect could be individually trained and thus language would improve in a commensurate manner. Hammill and Larsen (1974) reviewed thirty-eight different studies that measured the effectiveness of such training, and the results did not support this contention. A child like Abel (Pattern A), who demonstrated a serious perceptual discrimination problem, does not need drill on discrimination. Rather, the first step should be to modify the environment so that he can hear speech spoken at a slower rate in quiet surroundings. If he fails to understand, utterances should be reworded to further assist him in compensating. As the child gets older, his perceptual problem can be explained to him, and he can participate in efforts to modify his own listening environment.

Pattern B illustrated the type of child who could not be expected to benefit from specific drill on memory. Such children need to be taught better ways to attend, where to sit in class, and how to compensate. For example, they may be taught to take very simple notes on assignments, to ask the teacher to check these notes, and/or to enlist the help of a friend to take notes. In addition, they might be helped to learn to visualize messages and recall pictures instead of words.

During assessment, Carl (Pattern C) was identified as having symbolic problems that resulted in certain morphosyntactic errors. Despite the prevalence of language programs designed to drill on the use of these forms in sentence slots, such an approach would not be the most beneficial one for a child like Carl, who needs to develop the concepts underlying time and space. Instead of teaching prepositions of location, intervention might focus on body image and developing awareness of sidedness, directionality, space, and distance. Space and time are dynamic and relative concepts that cannot be memorized and are best learned in functional situations. As deAjuriaguerra et al. (1976) indicated, the rates of improvement of language-disordered children were more dependent upon the functional utility of the skills than upon the intensity of the exercises in a training program.

Some children with clinical language disorders (Pattern D) require a structured program of semantic development. Based upon the child's pattern of language disorder, this structured program should concentrate on the direct and immediate pairing of a word with a corresponding experience. A program that utilized modeling or imitation would not be as effective.

Programs of intervention need to demonstrate to the child the functional benefit of communication. There is evidence (Hubbell, 1977) that highly constrained therapy situations focusing on questions and commands tend to inhibit rather than encourage talking. Experience has suggested that the pragmatic rules of language are as likely to be impaired as are other systems, so emphasis on the functional use of language allows practice in these areas. The language specialist using an integrative approach would begin intervention with a knowledge of the units of language showing the most impairment and with the goal of maximizing the child's performance in all dimensions of language.

It has now been almost 40 years since Strauss and his colleagues began to develop intervention programs for the "brain-injured child." Although, follow-up studies are still very limited, deAjuriaguerra et al. (1976) completed an extensive follow-up of children over a period of 2 to 4 years. Their study revealed continuing deficits in intellectual and academic development. P. R. Hall and Tomblin (1978) did a retrospective study of 36 of 281 children previously seen at the University of Iowa Speech and Hearing Clinic. Parents of the eighteen children in the language-impaired group agreed that their children continued to exhibit some deviations in either language or articulation. They also displayed a lower level of achievement in reading. Reading problems in this group have been predicted by other researchers (Johnson & Myklebust, 1967; Wiig & Semel, 1976). Researchers and educators are clearly faced with continuing challenges in the area of intervention.

outline

ASPECTS OF THE RELATIONSHIP BETWEEN READING AND LANGUAGE

Oral Language Prerequisites for Reading
Comparison of Graphic and Oral Language
Reading and Speech Behavior
The Oral and Graphic Codes
Perception in Written and Spoken Language

THE PROCESS OF READING

The Role of Vision in Reading
Reading and Auditory Processes
The Subvocalization Hypothesis
The Direct Access Hypothesis
The Phonological Recoding Hypothesis

LEARNING TO READ

The Reading Tests
Developmental Aspects of Reading

READING DISORDERS AND GENERAL LANGUAGE PERFORMANCE

Phonetic Skills in Reading Disorders
Reading and Linguistic Knowledge
Syntactic and Semantic Processing and Reading
Oral Language Performance of Poor Readers

READING DISORDERS AND THE DIMENSIONS OF LANGUAGE

THE LANGUAGE SPECIALIST AND READING DISORDERS

reading disorders and language disorders

14

THE INCLUSION OF a chapter on reading and reading disorders in a text on language disorders is rare; however, the integrative approach demands that such a chapter be included. Reading is an aspect of language and it follows that reading disorders can be validly interpreted if viewed within the framework of clinical disorders of language.

Since learning disabilities are ordinarily characterized by reading problems, and if reading problems are in fact disorders of language, language disorders and learning disabilities may be the same behaviors. Perhaps *language disorder* is more appropriate for describing preschool oral language problems and *learning disability* is more appropriate for the description of school-related problems.

Historically, the reading process has been the primary concern of curriculum specialists in primary and elementary schools. As a result, reading has been viewed in terms of a subject to be learned in the same manner that history, math, and science are learned. Reading programs have been developed as separate all-inclusive units; reading teachers have been prepared to teach the reading curriculum, and reading specialists have been responsible for the diagnosis and remediation of reading problems. Within this approach, reading has been considered to be primarily a visual skill, comprised of learning visual characters that are associated with sounds. As a consequence, problems in learning reading skills have been most frequently studied in relations to problems in visual perception.

As a result of developments in psycholinguistics, a surge of theoretical and practical insights about reading has changed the visual perspective of reading to a language perspective. It appears that the broad perspective, which considers reading an aspect of language, is beginning to provide answers to questions regarding reading failure. An understanding of the nature of the reading behavior process in terms of its place in the communication-cognitive-linguistic-performance model of language may yield teaching approaches that take into account these factors.

This chapter provides a description of reading from the perspective of language as well as a description of reading disorders from the perspective of language disorders. Neither descriptions of nor labels for reading disorders, their causes, or the controversy over the merits of various methods of teaching are presented, except as they pertain to the relationship between reading and language.

ASPECTS OF THE RELATIONSHIP BETWEEN READING AND LANGUAGE

Oral Language Prerequisites for Reading

A child entering first grade has already mastered many language development skills. Ruddell (1976) listed five language behaviors important to the success of the beginning reader: (1) recognizing and producing novel sentences; (2) discriminating between grammatic and nongrammatic sentences; (3) utilizing context and prosodic clues to discover the meaning of sentences having the same surface structure; (4) comprehending sentences that possess different surface structures but have identical underlying meaning; and (5) comprehending sentences with identical constituent structures but different deep structures.

Samuel Torrey Orton

In 1925, Samuel Orton, a neuropathologist, published an article entitled "Word Blindness in School Children," which described a group of children who had reading disorders that were qualitatively different from problems caused by environmental factors. This historic essay initiated study into what is today called *dyslexia*. Although Orton's description of these disorders focused on the visual-spatial problems that characterized them, he thought that the cause of such problems is related to a developmental delay that defers the normal establishment of hemispheric dominance for language—thus implying that the reading function was a part of the language function. According to Orton, the view of reading as a language-specific function was further supported by the fact that visual-spatial confusions occurred only in language-coded information and not in other visual-motor activites.

Orton's views were elaborated in a book published in 1937, entitled *Reading, Writing and Speech Problems in Children*. Evidence of his continued influence in the area of reading disorders is the Orton Society, founded in 1949, an organization of individuals devoted to the understanding and improvement of dyslexia.

The basic structure of the oral language used by the child will be used for writing and reading. The child's mastery or lack of mastery of specific syntactic structures and word meanings will be reflected in his understanding of what he reads or in the lexicon and grammar of his written language. Frequently, when a child's oral language behaviors are disordered, his reading performance is also frequently affected.

Comparison of Graphic and Oral Language

Reading and Speech Behavior

The primary purpose of both graphic and oral language is communication. The written and oral forms of language are based on the same linguistic foundation, and, except for the peripheral aspects of the processes, the stages through which a spoken or written sentence must pass on the way to being comprehended are the same. The stages through which an idea must pass on the way to being spoken or written are also the same. Comprehension must ultimately be represented in the same mental symbolic system.

Wardhaugh (1976) identified some of the differences between written and spoken language: Whereas oral language is acquired gradually, the ability to read often occurs in a relatively short span of time. The process of learning to comprehend and speak is not accomplished through conscious effort; reading is taught formally and needs awareness on the part of the child. Children begin using oral language at different ages, and the differences among children in age and stage of development are accepted by parents and others; in learning to read, all children are expected to perform successfully within a 6- to 8-month period, regardless of chronological age, mental age, or any other factor.

Mattingly (1972) reported that adult reading is a faster process than listening; some people can read over 2000 words per minute, whereas the maximum possible rate of listening is 400 words per minute. Also, the reader has access to a more or less permanent graphic input, whereas the listener has input that in most cases perishes as it is produced (Goodman, 1970).

The Oral and Graphic Codes

In English, reading begins with graphic characters, which symbolize the sounds of English, which in turn form the grammatic structures, which in turn symbolize meaning. As is true of the vocal code, the written code is arbitrary; i.e., the characters that represent the sounds have no intrinsic meaning or relationship to the sounds. There are rules of correspondence (although not perfect ones) between the graphic symbols and the phonemic ones. The linear stream of phoneme sequences that makes up oral language is converted into written language by graphic representations of the phonemes arranged from left to right on a line, and from top to bottom in successive lines.

The spoken stream of sounds utilizes pauses, vocal intonation, and stress to provide meaning although there are no divisions between individual words. The units of spoken language are syllables. Each syllable contains a vowel or vowel-like sound that may or may not have modifying consonants preceding or following it. Syllables follow one another in temporal sequence—we utter them one at a time. Words or bound morphemes may be composed of one or more syllables, so the ability to identify them depends on the listener's knowledge of the language.

In many languages, the boundaries for written words are marked by space, and the boundaries for ideas and transformations are marked by punctuation. In writing, language information, which is primarily temporal and housed in the auditory system, must be converted to written forms, which are primarily spatial and housed in the visual system.

Perception in Written and Spoken Language

The point of contact in spoken language is the auditory processing system, whereas the point of contact in written language is visual perception. In both instances, the information provided to the listener/reader may be ambiguous, imperfect, and unclear; the listener/reader must provide information that makes it possible to understand the message of the stimulus.

In listening, sounds are frequently fleeting, distorted, or follow each other so rapidly that each cannot be fully perceived and identified; the knowledge and flexibility of the human processor makes compensations and fills in what is missing. Similarly, the reading text can be transformed through inversion or rotation of letters or transposition of letter and word order without destroying its readability by skilled readers (Geyer & Kolers, 1976). Goodman (1967) has called reading a psycholinguistic guessing game, since efficient reading does not result from precise perception but from skill in selecting the fewest most productive cues necessary to produce guesses that are right at the first contact with the input.

THE PROCESS OF READING

The Role of Vision in Reading

Reading begins with eye fixation. The reader's eyes focus on a point slightly indented from the beginning of the line of print and remain there for about 250 milliseconds; the eyes then move to the right to a new fixation (Gough, 1972). There are differences among adults, however, in the rate and duration of fixation. Brewer (1972) suggested that there is interaction between higher linguistic processing and the control of eye fixations; therefore, the characteristic of the linguistic material influences the fixation. Evidence in the literature on visual perception, reported by Gilbert (1976), indicates that in reading simple prose, slow readers use a smaller span of visual perception and a longer fixation pause than do faster readers.

Gilbert (1976) suggested three purposes for the fixation pause in reading: (1) when at rest, the eyes are more efficient in transmitting visual stimuli to the brain; (2) maximum functional efficiency in processing is achieved when the retina or cortex can have an interval of time free from interfering visual stimuli; and (3) the fixation provides time needed to comprehend the ideas and relationships involved in the passage read.

When the initial fixation takes place, a visual pattern is reflected onto the retina, which sets in motion a sequence of activity in the visual system that culminates in the formation of an *icon* (Gough, 1972), a relatively direct representation or image of a visual stimulus that persists for a brief period after the stimulus vanishes. It is an unidentified precategorical visual representation of strings of printed words, which may appear as bands, curves, angles, etc. (See Chapter 4 for an analogous description of speech perception.) According to Gough, the icon buffer has a capacity of at least seventeen or eighteen letters presented in three rows of six each. The useful content of the icon is about twenty letter spaces of a line under fixation. It is believed that letters are received all at the same time, rather than in sequence as in auditory perception (Brewer, 1972). The icon persists for less than half of a second in light and remains until displaced by the icon arising from the second fixation.

The method of analysis of the letters in the icon is not clearly understood (Foss & Hakes, 1978). The letters may be identified serially—one at a time and in a left-to-right order, or the letters are all worked on at once in a parallel manner. Feature theorists claim that the contents of the icon are analyzed for features of graphemes (abstract representations corresponding to letters) or that significant groups of graphemes are reconstructed (Foss & Hakes, 1978). Once letters are recovered from the icon, the reading process involves higher levels of linguistic organization for word recognition and comprehension.

Reading and Auditory Processes

It is generally accepted that reading uses some of the same processes as listening. Most theorists agree that once the syntactic units are identified, the process of decoding these units and arriving at the meaning of an utterance is the same for both reading and listening. There is disagreement, however, regarding the stage at which the visual and auditory systems merge and the inputs from both systems pass through a common pathway. Some believe that the characters of reading must first be converted into abstract sound units and that the process of reconstruction then follows the same lines as the sounds received in listening. Crowder (1972) stated that visual input in reading passes through a visual store and is then recoded into auditory form before it can be understood. Others (Conrad, 1972; LaBerge, 1972) believed that the comprehension of printed material may take place directly from the visual input. LaBerge (1972) considered it conceiveable that both the auditory and visual codes may be involved with the comprehension process in a parallel manner during the reading. Foss and Hakes (1978) organized the points of view regarding the relationship between listening and reading into three major hypotheses, the subvocalization hypothesis, the direct access hypothesis, and the phonological reading hypothesis.

The Subvocalization Hypothesis

The subvocalization hypothesis asserts that reading involves actually talking to oneself, i.e., converting the graphic material into subvocal speech and listening to what one says. Once the graphic signals are translated into subvocal speech signals, the reader translates them into lexical representations as in speech perception and then into the states through which speech ordinarily passes on the way to being understood.

The major objection to this theory is that it does not account for high reading rates as compared to listening rates. The time it takes to say the words, listen to them, and comprehend would be much longer than it is for fast readers.

The Direct Access Hypothesis

The direct access hypothesis states that the printed material makes direct contact with the mental lexicon. The reading input does not pass through a speech processing unit but converges with the speech process *after* the word meanings have been recovered and the process is no longer bound to a specific input modality. This theory considers every word to be like a logogram, in which the graphic signs do not relate to spoken sounds. The reader would have to learn an association between each separate word and its meaning—there would be no coding of the written word. This would place a greater burden on visual memory. Foss and Hakes (1978) stated that this would require 50,000 to 100,000 new connections for highly literate people.

The Phonological Recoding Hypothesis

This hypothesis states that the reader recodes the graphic representation of letters into the representation of systematic

The subvocalization hypothesis in lay terms. (The Lockhorns by Bill Hoest, reprinted courtesy of King Features.)

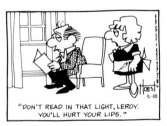

"DON'T READ IN THAT LIGHT, LEROY. YOU'LL HURT YOUR LIPS."

READING DISORDERS AND LANGUAGE DISORDERS

phonemes. Systematic phonemes are underlying abstract en-
tites, which are related to the sounds of language because they
form an internal representation of these sounds. In spoken language, the lexical store contains the phonological representation of each entry. In reading, the phonological representation
is assigned to the printed word, and the reader thereby has access to the lexical store without going through the speech loop
at all (Gough, 1972). The lexical storage contains the syntactic
and semantic information needed for reading comprehension.
Thus, the retrieval mechanism used for speech is employed by
recoding graphic characters to phonological ones. (N. Chomsky
[1970] suggested that the recoding is from the visual units to a
lexical representation—to phonological units that have meaning.)

   There are numerous arguments and evidence available to
support and refute the phonological recoding hypothesis (Foss
& Hakes, 1978, pp. 336–341.) It appears that this hypothesis
cannot be accepted as the only explanation of the reading process.

   A number of theorists believe that the reader probably uses
more than one approach, gaining access to mental lexicon by either the direct route or phonological recoding, and therefore
probably uses both approaches at the same time or one at a time
by fluctuating in some fashion between the two modalities (La-
Berge, 1972). Perhaps the phonological recoding approach is
used in recognizing new or difficult words, whereas words or
phrases that occur often may acquire a direct route from the letter pattern to the lexicon (Fig. 14-1).

Figure 14-1
Three major hypotheses of
the relationship between listening and reading: (1) the
direct access hypothesis; (2)
the subvocalization hypothesis; and (3) the phonological
recoding hypothesis.

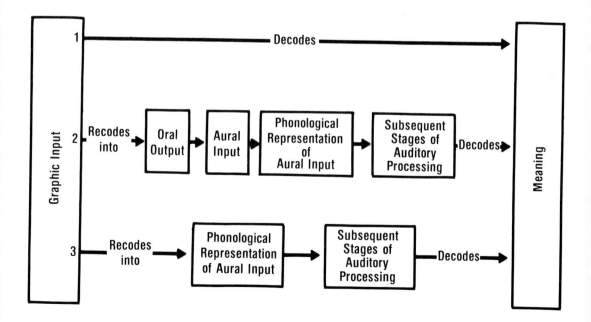

LEARNING TO READ   When a child begins to read, his entire experience with language thus far has been with the spoken form. During the early months of reading, the child can understand only if he reads aloud. As the child's reading improves, he relies less and less on vocalizing or subvocalizing.

The Reading Tasks

The importance of oral language to the adult reader can in no way be compared to the basic dependence of the child on his language skills when learning to read. Many children learn to read with ease, regardless of the method of teaching that is used. The cognitive systems of these children discover the code, and they generalize quickly from a few presentations of sounds or words to the recognition of new words. Because learning to read is easy for many children, it is considered to be an essentially simple task. When some children do not learn to read, many parents and teachers cannot understand why. An insight into the nature of the reading task may help to explain why, at least in some cases, learning to read is difficult. Breaking down the reading process into its behavioral components will also provide understanding of the roles of auditory and visual perception in reading.

The tasks a child must accomplish in learning to read are as follows (Carrow-Woolfolk, 1980):

- The child must hear and recognize spoken speech sounds and perceive minimal differences between these sounds. He must, for example, be able to hear that /ɛ/ and /æ/ sounds are different in order to "read" them correctly.
- The child's visual-perceptual skills must be adequate to recognize slight differences in shape, size, direction, or position of forms or letters. This is counter to all the previous perceptual experience of the child in which objects differing in orientation are equivalent, and such equivalence is deeply rooted in the bilateral symmetry of human anatomy (Gough, 1972).
- The child must be able to store a sequence of sounds and syllables in the order in which they occur. If he does not store the sounds or syllables in the right order, he will read the word and sentences incorrectly, thereby interfering with reading accuracy and comprehension.
- The child must learn to associate nonmeaningful abstract letters with nonmeaningful speech sounds. This is a major task in itself and needs to be broken down into subcomponents:
  - He must learn to associate the printed small case letters of the alphabet with their associated sound(s), e.g., *a* is /æ/.

- He must learn to associate the manuscript letters, those used in early writing, with the speech sound, even in cases where these differ from the printed letters, e.g., *a* and *α* or *g* and *ɋ*. He must also learn to associate cursive letters with the sounds.
- He must learn to associate the capital letters with the sound. Thus far he has five visual signs to represent the /æ/ sound: the printed *a*, the manuscript *α*, the cursive *α*, and the capitals *A* and *A*.
- He must learn that some single sounds are represented by two letters, e.g., /θ/ is *th*, /ɔ/ is *aw*.
- He must learn that some letters represent many different sounds, e.g., the letter *a* may represent an /æ/, /eɪ/, or /a/ sound. He must also learn to identify the environment in which these various sounds occur.
- He must learn that some sounds are associated with many different combinations of letters, e.g., /i/ with *ee*, *e*, *ei*, *ey*, *ea*.
- He must learn the names of letters. (An unfortunate procedure in early reading.)

• The child must know left and right directionality as it relates to his own body position.
• The child must be able to relate the order and position of sounds and syllables in words to the ordering of letters in a left-to-right direction, on a line, on a page, and he must be able to translate back and forth from visual to auditory and from auditory to visual as he tracks the letters from left to right.
• The child must learn the significant differences in letters, that differences between and *A* and *a* or *H* and *h* are unimportant but that differences between *b* and *d* or *p* and *b* are important.
• The child must learn that how a letter is situated or positioned relative to other letters on horizontal lines makes a difference, e.g., *P* (beginning of a sentence) and *p* (within the sentence).
• The child must learn that size makes a difference, as in the *e* and *l* in cursive writing.
• The child must be able to get meaning from words as he reads them (usually aloud). Each word must be successfully transferred and reconstructed through all the processing stages, including perception and memory, to reach the level of comprehension.
• The child must know the grammar, the syntax, and the semantics of the language, so as to correctly structure and interpret the incoming written messages.
• The child must learn to interpret the punctuation marks in reading *as he reads*.

It's a good thing she doesn't know what's ahead! (The Family Circus *by Bil Keane, reprinted courtesy of The Register and Tribune Syndicate, Inc.*)

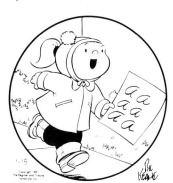

"We learned how to make an A in recl grown-up writing."

- The child must learn the rule relationship between the grammar of the language and the sounds that particular written letters and letter combinations make; e.g., when the syllable *ed* is at the end of a verb, marking past tense, and follows a voiceless consonant, such as /p/, the syllable *ed* is pronounced as /t/.
- When reading aloud, as he is often required to do, the child must pronounce the words correctly, read without false starts or hesitation, and read with vocal inflection.

Usually the child is taught writing and reading at the same time, which requires additional skills. Even a cursory review of the necessary reading skills is sufficient to realize the enormity of the task of learning to read, this enormity explaining at least some of the reasons that a child may not learn quickly and with accuracy. If, in addition, the child is suffering from the effects of poor teaching or a dysfunction of the central nervous system, it is easy to understand why he will be a poor reader. In fact, it is probably more difficult to understand how so many children learn to read *without* problems.

Developmental Aspects of Reading

Gibson and Levin (1975) emphasized the developmental changes that occur in the processing capacities of the child as he progresses in his reading skills. These developmental changes are in part related to the reader's overall ability to handle longer and more complex reading material.

One difference between the beginning reader and the more advanced reader is the cues used for retrieval and storage of linguistic data. Hagen, Jongeward, and Kail (1975) have proposed that children at different ages may form memories based on different attributes. In younger children, the acoustic and spatial

Eleanor Jack Gibson

Eleanor Gibson, professor of Psychology at Cornell University since 1949, received her highest academic degrees at Yale and Rutgers Universities. From that time, Gibson has concentrated her research interests on the study of perceptual development and the basic learning processes in the acquisition of reading skills.

Gibson's contribution to the understanding of the reading process is feature theory, which states that the visual and other types of information about words are stored in the form of features, and these features (graphic, phonological, semantic, syntactic) are attended to in a sequential and hierarchical manner. Although much of Gibson's research has been on the visual aspects of reading, she recognizes the linguistic base upon which the reading task is built.

Gibson has written many professional articles; her two major books are *Principles of Perceptual Learning and Development* and *The Psychology of Reading* (with Levin). For these and her many contributions, Gibson has been honored with numerous awards.

attributes of the reading input is dominant, whereas older children form memories based on higher order linguistic attributes (syntactic and semantic characteristics), which help organize information in larger units for efficient storage. The differences reflect the child's developing capacity to abstract meaning from the text. LaBerge and Samuels (1974) suggested that the early processes used in reading (strategies for decoding single words) become automatic, with the result that attention can be given to higher-order linguistic units. Thus, when a child can process larger units of information, reading ceases to be a word-for-word process.

Studies of differences in linguistic processing of reading disordered and nondisordered children have strengthened the position supporting a relationship between general linguistic abilities and reading. Two aspects of reading have received considerable attention in relation to linguistic attributes: word recognition and comprehension. The studies of word recognition abilities in reading have focused on such aspects of linguistic processing as phonetic segmentation and phonetic recoding. Investigations of the relations between linguistic attributes and reading comprehension have focused on levels of grammaticality of the reading text as well as general ability of readers in oral language skills.

READING DISORDERS AND GENERAL LANGUAGE PERFORMANCE

Phonetic Skills in Reading Disorders

Numerous authors have hypothesized that in the establishment of the link between oral and written language, a child applies his understanding of the acoustic structure of speech to the phonological correlates of letters and words. Consequently, insufficient or inadequate development of the child's knowledge of the acoustic character of speech might hamper his ability to recognize words. I. Y. Liberman and her associates (Liberman & Shankweiler, 1976; Liberman et al., 1977) acquired considerable data on phonetic segmentation and phonetic representations in short-term memory, and found that some children with reading problems are not sufficiently aware of the phonetic structure of spoken language. These children have difficulty in relating a series of letters to the phonological representation of a syllable, which is the unit of spoken language. The inability to analyze the phonetic structure in spoken words—to detect the number of phonemes in words—appears to be related to poor achievement in reading.

A second group of studies was made by Liberman and colleagues (Liberman & Shankweiler, 1976; Shankweiler & Liberman, 1972) to determine if poor readers are less efficient than normal readers in phonetic coding. They found that good readers responded differentially to phonetically confusable (rhyming) letter strings than to nonconfusable (nonrhyming) strings, indicating that good readers were more sensitive to the acoustic constituents of words than were poor readers. These findings were true whether the stimuli were presented auditorially (Shankweiler & Liberman, 1972) or visually (Liberman & Shankweiler, 1976). These studies have led to an increased interest in the role of phonological factors in reading. They also lend support to the hypothesis that reading consists, at least in part, of auditory recoding of the visual input.

Reading and Linguistic Knowledge

Investigations have also been made of differences in these reader groups in aspects of verbal learning, namely, the semantic and syntactic systems. The semantic and syntactic systems need to be intact for comprehension to take place in reading. It is not sufficient for the child to recognize words; he must also be able to reconstruct segments of written script and discover their meaning.

Syntactic and Semantic Processing and Reading

The ability to organize verbal input syntactically permits the memory storage to retain larger chunks or segments of information and thereby improve the efficiency of the processing and comprehension of the material read. Studies on eye-voice span (reviewed by Gibson & Levin, 1975) indicate that older good readers have larger eye-voice spans than younger and/or poor readers. The older reader tends to use the clause (a syntactic unit) as the basic unit of processing, while the younger reader uses the phrase. In a study by Isakson and Miller (1976), the errors in two groups of fourth-grade children differing in reading comprehension were analyzed. They found that poor comprehenders were less disturbed than good comprehenders by syntactic violations of sentence structure.

Several studies have investigated the role of semantic organization in distinguishing between poor and good readers. One explored the differences between poor and good readers in recall of meaningful and nonmeaningful material and found that the organized material facilitated recall only for the good readers (Parker, Freston, & Drew, 1975). In a sentence-recognition task, Paris and Carter (1973) found that poor readers were not as effective as normal readers in retaining verbal details such as grammatic markers and specific word strings. Richman (1979) found that poor readers were less proficient than normals in use of verbally mediated responses.

These studies support the thesis that at least some poor readers have generalized difficulty in the verbal coding process, which affects their performance in reading. The problem is exemplified in problems of syntactic organization, semantic categorization, and the use of semantic cues in reading (Fletcher, 1980). Reading errors may be due to a large extent to malfunction of phonetic, semantic, or syntactic processing.

Oral Language Performance of Poor Readers

If relationships are found between reading disability and generalized language disability, further support is given to the argument that the reading disorder should be viewed as one type of disorder of language.

A summary of the findings of studies of language performance indicates that there also appears to be a relationship between oral language and poor reading for at least some children. Compared to good readers, poor readers have been found to have (1) smaller speaking vocabularies (M. A. Fry, Johnson & Muehl, 1970); (2) less appropriate use of grammar and syntax (Calvert, 1973; Vogel, 1975); (3) poorer verbal fluency and organization of verbal concepts (Vellutino, 1978); (4) poorer word retrieval (Denckla & Rudel, 1976); (5) history of oral language problems (T.T.S. Ingram, Mason, & Blackburn, 1970; Lyle, 1970); (6) differences in morphological usage (Vogel, 1975; Wiig, Semel, & Crouse, 1973); (7) slower response time in vocalization (Eakin & Douglas, 1971; Spring, 1976); and (8) poorer listening comprehension (Wiig & Semel, 1976a).

By interpreting the literature supporting the thesis that reading is a decidedly linguistic function, Vellutino (1978) decided that most reading problems may be associated with specific language disorders. Fletcher (1980) preferred to interpret the findings to mean that only *some* children with reading problems (particularly older children) have associated linguistic disorders. He concluded that younger readers may have difficulty in phonological coding, whereas older readers' difficulties are semantic and syntactic processing. In spite of the close association between reading and general language abilities, Fletcher suggested that the unitary deficit interpretation of reading problems is an inadequate characterization of disabled readers. Blank (1978) concurred, stating that although the major difficulties of most retarded readers are in language, some groups of poor readers have been found to have problems in the visual-perceptual areas.

It may be of value to view the reading system as a representation of the vocal system and, in so doing, to consider the graphic letters that correspond to the phonemes as part of the total linguistic system. This approach would consider the visual aspects of the letters as linguistic in the same way as the acoustic aspects of sounds are linguistic. This would make reading a part of the language system and the visual perception of letters a language-specific function. The findings regarding the co-occurence of various linguistic disorders may not indicate a cause-effect relationship between language disorders and reading; however, these findings do support a hypothesis that reading and other linguistic problems may stem from a common source.

READING DISORDERS AND THE DIMENSIONS OF LANGUAGE

The behavioral function of reading can be easily integrated into the four-dimensional integrative structure by adding graphology to the elements of the linguistic code, visual perception to auditory perception, and reading and writing, as parallel functions, to listening and speaking (Fig. 14-2). The model, thus adapted, does not clearly illustrate that graphic symbols are recoded into phonemic ones in reading, but it does show the place of reading within the total language system. From the model, it is obvious that a disorder of reading at the performance level may be related to problems in other dimensions and levels,

Figure 14-2

The role of reading and writing in the four-dimensional model.

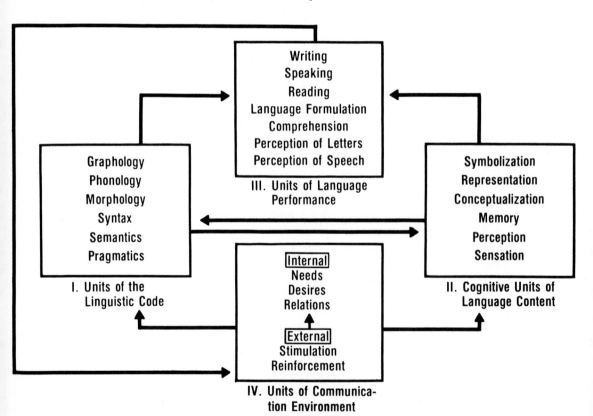

through the dependency effect, through the interaction of cumulative effects, or as effects of a common source. In fact, many of the disorders described in previous chapters may affect the reading process in some way. For example, what appears to be poor short-term memory for verbal material may be a function of inadequate syntactic organization, which interferes with the length of the segment (spoken or written) that can be analyzed and stored, which in turn may affect both listening *and* reading comprehension. A semantic disorder may influence listening and reading comprehension as well as speaking and writing; cognitive problems of conceptualization will also be reflected in reading. Consequently, an adequate analysis of a disorder of reading must take the total language system into account.

Disorders of reading are affected by problems in visual perception and memory as well as in auditory perception and memory. For the written linguistic units to be processed adequately, they must be received accurately by the cognitive system through both sensory channels. Once received, the processing of the written word depends on the integrity of all of the other dimensions of language, as does oral language. In the model adapted for reading, visual perception of letter strings is added to speech perception. Reading, like speech, can be purely a performance phenomenon. Just as there is echolalia in speech, there is the ability to "rote" read by autistic children. Children can learn to see and say words without deriving any meaning from what is "read." This supports the strong relationship between visual and auditory factors in reading.

A linguistic theory of reading disorders must include a description of the role of each of the four dimensions in the reading process. It must focus on the varied factors that may produce reading disorders but must also stress the fact that all of these factors may be viewed within the framework of language and its disorders.

THE LANGUAGE SPECIALIST AND READING DISORDERS

The view of reading as a component of the linguistic system has implications for the language specialist. If the phonological, semantic, and syntactic aspects of the language code, as well as auditory perception and memory, play a role in learning to read, and if dysfunction of these processes is related to reading disorders, the language specialist will have an important role in the identification of reading disorders, in their assessment, and in remediation.

Delayed articulation and language development and a history of poor response to sound are among early indicators of future reading problems in the child. The histories of poor readers typically reveal the mother's concern with the child's inattentiveness and misunderstanding of instructions, and the mother's consequent suspicion of hearing loss. The child's speech often contains words with transferred sounds such as *eslacator* for *escalator* and *emeny* for *enemy*. Repeated visits to the otolaryngologist or audiologist indicate normal peripheral hearing. If an articulation problem exists, it is usually corrected before the child starts school. In many instances, no further help is obtained until the child begins exhibiting marked reading failure in the second or third grade.

If the language specialist watches for early signs of linguistic difficulty in children, some reading problems may be avoided by early teaching of phonological and linguistic skills. If a reading problem is identified early and remediation provided, the child can "catch up" and not be penalized in other subjects to any great extent. If the child enters third grade with a reading disorder, he suffers not only in reading but also in all subjects dependent upon reading, such as science and math. Remediation at third grade and later on may bring him up to grade level in reading skills, but may not be able to close the gap in other subjects, such as vocabulary that has been missed.

Prereading skills (Carrow-Woolfolk, 1980) that may be taught to children include (1) auditory awareness, recognition, and discrimination of environmental sounds, speech sounds, and sound sequences; (2) recognition of the position of sounds in words; (3) sound-letter associations; (4) visual discrimination of letters; (5) left-to-right directionality; (6) relation of the temporal sequence of sounds; (7) translation of sounds and syllables to letters; (8) translation of letter groups to sounds; (9) phonetic segmentation of words through audition; and (10) syllabic identification of words through audition.

The language specialist can contribute to the assessment of the reading-disordered child by providing procedures that evaluate the linguistic process. In general, the procedures described in Chapter 11 apply to the evaluation of cognition and linguistic structure in children with reading problems. There are a few additional procedures that will assist in studying the child who is having difficulty in learning to read and that the language specialist can administer.

Of particular interest are special tests that measure aspects of phonological processing that are not included in the standard language battery. The standard measures of auditory processing include tests of auditory discrimination, auditory blending and auditory memory. For the child with a reading disorder, additional tests may be useful, such as tests of phonetic segmentation and syllabication, which involve the ability to identify the phonetic parts of words either by individual sounds or by syllables.

Although, historically, concern for language disorders in children has not included concern for reading disorders, it seems apparent that the language specialist can no longer neglect her responsibilities to children who have such problems. Since the academic background of the language specialist emphasizes the oral language code and its auditory undergirdings, she is well suited to provide assistance in the development of prereading skills.

acquired aphasia in children

15

THIS CHAPTER CONCERNS only a very small number of children, who generate virtually no controversy regarding either the etiology of their language disorder or the terminology with which to describe it. These are the children who sustain brain trauma following a period of normal development. They are labeled *aphasic,* as are adults who have lost language due to stroke or trauma. To clarify the distinction between the children and adults, the children are sometimes described as having *acquired aphasia* (Hécaen, 1976). The previously normal language of the child with acquired aphasia has been interrupted and adjectives such as *delayed* or *deviant* are not used to describe it. These unique "experiments of nature," as they have sometimes been called, are worthy of special study by language specialists for several reasons. Primarily, it is of interest that children who sustain sometimes dramatic brain injury can recover language so well, whereas other children with no overt sign of brain injury demonstrate persisting language disorders.

This chapter also describes certain children with acquired aphasia in detail so that the language specialist will have a frame of reference for assessing or intervening with such children. Many of these children are referred to language specialists during the acute stage of their illness, and many others are referred for special remediation after they return to school. However, most texts on language disorders tend to omit this group entirely or dismiss them with statements such as "Children with acquired aphasia make remarkably good recovery" (Eisenson, 1972, p. 61).

The final purpose of this chapter is to provide additional information about the relationship of cerebral dominance and language development. In addition, the concept of the "critical period" of language development is discussed. The relevance of a critical period is of particular importance to programs of early intervention, as well as to planning for the language habilitation of teenagers and older individuals with conditions of mental retardation, emotional disturbance, deafness, and various multiple handicaps.

COMMON ETIOLOGIES

Acquired aphasia results from focal cerebral lesions occurring during childhood as opposed to suspected injury occurring before or at birth (Alajouanine & Lhermitte, 1965). Normal children may acquire aphasia in several ways. The most obvious is traumatic injury—a blow to the head leading to contusions, lacerations, hemorrhage, and/or edema of the brain with or without skull fracture. For a number of children, brain surgery is required, and thus some estimate of the site and extent of damage can be made (Ford, 1973).

Some children develop brain tumors, which may ultimately result in hemispherectomy (surgical removal of an entire hemisphere) (Gott, 1973). It was once customary to regard brain tumors in children as a great rarity, but due to better diagnostic methods, it is now estimated that brain tumors in children are as common as in adults (Ford, 1973, p. 1065). However, brain tumors in children have a higher rate of malignancy than in adults. Most symptoms occur prior to 15 years of age. About 65 percent of childhood tumors are of the cerebellum.

A few children with intractable epilipsey that cannot be controlled by medication may require brain surgery. These children often show behavioral disorders, including outbursts of temper, that are sometimes severe in nature (Basser, 1962; A. Smith, 1974). Some of these children may ultimately undergo hemispherectomy.

CHARACTERISTICS OF ACQUIRED APHASIA

The children who sustain brain injury after speech has been acquired have a peculiar and characteristic style of speaking. In the past 30 years, there have been several large reviews of cases of cerebral damage in children who had already begun to speak. Four of these reviews have been summarized in Table 15-1. A problem with such reviews is that characteristics of the cases must be presented only in general terms because of the great variation in case reporting. The majority of cases were reviewed from hospital charts, which focused primarily on physical recovery from life-threatening events. At times, follow-up has been retrospective, often relying upon letters written by parents to the primary physician. The few well-documented cases are cited by so many authors that they keep reappearing in the literature like old friends.

Table 15-1

Language Observed in Children Following Brain Injury

Study	Number of Cases	Age at Onset	Verified Causes*	Language Observed
Guttmann (1942)	30	2–14 years	Trauma, 6 tumor, 6 abcess, 12 thrombosis, 1	16/30 had aphasic symptoms: 14/16 were initially mute; 14/16 used telegraphic speech; 9/14 were dysarthric.
Basser (1962)	30	After speech developed	Left hemisphere lesion, 15 Right hemisphere lesion, 15	20/30 had aphasic impairment: 19 were initially mute; Duration of impairment was from days to 2 years.
Alajouanine and Lhermite (1965)	32	6–15 years	All left hemisphere lesions: trauma, 13 vascular disease, 10 tumor, 2 other, 7	32/32 had aphasic symptoms: 32/32 were initially mute; 22/32 had dysarthria; 10/32 had comprehension problems; 27% had normal speech at 6 months, 75% had normal speech at 1 year.
Hécan (1976)	26	3½–15 years	Trauma, 6 hematoma, 6 tumor, 2	88% of left hemisphere lesions had aphasia and 33% of right lesions had aphasia: 33% had loss of comprehension; 33 % had naming impairment; Acalculia was "common."

*In some cases the cause was not specified.

Aphasia in children has certain characteristics. First of all, some researchers found that disorders of comprehension tended to be uncommon (Alajouanine & Lhermite, 1965; Guttmann, 1942). Hécaen (1976) reported more common loss in comprehension with one out of three children he studied showing some loss in receptive language.

There is almost universal agreement that the most common verbal symptom initially following injury is mutism (Alajouanine & Lhermitte, 1965; Basser, 1962; Guttmann, 1942), which may last from days to months. A purely psychological explanation has been offered for this mutism by Alajouanine and Lhermitte (1965). They observed that, in their reactions to all overwhelming conflict or difficulties, children tend to isolation, refusal, and silence. The few reluctantly produced words of aphasic children are reminiscent of the behavior of normal children when faced with problems that they cannot possibly solve. The summaries of the 118 children reported in Table 15-1 indicates that initial mutism is the most universal symptom. Following onset of speech, a kind of verbal inhibition is commonly observed in these children. To get them to say even the few words they were capable of producing required unusual incentive and encouragement. It appeared necessary to "gear" children into action through prompting, coaching, repetition, and much encouragement. It was hypothesized that language has a different function for children and that it is only in adults that language has taken over as the most likely response to almost any situation.

Another characteristic of the aphasic child is the lack of a consistent association between aphasia and brain injury. As Table 15-1 indicates, aphasia may not always be present, regardless of whether the injury is to the left or the right side of the brain. Aphasia is more likely, however, with damage to left side of the brain. Alajouanine and Lhermitte (1965) reported the occurrence of aphasia in all thirty-two cases of left-hemisphere lesion that they studied. Hécaen (1976) reported aphasia in 88 percent of the left-hemisphere lesions and in only 33 percent of the right-hemisphere lesions.

PERIOD OF IMMEDIATE RECOVERY

It is very difficult to generalize about the course of recovery of these children. For this reason, the period of immediate recovery is illustrated here primarily through case presentations. The first three cases were originally described by Guttmann (1942) as a part of his study of 30 cases. Cases 1 and 3 sustained accidental head injury, and case 2 sustained injury due to infection.

Paul Broca

Paul Broca was the most distinguished French medical scientist and surgeon of the mid-1800's. In 1861, the most popular topic for scientific discussion was the theory of cerebral localization; Broca expressed his support of this theory and presented as evidence the report of one of his patients who had lost his ability to speak and whose right side was paralyzed following injury to his left cerebral hemisphere. Upon autopsy, Broca found a lesion in the left frontal lobe in the brain. This area of the brain is now known as "Broca's Area."

Broca's undergraduate work was completed by the time he was 16 years old, when he entered the University of Paris to study medicine. His doctoral dissertation was on cancerous tumors—a topic on which he published widely. Broca rose quickly to Chairman of Surgery and was appointed to the Academy of Medicine. In addition to his academic work, he continued seeing patients in surgical clinics and became increasingly active in research in the field of anthropology. His reports regarding the localization of function and his discussion of the syndrome of aphasia (aphemia) were made to the Institute of Anthropology.

During his professional life, Broca contributed more than two hundred scientific articles as well as textbooks on tumors. France honored him by electing him to the Senate of the French Republic in 1880. In a subsequent public announcement Broca stated that this election had fulfilled all of his dreams. He died of a heart attack during a session of the Senate later that same year.

The descriptions of recovery in cases 1 and 3 are reported using the type of brief phrases that might be entered on a hospital report.

Case 1

A 6-year-old boy who sustained a compound fracture of the left frontoparietal region in a bicycle accident. Never lost consciousness. Day 2: awake and alert. Mute. Carried out simple instructions. Day 4: still mute. Could nod head "yes" or "no." Could hum. Day 6: repeated simple words. Counted with much urging. Speech hard to understand. Day 9: counted and named on request. Gave single word responses to questions. Still very hard to understand. Day 10: said first spontaneous words. Day 16: spoke spontaneously but less than expected for his lively, well behaved manner. Speech slow and slurred, with very short sentences.

Case 2

An 11-year-old boy who sustained temporal lobe abscess following ear infection. He lost consciousness, and surgery was performed. Subsequently he could follow uncomplicated commands and produced no spontaneous speech. When strongly urged to speak, he displayed marked naming difficulties. Weeks following his first surgery, his speech was still telegraphic. A second operation was performed in an attempt to control continuing infection. Some 2 years later he was again speaking freely, but his speech was slow and he made a number of syntactic errors. Three years later his speech was still slow with some articulation errors.

Case 3

A 10-year-old boy who was struck in the temporal area by a cricket ball. Never lost consciousness. Day 1: some problem in understanding what was said to him. Produced some spontaneous speech, which was very slow. Could not name common objects nor form sentences. Day 6: comprehension improved. Still had trouble naming. Day 60: comprehension intact. Spontaneous speech and naming returned to normal.

Case 4

A 10-year-old girl who had a hemispherectomy because of a tumor in the parietal area (Gott, 1973). The presence of this tumor had been suspected for 2 years prior to this radical surgery, so it may be presumed that a gradual transfer of function from the diseased left hemisphere to the right hemisphere may have occurred prior to the surgery. On the day after surgery the girl was able to sing and speak the names of family members. Two years following surgery, her comprehension on the Peabody Picture Vocabulary Test yielded an IQ of 70. She could correctly follow verbal directions and respond to yes/no questions, but could not answer questions about a paragraph read to her. Her responses to the vocabulary test (Wechsler Intelligence Scale for Children) placed her in the "dull-normal" range and her speech was limited to single words or short phrases. Her visual perceptual skills were limited.

Case 5

A 7-year-old boy who sustained brain injury when he fell 30 feet from a footbridge onto a rocky stream bed was reported by Lynch (1972). Surgery was performed, and a portion of the left temporal lobe was removed. At the time of the accident he was an average student in the third grade with no reported developmental problems. He was left handed, as were several other members of his family. For 1 month following surgery, he was comatose, and severe right hemiplegia developed. His language recovered in the following sequence. Month 3: could recognize familiar people and objects. Attended to the television but paid no attention to the radio or environmental sounds. Mute. Month 5: still mute. Even laughing and crying were silent. Month 6: began to use sound projectively to gain attention. Imitated a few sounds. Month 7: said his first words since the accident. The following utterances were recorded by his parents: Dec. 12: "Mama" (his first articulate word); Dec. 14: "Papa"; Dec. 15: "Orly" (his nickname) "is good," "Me hungry," "Mama gone home," "Orly sick," "Daddy, Orly need you"; Dec. 24: "Let me put decorations, too."

During month 8 his description of pictures was recorded. In response to two pictures he produced a total of 16 words. Two months later he produced a total of 31 words in describing the same two pictures.

The primary change in picture description during this 2-month period was in the number of words produced. This boy was able to correctly express the point of the picture as soon as he could undertake the task. Between months 7 and 10 following his injury, this 7-year-old boy progressed from his first words to functional ability to communicate verbally. His most rapid progress occurred in the first month he spoke. Tests for language indicated that his vocabulary was superior to his syntax. Comprehension of content words, as measured by the Peabody Picture Vocabulary Test, remained fairly appropriate for chronological age, with an IQ of 90 obtained 7 months following injury. Vocabulary definitions on the Stanford-Binet L-M were at the VI to VIII year level, which was within normal limits. Approximately 1 year following injury, his syntactic ability as measured by the Northwestern Syntax Screening Test fell below preschool norms by 2 standard deviations. Ability to read returned with no instruction, and 8 months after injury he could read at the second-grade level (Lynch, 1972).

In one of the larger series of cases reviewed, Basser (1962) reported on 102 patients with early hemiplegia or hemispherectomy. However only 30 of these patients were speaking prior to their illness (see Table 15-1). Basser's case summaries illustrated recovery from both left and right hemisphere damage. He reported on a 2-year-old boy who sustained left hemisphere damage following viral infection. This boy lost his speech for six months, and once he began to speak again he was reported to be making "normal" progress. A 9-year-old who sustained left hemisphere damage following convulsions lost her speech completely for 2 months. Even after her recovery was considered complete her speech was considered "imperfect." A 5-year-old who sustained right hemisphere damage from unknown causes was mute for 18 months. Once she began to speak she regained "normal speech" with the next six months. In his summary of cases, Basser observed that, despite initial muteness in 19 cases, total loss of speech was never permanent. The course of speech recovery could progress very quickly following the onset of the first words, or the patient might pass slowly through the usual stages of initial language acquisition. Basser (1962) concluded that children who sustained cerebral damage before 2 years of age were without speech for a significantly longer time than those who were over 2 years at the time damage occurred.

Speech and Language Recovery

Once the period of mutism has passed, injured children tend to have specific disorders of naming, and their syntax is simplified and telegraphic in style. Several authors noted that such children may relearn language in stages comparable to those of an infant learning language. Dysarthria may or may not be present, with only one research team (Alajouanine & Lhermite, 1965) noting a positive correlation between dysarthria and the severity of the hemiplegia. There are specific reports of dylexia (reading/writing disturbances) in the surveys of some researchers (Alajouanine & Lhermite, 1965), while in other reports (Hécaen, 1976) the most common academic problem was acalculia (inability to do arithmetic).

A child under 10 years of age has a good chance of reacquiring lost verbal skills within 1 year, but this reacquisition may be at the expense of other nonverbal skills (Penfield, 1965; Rosenberger, 1978). Once recovery of speech begins, it is usually quite rapid, often within 4 weeks. The brain of a child has tremendous capacity to recover from injury.

Differences Between Aphasia in Children and Adults

The aphasic child differs from the aphasic adult in several obvious ways. In contrast to adult aphasics, children are uniformly shy and quiet, with an initial absence of spontaneous speech. Children never have logorrhea or jargon speech, nor do they produce frequent automatic or stereotyped phrases (automatic speech consists of greetings, profanity, etc., and stereotyped phrases include utterances such as "I see" or "I don't know"). Once speech begins to re-emerge, children may have name-finding problems, but they do not display the paraphasic or misnaming symptoms characteristic of adults. Finally, most children, in contrast to most adults, retain fairly intact receptive language. Apparently, the main forte of the aphasic adult is her past experience as a language user, whereas the child's advantage is youth and a still-growing brain with its proclivity for acquiring new symbol systems (Gardner, 1978).

PROGNOSIS OF CHILDREN WITH ACQUIRED APHASIA

Guttmann (1942) made some tentative conclusions about children who were over 2 years of age at the time of their injury. Unfortunately, he administered no formal tests, basing his impressions entirely on parental reports. Samples of these reports illustrate their subjective nature.

> "Still in infant school at age 6. An intelligent boy, but with such a handicap."
> "A fine girl. Can't do hard work."

Guttmann concluded that regardless of the outcome of the language impairment, intellectual and emotional disturbances were a likely result of the injury.

There is also a tendency for IQ scores of brain-damaged individuals to deteriorate. Formal intelligence testing was carried out in cases reviewed by Basser (1962), showing that 64 percent of children with left-hemisphere damage and 56 percent of those with right-hemisphere damage had subsequent IQ scores below 80. Basser felt that it was possible that some delay in recovery of speech might be related to reduced intelligence. However, he pointed out that aphasia and intellectual impairment are not necessarily related; Some children with no aphasia show intellectual impairment.

The review of cases by Alajouanine and Lhermite (1965) focused on school follow-up. They found that none of the 32 children they followed could keep up with a normal school program. Children with left-hemisphere damage showed more problems with language arts than with mathematics. It seemed to these researchers that the children could regain the language they had lost but had particular difficulty in acquiring new data. They agreed with Basser that intellectual and aphasic impairment were distinct from each other. In the single hemispherectomy patient reported by Gott (1973), school records showed a Kuhlman-Anderson IQ of 100 prior to the development of a tumor at age 8. Following initial surgery, a Stanford-Binet IQ of 86 was obtained, and after the hemispherectomy, the WISC IQ was 55. Although this girl's right hemisphere had obviously taken over language function, there were permanent language abnormalities, and visual perceptual functions (usually subserved by the right hemisphere) were significantly limited. Hécaen (1976) found that although five of fifteen aphasics in one sample had recovered language completely, their verbal IQ scores remained below their performance scores. These particular patients showed no visual-spatial defects. The consensus of the studies show that damage to either hemisphere may cause a change in intelligence (Dennis & Whitaker, 1977).

A follow-up study was completed on the 7-year-old boy discussed in Case 5 (Lynch & Hayden). At the time of the follow-up Orly was 15 years old and enrolled in a special education program in junior high school. He walked with a cane and had limited use of his right hand. Vocabulary as measured by the Stanford-Binet Vocabulary definitions was at the X- to XII-year level with a chronological age of 15 years. Logicogrammatic errors were apparent on the Wiig and Semmel tests of linguistic concepts. Reading of single words was at the eighth-grade level, but comprehension of a text was only at the fifth-grade level; logicogrammatic confusions appeared to affect this score. Neuropsychological testing revealed that verbal memory and learning were surprisingly intact considering the injury. The WISC Verbal IQ was 82, performance IQ was 68, with a full-scale IQ of 73 (borderline). Interpersonal responses were immature for chronological age. This young man suffered an obvious intellectual impairment following his injury, impairment being most obvious in the realm of judgment. Although he appeared to regain the oral and written language skills that he had had prior to the injury, he continued to have difficulty acquiring new skills.

A 6-year follow up of 307 children who were brain injured between birth and 14 years showed that 11 percent developed seizure disorders (P. Black, Shepard, & Walker, 1975). Another longitudinal study, of 98 children who had localized head injury, explored possible effects on personality and adjustment. Parents and teachers were interviewed, and the results showed that these children are at higher risk for psychological problems; this likelihood is markedly increased by adverse home conditions (Schaffer, Chadwich, & Rutter, 1975).

ASSESSMENT

As a member of the rehabilitation team, the language specialist has several contributions to make to the overall assessment of the child with acquired aphasia: (1) to assist in establishing the child's current condition; (2) to chart progress; and (3) to contribute to determining the mode of intervention to be used.

The earliest observations following injury begin with monitoring states of consciousness, for which organized test instruments may be used. Comprehension tends to emerge well before verbal expression in children with acquired aphasia; at the first stages of recovery, comprehension may be estimated by carefully observing the child's nonverbal expressions of attention, interest, and/or excitement as favored or nonfavored persons come and go or certain activities take place. As the injured child's physical condition improves, it is possible to ascertain if he can look at or point to objects. Standard tests of language comprehension may then be used.

Any child with brain trauma, and especially with damage to the brainstem, may display motor speech problems. It is vital to

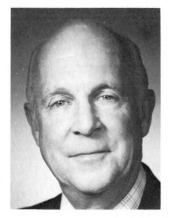

Frederic L. Darley

Darley has come to exemplify the clinically competent speech pathologist, particularly in the area of diagnosis. When he was awarded the Honors of the American Speech and Hearing Association in 1970 his colleagues noted that his "imposing productivity and unfailing lucidity as a writer . . . epitomized his belief that clinical acumen and scientific rigor were philosophically and intellectually inextricable."

Darley's pioneer contributions to diagnosis began in the 1950s with publication of the *Diagnostic Manual in Speech Correction.* This volume (and the 1963 revision) remained one of the very few diagnostic texts of the time. The most recent revision (1978) emphasized the need for professionals to understand normal development and behavior prior to attempting to identify the disordered. Darley's other contributions include his work in the field of motor speech disturbances. He has clarified the areas of dysarthria and apraxia through numerous publications. He is also the co-author of the *Templin-Darley Test of Articulation.*

A graduate of New Mexico State Teachers College, Darley received an M.A. in speech from the State University of Iowa in 1940. He began his teaching career as an instructor of public speaking and English at the University of Arkansas in 1940, and also taught public speaking at the University of California at Berkeley. In 1950, he obtained his Ph.D. from the University of Iowa and was an associate professor of Speech Pathology and Director of the University Speech Clinic there. He joined the staff of the Mayo Clinic in 1961, where he continues as a consultant in Speech Pathology and professor of Speech Pathology in the University of Minnesota's Mayo Graduate School of Medicine.

distinguish between mutism due to linguistic deficit and mutism due to dysarthria or apraxia of speech. In their extensive study of motor speech problems, Darley, Aronson, and Brown (1969, p. 246) defined dysarthria as referring to a group of speech disorders all of which resulted from disturbances in mucular control over the speech mechanism, caused by damage of the central or peripheral nervous system. These disorders are characterized by paralysis, weakness, or incoordination of the speech musculature.

Apraxia of speech is an articulatory disorder, resulting from brain damage, which impairs the capacity to program the positioning of speech musculature and the sequence of movement (Chapter 13). These same structures do not show weakness or incoordination for reflex or automatic acts (Deal & Darley, 1972).

A child who has begun speaking again can be tested with the same instruments used with any other child. Other techniques are necessary for the child who is not yet speaking: the integrity of the speech mechanism may be judged by evaluating feeding procedures, the presence or absence of oral reflexes, the existence of drooling, and attempts the child may be making to vocalize.

INTERVENTION

The choice of intervention techniques must be guided by the recovery pattern of each individual child. There is no standard curriculum for these children. Most will be seen initially while they are hospitalized; others will be followed by tutors at home; and a lesser number will be referred for continuing therapy once they have returned to school. Intervention must be planned with the child's other therapy schedule in mind and must allow for the fatigue that follows serious head trauma.

During the period of recovery, some of the techniques now gaining popularity with the severely and profoundly handicapped might be applicable to facilitate communication prior to the emergence of speech. If the child has sufficient alertness, comprehension, and eye-hand coordination, a simplified communication board might be used. In a case known to the authors of this volume, sign language was successfully introduced to a school-aged boy who had such severe dysarthria that he was prevented from attempting verbal language.

The studies reported in this chapter suggest that time and physical recovery work strongly for the child with acquired aphasia. The majority of these cases make a marked recovery. A review of the studies suggests that the recovery period may extend up to 5 years.

CEREBRAL DOMINANCE AND LANGUAGE THEORY

As discussed in Chapter 3, evidence of handedness has importance for the study of language because some 99.6 percent of right-handed people are left-cerebral-dominant for language (J. Levy, 1974). However, when brain surgery is contemplated, the determination of cerebral dominance for language is too crucial to be left to simple verification of handedness. One method of determination is to inject sodium amobarbital into the carotid artery in the neck. When this substance flows into the side of the brain dominant for language, obvious aphasic symptoms appear.

Undoubtedly, the ultimate experiment in cerebral dominance can only be observed in those patients who, in a final attempt to control tumor or constant seizures, undergo hemispherectomy. A. Smith (1974) reported on twelve cases of hemispherectomy performed in an attempt to control epilepsy. These children were between 8 months and 21 years of age. Ten of the twelve were left-handed. An important caution in reviewing these studies is that this radical surgery is performed only following long-standing disease, and language may already have transferred to the other hemisphere. In these twelve cases there was no apparent worsening of language following surgery. In some cases of severe seizure disorder, there is a report of a general improvement in IQ. Dennis and Whitaker (1977) followed three children (one right-handed and two left-handed) who had complete hemispheres removed to control seizures while they were infants. These children were tested at 9 years of age and all had IQ scores in the 90s. The right-handed child had more difficulty with visual than with auditory tasks, and also had some difficulty with language structure.

Certain generalizations concerning the possible role of the hemispheres emerge from these studies. The two hemispheres of the brain are not just mirror images of each other. There are anatomical differences between the left and right hemispheres, with some size and complexity advantage to the left hemisphere (Geschwind, 1974). Damage to the left hemisphere occurs four times more frequently in children then does damage to the right, according to some researchers (Annett, 1973). Even with damage in infancy, an impaired left hemisphere tends to cause more language disturbance than a damaged right hemisphere (Dennis & Whitaker, 1977): left-hemisphere damage delays the acquisition of language, with syntax significantly more impaired than semantics.

Comprehension of language seems most resistant to damage in children. However, damage to *either* hemisphere may be expected to cause both language and intellectual impairment. Therefore, it is felt that in the young child, the right hemisphere contributes to early language and cognitive development. However, Moscovitch (1977) has made the point that transfer of language function to the right hemisphere is at the expense of the various nonverbal functions usually subserved by the normal right hemisphere. This theory helps to explain the uneven test performance of injured children who regain their language but fail to develop certain nonverbal skills. In other children with acquired aphasia, there is no improvement in language, and it has been hypothesized that when the left hemisphere has been badly damaged it may actually inhibit or prevent the right hemisphere from assuming language functioning. Consequently, there are reports of apparent remarkable "improvement" following removal of the damaged left hemisphere. Rosenberger (1978) agreed that hemispheric dominance may be just that—a suppression of one hemisphere by the other.

CRITICAL AGE FOR LANGUAGE ACQUISITION

The concept of "critical periods" was originally put forward by biologists who observed that certain birds, such as goslings, were "imprinted" by the sight of a moving object during the first several hours after hatching; that is, whatever object they saw and followed at that critical time became "mother." If correct imprinting did not occur in that period, it would never be established.

In studying humans, Lenneberg (1967) put forward his hypothesis of a critical period in language learning. He contended that a prepubescent child could relearn language following injury because "dominance" was not firmly established until about age 12 and prior to that time the right hemisphere could take over. This hypothesis affected not only the study of language recovery in young children, but also contributed to the nationwide pressure to establish programs of early language intervention.

Some researchers suggested that the cerebral hemispheres are already lateralized for language at birth (Kinsbourne, 1975). Children during the first years of life learn language with an ease and speed that testifies to what some neurologists have referred to as a "biological clock." If a child less than 10 to 12 years of age sustains injury to the language area of the cortex, this biological clock enables him to recover (Penfield, 1965). Children who sustain damage prior to the age of 3 seem to follow the normal course of language acquisition after an initial pause in all language development (Yeni-Komshian, 1977). Up to age 5 there is interference in language following injury, but the recovery period does not necessarily mirror normal acquisition. Krashen (1975) believed that lateralization for language may be completely established by age 5 and so may not be associated with a critical period.

Obviously, there are no laboratory experiments with which to answer these questions, but adverse circumstances provided a natural experiment (Fromkin et al., 1974) that has been widely quoted in the literature.

Case 6

Genie was discovered by the California police when she was 13 years, 9 months of age. She was a tiny, undernourished child unable to stand erect or chew, incontinent, and totally mute. There was evidence that from age 20 months until she was found she had been kept tied in a chair or crib in a dark, silent room and severely punished if she made any sound. It seemed that Genie was a normal child of psychotic parents. In the two years of care and training that Genie received prior to publication of this report, it was apparent that she was learning language despite her age; slow, but steady, progress was taking place. Comprehension was obviously ahead of production and 8 months after she was found, Genie began to speak, producing two-word utterances like "more soup," "yellow car," and "Genie purse." Two months later verbs emerged and then three- to four-word "sentences" with subject + verb + object or subject + object. Her language development in many ways paralleled normal development, with the exception that her vocabulary was much larger than that of normal children who had comparable syntactic development. The cognitive nature of her speech appeared considerably in advance of what would have been expected from her current syntactic stage.

Genie obviously learned language beyond the so-called critical period. Both language and nonlanguage functions seemed lateralized to the right hemisphere. The theory is that because of her extreme environmental isolation, the left hemisphere had a kind of functional atrophy of the language centers, and her current achievements in language are occurring in the hemisphere (right), which somehow did mature more normally. If this theory is true, it modifies the concept of the critical period, suggesting that the left hemisphere must be linguistically stimulated during a specific period of time for it to participate in normal language acquisition. The authors of this study concluded that despite the extensive research into the questions of lateralization, cerebral dominance, and the critical age for language acquisition, there are still more questions than answers.

outline

DEFINITION

CAUSES OF MENTAL RETARDATION

Organic Causes
    Genetic Conditions
Other Congenital Disorders
    Postnatal Disorders
Environmental Causes

MEASUREMENT OF INTELLIGENCE AND ADAPTIVE BEHAVIOR

Intelligence Tests
Measurement of Adaptive Behavior

LANGUAGE AND MENTAL RETARDATION

Prevalence of Language Impairment
among the Mentally Retarded
The Cognitive Dimension
    Sensation
    Perception and Memory
    Conceptualization and Representation
The Communication Environment
The Linguistic Code: Delayed or
Deviant Development
Speech Performance

THE INTEGRATIVE APPROACH

ASSESSMENT

INTERVENTION

language disorders among the mentally retarded

16

T HE OBSERVATION THAT individuals differ in their intellectual abilities is so commonly accepted today that it is surprising to realize that as recently as the last century intelligence was viewed in a binary manner: either one was an "ament" and lacked intelligence or one was "normal." Despite our current acceptance of differences in intelligence among "normal" individuals, many people still view the retarded as a homogenous group. As the drive to provide services for the retarded increases, the question of "Who is retarded?" becomes increasingly relevant and will be discussed in this chapter.

One service that receives high priority from parents and educators of retarded individuals is language intervention. This chapter describes for the language specialist both mental retardation and the language observed among the retarded. Obviously, mental retardation is not the cause of the language disorder; rather it is the language disorder that is one of many symptoms of the retardation. However, if the language specialist is to effectively intervene with the child who is retarded, then that specialist must understand the condition affecting the child as well as the characteristics of his language.

Until the last several decades, the language of the mentally retarded received minimal attention in the research literature, and techniques of evaluation were viewed by professionals, much as they are viewed today by the general public, as reflecting a lack of thought or reason. As Ryan (1977) noted in "The Silence of Stupidity," if one assumes that the silence of the retarded results from a lack of ideas and that only ideas require language, then there is no point in attempting to teach the retarded to speak. Obviously, the assumption that the retarded have few if any ideas to express is no longer acceptable, yet the assumption that to be unable to speak is to be "stupid" is perpetuated in our language, which provides as the first definition for the word *dumb,* "devoid of the power of speech" (Webster's New Collegiate Dictionary, 1974).

The study of the language of the mentally retarded has followed the trends of the psycholinguistic investigation of normal language acquisition. Early studies explored the development of the syntactic system, and later research focused on semantics and analysis of semantic intentions. Currently, investigation of the pragmatic system and the use of language is popular. One of the more complete reviews of the early literature concerning the language of the retarded (Spreen, 1965a, 1965b) concluded that there was no one specific type of language impairment that could be represented as "typical" of the retarded. All types of impairment and degrees of severity were observed. The continuing equivocal nature of our conclusions about the language of the retarded appears related to the tendency of researchers to try to generalize about the retarded without first carefully defining the population under study. The mentally retarded are a diverse group, and retardation may be caused by many factors. In a great number of cases, the exact etiology may never be known; an estimated 80 percent of retarded individuals have retardation of unknown etiology (K. G. Scott, 1980). In addition, the consequences of retardation differ widely in terms of family life and educational opportunities.

This chapter begins with a definition of mental retardation, including a presentation of some of the clinical syndromes associated with retardation, their range of severity, and the tests commonly used to identify the developmental disorder known as mental retardation. Following this discussion, the effect of mental retardation on the dimensions of language is presented. Finally, the integrative view of language disorders in the mentally retarded is presented, along with implications for assessment and intervention.

DEFINITION   It is customary to view mental retardation as a classification based on some organic characteristic, yet operationally the term mental retardation is a diagnostic label used to describe the lack of the capacity to adapt to one's social and educational environment. A close look at both intelligence tests and scales of adaptive behavior shows that a high reliance on language skills exists in these measures of intelligence. There is a clear overlap between the behaviors used to classify a child as mentally retarded or language-disordered. In addition, the emergence of these behaviors is subject to environmental control.

Mental retardation occurs on a continuum of severity, and the language disorders associated with retardation also vary widely on this continuum. As with other handicaps, the identification of one disorder does not preclude the occurrence of others. Thus, a child may be deaf and emotionally disturbed, for example, as well as mentally retarded.

Despite the diversity of opinions about intelligence, the majority of definitions of retardation include one or more of these principles: (1) capacity to learn, particularly as judged by developmental standards or by comparison to developmental norms; (2) knowledge acquired, often measured by many items on intelligence tests; and (3) ability to adjust or adapt to the environment and to novel situations in that environment, measured by scales of adaptive behavior or social competence.

Over the years, an influential group devoted to the study of mental retardation, The American Association on Mental Deficiency (AAMD), has compiled and updated its definition of mental retardation. In 1973, AAMD issued a manual on terminology and classification (Grossman, 1973). The definition indicated that mental retardation refers to significantly impaired intellectual functioning, without reference to etiology, occurring during the developmental period—under 18 years of age. It may be due to social, genetic, environmental, nutritional, or biological factors. The term is descriptive of current functioning only and carries no implication about prognosis for future functioning. Intellectual functioning may be evaluated by any one of a number of tests and is commonly expressed in terms of IQ, with IQ scores under 70 on the two most commonly used tests (Stanford-Binet and WISC) as the cut-off point. The classification of mental retardation must also include adaptive behavior, which is the effectiveness of the individual's ability to cope with personal independence and social responsibility as expected in his culture for his age. The definition emphasizes that IQ alone is *not* sufficient to make a diagnosis of mental retardation (Robinson & Robinson, 1976). The addition of adaptive behavior is important because of the severe criticism leveled at the psychometric model of intelligence as measured by IQ tests.

CAUSES OF MENTAL RETARDATION

The cause of retardation may be organic, environmental, or an interaction between the two. Debate over the relative importance of each factor has been reported in the literature for decades and still continues without resolution.

Organic Causes

The study of genetics has contributed to our understanding of the causes of retardation. The earliest attempts to test for intelligence were apparently undertaken to demonstrate that genius was common in certain families. This simplistic desire to prove scientifically the superiority of a certain family (usually the investigator's), was doomed to failure. Although intelligence is influenced by inheritance, it is most likely the result of cumulative contributions from a number of genes and so is a form of "polygenic" inheritance.

Genetic Conditions

The addition of part of a chromosome, or a defect in a single gene or a pair of genes, can make it virtually impossible for the affected individual to develop normally. Profoundly retarded children are often impaired because of overriding damage to their genetic makeup. Brief and relatively nontechnical reviews of the process of genetic inheritance are contained in various introductory texts (Apgar & Beck, 1972; Menolascino & Egger, 1978; Robinson & Robinson, 1976) and will not be discussed here.

The most common and extensively researched genetic form of mental retardation is Down's syndrome, which is the result of an extra set of genes on chromosome number 21. Thus it is called Trisomy 21. This syndrome was previously known as "mongolian idiocy" and was first identified and described by an English physician, Langdon Down, in 1866. In his brief but remarkably accurate description, he noted the outstanding symptoms, including the unusual "oriental-like" slant of the eyes from which the term "mongolism" was coined. Approximately 9 to 10 percent of all retarded children have Down's syndrome (Coleman, 1980).

Other abnormalities of the chromosomal material have also been observed. Trisomy 13 and 15 (D Group) tend to be associated with severe physical and mental defects, and most children so affected die within the first few months of life. Trisomy 16 and 18 (E Group) have also been identified, but the number of recorded cases remains very few and most of these infants die early. Other syndromes may be associated with abnormalities of the sex chromosomes. These include Turner's and Klinefelter's syndromes as well as ten to thirteen other conditions (Zellweger & Ionasescu, 1978). Retardation ranging from moderate to severe is common in afflicted individuals.

Another group of genetic disorders results in biochemical dysfunction and is often called "inborn errors of metabolism." The biochemical imbalance causes the production of toxins,

which may affect the brain. One such disorder is phenylketo-
nuria (PKU), for which mass screening programs now exist.
Others, such as Maple Syrup Urine disease, Tay-Sachs disease,
Hunter's syndrome, and Hurler's syndrome are more common
examples of the several hundred syndromes that have been associated with mental retardation.

Other Congenital Disorders

Other *congenital* disorders may be apparent at birth, yet they
are not inherited. During some pregnancies, a blood incompati-
bility associated with the Rh factor may cause problems for the
infant resulting in cerebral palsy. Although some cerebral palsied children prove to be normal or superior intellectually, mental retardation is more common in this group than in the general
population. The best estimates are that about 50 percent have
IQs below 70 (Hutt & Gibb, 1976; Robinson & Robinson, 1976).

Maternal infections during pregnancy can cause many problems in the child although the mother may be aware of only mild
symptoms. Rubella, when passed on from the mother to her unborn child, can cause mental retardation, as well as hearing and
vision loss and other problems (Menolascino & Egger, 1978).
Ingestion of various drugs by the mother during pregnancy may
also result in damage to the unborn child, including symptoms
of mental reardation.

Postnatal Disorders

Some children who begin life with no impairment may later
sustain brain damge resulting in mental retardation. Diseases
that affect the brain, such as meningitis and encephalitis, can
cause some degree of mental retardation. In addition, ingestion
or exposure to toxins such as lead or mercury may also result in
retardation.

Environmental Causes

Although inheritance is determined by a single ova and a single sperm, the resultant individual is nurtured first within the
environment of his mother's body, then in the family, and finally
in the broader community. The importance of environmental influence is suggested by prevalence figures. Some three percent
of the general population are commonly said to be mentally retarded. Bensberg and Sigelman (1976, p. 64) suggest that the
figures may run as low as two percent in middle- and upper-in-
come neighborhoods; five percent in rural areas; and seven per-

cent in lower-income neighborhoods. Surveys (Mercer, 1972; Robinson & Robinson, 1976) of all of the children labeled as mentally retarded in one community in California indicated that the label of retardation does not cut evenly across social and ethnic groups. There were 300 percent more Mexican-Americans and 50 percent more blacks than would be expected from their proportions in the community, and 60 percent fewer Anglos. These figures were not simply a local phenomenon as shown by a survey of the rest of the state. This study further indicated that the public schools were the primary labeling agency; therefore, it was not surprising to find that the great majority of the identified cases were of school age.

The undeniably higher rate of retardation among the poor and disadvantaged has resulted in heated and emotional discussions regarding the relationship of genetic inheritance and environmental factors. Children born into poor environments have greater birth risks including prematurity and resultant low birth weight (Menolascino & Egger, 1978). Many factors have been associated with low birth weight, including inadequate prenatal diet, inadequate maternal care, number of previous children, overall health of the mother, and young age (especially teens) of the mother. All of these factors are most likely to occur among mothers from low socioeconomic areas. Low-birth-weight infants are born almost twice as often in nonwhite as in white areas (13.6 percent versus 7.1 percent; Robinson & Robinson, 1976). Not only are poor children exposed to greater risks surrounding their birth, but during childhood they are at greater risk for bacterial and viral infections and exposure to toxic substances. Their subsequent health care is often inferior to that of children from more affluent families.

MEASUREMENT OF INTELLIGENCE AND ADAPTIVE BEHAVIOR

The two most common measures of intelligence are intelligence tests that yield an IQ, and tests of adaptive behavior.

Intelligence Tests

During the past century, various attempts were made to devise a measure of intelligence, but none succeeded until Alfred Binet and Theodore Simon suggested that intelligence might be age-related and could be measured by administering a large number of questions to children. The 1905 Binet-Simon Scale proved successful not only in identifying retarded children but also in measuring the capacity of normal and superior students. The scale was adopted for use in the United States; the 1973 revision is currently in use.

Only after the publication and widespread use of this "intelli-

Alfred Binet

Alfred Binet was the most prominent French psychologist of the late 1800s. After studying both law and medicine in Paris, he founded the first psychological laboratory in France at the Sorbonne in 1889. When the Paris school district was faced with the problem of identifying those children who could benefit from an education from those who could not, they went to Binet for assistance. Binet, with his colleague, Theodore Simon, designed a test to divide individuals on the basis of intellectual capacity. To do this, they invented a large number of questions that they hoped would separate normal from retarded children. To their surprise, these questions also separated children with various degrees of normal and superior intelligence. As a part of this work, they developed the concept of mental age.

The Binet-Simon test of intelligence proved so popular that it was translated into a number of languages. The English translation was done at Stanford University and became known as the Stanford-Binet Test of Intelligence. It is still widely used as a measure of intelligence. The latest revision of the Stanford-Binet was done in 1960. The resulting L-M Form extends from age 2 to 14, with additional items at the Average Adult and Superior Adult I, II, and III levels. The items on this scale are highly verbal in nature, and a majority of them require an ability to use words, define words, or solve verbal problems.

gence test" did serious research into the structure and nature of intelligence begin. In 1927, Spearman described a unitary concept of intelligence, while Thorndike and Thurston proposed an aggregate of specific abilities; Wechsler deplored what he termed this artificial disagreement (C. G. Morris, 1979). Wechsler felt that intelligence was a global capacity allowing people to act purposefully, think rationally, and deal effectively with the environment. His intelligence scales have come to be the most widely used tests in the United States and include the Wechsler Preschool and Primary Scale of Intelligence (WPPSI), the Wechsler Intelligence Scale for Children—Revised (WISC-R), and the Wechsler Adult Intelligence Scale (WAIS). All of these consist of a performance scale including items such as copying patterns with small blocks or cubes, and a verbal scale with items such as defining words or giving explanations. They yield separate scores as well as an overall IQ.

Once an intelligence test has been administered, the score may be expressed in terms of mental age (MA) if tests such as the Stanford-Binet have been administered. Scores are then converted to an intelligence quotient (IQ) by employing a formula:

$$IQ = \frac{\text{mental age}}{\text{chronological age}} \times 100$$

These scores have a normal and expected variation of as much as 15 points. A serious concern of test designers, test administers, and, more recently, legislators, is the realization that the most common tests reflect the white, middle-class culture of their designers. Such bias puts individuals from other races, language backgrounds, and cultures at a disadvantage, and at-

Table 16-1
Classification of Mentally Retarded by IQ

IQ Range	Descriptive Term	Percent Affected	Skill Potential
55–69	Mild retardation	89	Simple productive work
40–54	Moderate retardation	6	Routine tasks; supervised self-care
25–39	Severe retardation	3.5	Supervised self-care
Below 25	Profound retardation	1.5	Needs major care throughout life

tempts are under way to substitute certain untimed performance tests for verbal tests and to design new culture-fair tests.

Mental ages may be generated by a number of tests, and it is important for the language specialist to appreciate the role of mental age in determining the extent of a problem and the expected rate of change or prognosis. The mental age is commonly expressed in terms of months or years. For example, a delay of 9 months in a 12-month-old child indicates a mental age of 3 months. This constitutes a significant problem, and, if an appropriate test was administered, represents an IQ of 25. If that measure truly reflects the child's potential, the child's rate of change will be predictably slow, so that at 4 years he will have attained the mental age of 12 months, and at 12 years, his mental age will be 3 years. The same delay (9 months) discovered in a 4-year-old child would represent a variation in the range of low normal and would yield an IQ in the 80s. This child's development would be expected to continue at least at 80 percent of the so-called normal rate. A delay of 9 months in an 8-year-old child would obviously be within normal limits. The extent of delay is meaningless unless it is related to chronological age, and it is only then that it assumes any prognostic significance.

The American Association of Mental Deficiency has described the expected relationship of IQ to skill potential and has assigned descriptive terms that correspond to the IQ range. The percentages of the total retarded population that fall into each classification are also provided (Menolascino & Egger, 1978; Robinson & Robinson, 1976) (Table 16-1).

Measurement of Adaptive Behavior

As intelligence tests were administered to more and more children from nonmiddle-class and nonwhite homes, the validity of IQ scores came under increasingly sharp criticism. Users of intelligence tests appeared to lose sight of the fact that, beginning with Binet's test, such instruments were designed to predict how well a child would succeed in a school using a curriculum geared to the mainstream of the population. Such tests were *not* designed to predict how a minority child would succeed in his own environment nor how any child would succeed in adult life.

The first widely used adaptive scale was the Vineland Social Maturity Scale published in 1936 by Edgar Doll and revised in 1964. The 1964 scale consists of a series of age-related items ranging from birth through 25 years of age. The items are in the form of open-ended questions, which are asked of a person familiar with the behavior of the individual being tested. Based upon these responses, a social age and social quotient (analogous to MA and IQ) may be computed. This scale is currently undergoing extensive revision by American Guidance Corporation. The revision will not only reflect current research but will expand the overall usefulness of the scale.

As an outgrowth of the previously discussed California research that showed an abnormally high percentage of retarded in Mexican-American and black neighborhoods, Mercer (Soeffing, 1977) proposed a new assessment technique for mentally retarded and culturally different children. Called the System of Multicultural Pluralistic Assessment (SOMPA), it requires an interview with the child's mother or principle caretaker and two test sessions with the child. Preliminary data indicates that there is a separate group of culturally different children who have low scores on standard IQ tests but who score in the normal range using culturally appropriate norms. This suggests that their educational problems may be due to cultural differences (Soeffing, 1977, pp. 55–61).

Despite the clear need for good measures of adaptive behavior, some experts (Robinson & Robinson, 1976) in the field of

Edgar A. Doll

Edgar Doll's unique contribution to the evaluation and training of mentally retarded persons was the development of scales of social maturity. He correctly observed that scores on standardized intelligence tests did not necessarily predict how well an individual could care for himself or others nor how well he could function in society. He also observed that mentally retarded children were often difficult to test and that their performance in a testing situation did not always reflect their true potential. In an effort to provide a supplement or alternative to intelligence scales, Doll first published the *Vineland Social Maturity Scale* in 1936 and then the *Measurement of Social Competence*. His writing reflected his philosophy that all of life is a process of becoming.

A native of Cleveland, Ohio, Doll received his Ph.D. in psychology from Cornell University in 1912. Although he lectured for limited periods at a number of American universities, Doll spent the majority of his professional career as Director of Research at the Vineland Training School in Vineland, New Jersey, which was a facility for mentally retarded individuals. From 1935 to 1936, Doll served as president of the American Association on Mental Deficiency.

mental retardation conclude that assessment in this realm is even more primitive than intellectual evaluation; however, energetic efforts are underway to improve this situation.

Adaptive behavior refers primarily to the manner in which the individual *copes*. The concept of coping is represented by three major facets incorporated in Adaptive Behavior Scales (ABS; Kennett, 1976, p. 147): (1) independent functioning demonstrated by accomplishing tasks expected of age group; (2) personal responsibility for own behavior, and basic decision-making capacity; and (3) social responsibility, reflected in basic conformity, civic responsibility, and some economic independence.

In addition to these scales, there are over a dozen other scales of adaptive behavior on the market that evaluate skills deemed appropriate for various ages. For example, during infancy and early childhood, adaptation consists of development of sensory and motor skills such as sitting alone and walking; communication skills such as following directions and speaking; self-help skills such as feeding oneself and being toilet trained; and socialization, including ability to interact with others. During childhood and adolescence, social maturity is reflected by the application of basic academic skills to life, application of common sense to the mastery of the environment, and participation in the community.

LANGUAGE AND MENTAL RETARDATION

Impairment in the language of the retarded ranges from mild deficits resulting in generally reduced vocabulary to profound impairment resulting in the total absence of any means of communication.

Prevalence of Language Impairment among the Mentally Retarded

Summaries of various surveys suggest that virtually 100 percent of the profoundly retarded have impaired language, while 90 percent of the severely retarded (IQ between 21 and 50) and about 45 percent of the mildly retarded are so impaired (Gomez & Podhajski, 1978; Schlanger, 1973; Spreen, 1965a, 1965b). The extent of language impairment is greatest in those with the lowest IQ. However, in her review of the subnormal without speech, Ryan (1977) stressed that while the nonspeaking subnormals tended to be those with the lowest IQ scores, there were exceptions to this generalization in both directions. In her opinion, it was not possible to find any meaningful prevalence figures for the nonspeaking subnormals because few people have counted them, and also because the criteria vary so greatly. The total absence of speech may or may not co-exist with comprehension and the use of gesture, vocalization, facial expression, and other forms of reciprocal social communication. There is agreement, however, that the incidence of these nonspeaking persons is greatest in institutions. Many of the surveys did not mention how language was sampled or state the criteria for impairment. Most importantly, little or no mention is made of the willingness of the retarded individual to interact with the examiner. These surveys seldom consider the functional use retarded persons can make of their language.

The tendency to group mentally retarded persons is nowhere more evident than when attempting to present data on the prevalence of language impairment. Few studies use the same classification system, and the populations surveyed may be identified only with such a vague term as "institutionalized." The resultant confusion is illustrated by the fact that before the 1970s, many of the persons in institutions tended to be only mildly or moderately impaired, while more recently only the most profoundly impaired have been institutionalized. Thus, over a period of 10 to 20 years, the population represented by the term "institutionalized" has changed radically.

The Cognitive Dimension

Sensation

Information enters the cognitive system through the sensory channels. Audition is crucial for the development of the auditory-vocal code, and the relationship of reduced auditory sensation to langauge development is well known. Hearing loss has been extensively studied in the mentally retarded. Conservative estimates indicate that 15 to 20 percent of the mentally retarded have some hearing loss (Bensberg & Sigelman, 1976; Fristoe, 1976) and that 15 percent of the children in schools for the deaf are mentally retarded. Downs (1980) surveyed the studies of Down's syndrome individuals, and found that prevalence of hearing loss varied from 40 percent to 78 percent. (Hearing loss was judged by different criteria in different studies.) Downs' survey included 107 subjects between the ages of 2 months and 60 years. Seventy-eight percent had hearing loss of more than 15 dB in one or both ears, and 65 percent had significant loss in both ears. Of these, only 16 percent had received amplication—none at an early age.

A survey of diagnostic services provided in facilities for the retarded showed that speech and language services were available in 20 to 40 percent more facilities than were audiological services. With hearing loss as widespread as the above studies suggest, the lack of audiological services and remediation may be expected to significantly inhibit the effectiveness of speech and language treatment, particularly since present technology is capable of detecting at least middle ear pathology in virtually all retarded persons.

Perception and Memory

Other cognitive abilities, such as perception and memory, have been less well studied in the mentally retarded. Perception may be assumed to be affected by the hearing loss already documented in this population. A loss of immediate memory may further complicate the mentally retarded child's ability to hold the speech signal until it is decoded. The independence of these cognitive abilities may be illustrated by the particular ability of some retarded individuals to retain long strings of information in short-term memory and repeat them without demonstrating ability to comprehend the material. More characteristic, however, is the report by Rohr and Burr (1978) showing that Down's syndrome children, in particular, have a defect in auditory processes, especially in short-term memory as measured by the repetition of digits. Children with Down's syndrome also appear to be highly susceptible to auditory distraction. The ability to perceive and retain auditory information is essential to language development. These cognitive abilities require further study in well-defined populations of children.

Conceptualization and Representation

Conceptualization and representation have been more completely studied than memory and perception. Piaget's cognitive theory suggests that the appearance of language is dependent upon the cognitive structures achieved during the sensorimotor period, particularly the ability to classify objects and to relate objects to action (Sinclair, 1971). Until these concepts are achieved, any attempt to facilitate language acquisition is felt to be doomed to failure. A study (Greenwald & Leonard, 1979) explored the relationship of cognitive skills to language acquisition in nonretarded and Down's subjects. Specifically, they explored two types of prelinguistic behavior: (1) preimperative, such as looking at, reaching for, or pointing to an object; and (2) declarative, an imperative that consists of grasping, showing, or giving an object. The study confirmed a relationship between the sensorimotor stage and communication. This correspondence was closest at the younger ages. The effect of prolonged time spent in any one stage remains unclear.

Cromer (1974) pointed out that the possession of a certain level of sensorimotor intelligence cannot of itself guarantee the expression of that intelligence in language. One of the problems in attempting to explain failure of language development on the basis of the Piagetian model is the difficulty of applying tasks developed for infants to fully grown, often ambulatory, grossly retarded individuals. Such studies continue to fail in their attempt to clarify which levels are the necessary prerequisites to speech (Ryan, 1977). O'Connor (1975) reflected that language and thought in the very young child and the retarded child appear to have a differential development. At some point the two converge. Concepts become linked to the linguistic code and thought becomes verbal. The relationship between concepts and language is a reciprocal one. Language development is dependent upon the acquisition of concepts, yet language facilitates the categorization and storage of experiences that form the basis of concepts. It is possible that some retardates never achieve this association between concept and the linguistic code. In other retardates, it is possible that deficits in the areas of auditory sensation, memory, and retrieval may impede this convergence of thought with its verbal expression.

The Communication Environment

Recently, studies emerged that explored the language mothers use at home to their retarded children. Burium, Rynder, & Turnure (1974) suggested that the linguistic forms used with Down's infants were different than forms used with normal children, thus making the linguistic environment different. Gutmann and Rondal (1979) found differences, but felt that these differences were appropriate to the child's level of language.

Berry and Marshall (1978) found that mentally retarded children had difficulty using nonverbal signals. In addition, they observed that facial expression was less important to young mentally retarded children than it was to normal children. Based upon what is known about development in normal children, it would appear that the differences in the rate at which retarded children develop such interpersonal responses may modify their parents' responses to them. Possibly, at the age when the child is most ready to react, the parents have ceased the stimulation.

Bedrosian and Prutting (1978) commented upon the lack of literature on the use that mentally retarded persons make of their language. They explored dominant and submissive roles, specifically whether four mentally retarded adults would express verbal control or authority in *any* social situation. Their subjects interacted (1) with a speech and language pathologist, (2) with a peer, (3) with a parent, and (4) with a normal child. Normally, an adult is always dominant with a child; however, none of the subjects held a dominant position in any of the conditions, except for one subject who was dominant only with her peer and with the child. The authors concluded that it is as important to teach communication in various settings as it is to teach vocabulary or structure.

A child's awareness of the usefulness of language predates the onset of words. Preverbal children already display several communicative functions of language such as greeting and regulating the behavior of others. Fostering this awareness in mentally retarded individuals continues to be prerequisite to both verbal and nonverbal communication.

The Linguistic Code: Delayed or Deviant Development

The question of delay versus deviance extends beyond the area of clinical language disorder into the study of the mentally retarded. The traditional wisdom has been that the language of the mentally retarded developed in slow motion. Too often, that judgment was supported by vague references to language that was "sparse," "limited," or simply "defective for age." With increased linguistic sophistication in the study of normal children, it was possible to replicate these studies with the mentally retarded. Investigators like Lackner (1968) collected samples of spontaneous languages and analyzed the grammars. Other researchers studied the order of development of morphemes, sentence complexity, and many of the other variables previously charted for normal children. These studies are noteworthy for several reasons. First, they provide a description of the language of the mentally retarded, which is valuable in itself. Also, they investigate the question of whether the language of the mentally retarded differs from normal language quantitatively or qualitatively.

The theory of the quantitative delay of the language of the mentally retarded was clearly articulated by Lenneberg (1967), who associated the emergence of verbalization with the acquisition of key motor skills such as sitting and walking. He postulated that, as the brain matures, the growing infant successively attains various developmental milestones such as sitting, walking, and speaking. Cross-cultural studies showed that all children begin to stand and say single words around their first birthday. Lenneberg did not imply that the motor skill of walking, for example, was a necessary prerequisite to language, but that the emergence of both skills reflected growth in the complexity of the brain. In his 1967 study, Lenneberg investigated children with Down's syndrome. These children were more likely to begin saying words after gait was established than before.

Lackner's influential study (1968) matched five mentally retarded children with five normal children based on mental age.

The mental ages of the retarded were 2 years, 3 months to 8 years, 10 months, and their chronological ages ranged from 6 years, 6 months to 14 years, 5 months. The mental ages of the normals were the same, but their chronological ages were 2 years, 8 months to 5 years, 9 months. After obtaining samples of spontaneous language, he wrote grammars for the normal and the retarded children. Lackner's original assumption was that retardation does not result in a different form of language. The retarded simply develop language more slowly and terminate it at a stage below that of the normal child. His study confirmed this hypothesis. Another study (Yoder & Miller, 1972) explored the order of development of inflectional forms in both retarded and nonretarded groups. The order of development proved to be the same in both groups and thus supported the delay hypothesis. Other studies of the ability of the retarded to understand sentences of varying grammatic complexity (Semmel & Dolley, 1971) and to process different types of transformations (Gordon & Panagas, 1976) tended to confirm the "slow motion" hypothesis of language development.

The expression of semantic relations in the two-word utterances of Down's syndrome children was investigated (Coggins, 1979) in four subjects with mild intellectual deficits. The chronological ages of these subjects ranged from 3 years, 10 months to 6 years, 1 month, and they were in either early or late stage I grammar. The children concentrated on the same, rather small set of relational meanings as did normal children at the same linguistic stage. They identified regularities in experience, attributes of objects and people, recognized change in position, etc. This evidence supported J. F. Miller and Yoder's study (1974)

Reflections*

If you go away from me you look small,
Like a small standing doll in front of a mirror.
But when you come back to stay with me I want to
* say*
Your love is with me always. I can picture you in
My mind, the image of you, the likeness of you.
You're so beautifully made by God
That your love always stays with me, forever.

This poem was written by a mildly mentally retarded man, Roger Meyers, whose parents were told that he would never be able to learn to read or write. After years of effort Roger learned to do both, and this is only one of a number of his poems included in a book written about Roger's life by his brother (Meyers, 1978). Although the poem has no dedication, Roger may have been thinking of the woman who is now his wife. They met while both of them were living in a group residence for retarded adults. They learned to live independently in the community, got jobs and married. Their achievement is modest when compared to their normal siblings, but when compared to what society would have offered them in the past, it is worthy of recognition.

*From Robert Meyers: *Like Normal People.* New York: McGraw-Hill Book Company, 1978. Reprinted with permission.

---

that retarded children acquire language in a manner similar to normals except at a slower pace.

In contrast to the preceding studies, other researchers suggested that the language of the retarded differs in a qualitative manner from the normal. Their use of morphemes differs (Menyuk, 1971), and as mental age increased some differences are also observed in the use of inflectional forms (R.S. Schiefelbusch, 1972). It was suggested that these differences may be due to the tendency of the retardates to use only those inflections that they have learned from memory through constant usage rather than to generalize the rule as normal children appear to do. Ryan (1977) found that vocabulary improved more quickly in the mentally retarded than did grammar. A study of semantics (Semmel, Barrett, & Bennet, 1970) indicated that when retarded and normal subjects of the same mental age are compared on word association tasks, the retarded fail to shift from synonyms to antonyms at the same mental age as the normals. This indicates a deviance in language development that can not be explained on the basis of intellectual development above.

Bliss, Allen & Walker (1978) used a story completion task with 15 trainable (IQ 29 to 50) and 15 educable (IQ 51 to 78) mentally retarded children to study similarities and differences in their language behavior. This study revealed an obvious delay in development in that both groups showed a positive association between their intellectual functioning and their ability to produce the more complex grammatic forms. However the study also revealed signs of deviance; both groups of retarded mastered the simplest form, the imperative, but they were limited in the use of abstract and elaborate structures such as the future, embedded sentences, and double-adjectival noun phrases. The

Figure 16-1
Schematic representation of a developmental schedule comparing normal and mentally retarded individuals. The age at which a majority of the children may be expected to master a skill is indicated by the widest point in the diamond. The period of development is not only longer for the retarded, but some skills may never be accomplished by some retarded as indicated by the open diamonds. (From data of Gomez & Podhajski, 1978; Karlin & Strazulla, 1958; Lenneberg, 1967; and Robinson & Robinson, 1976.)

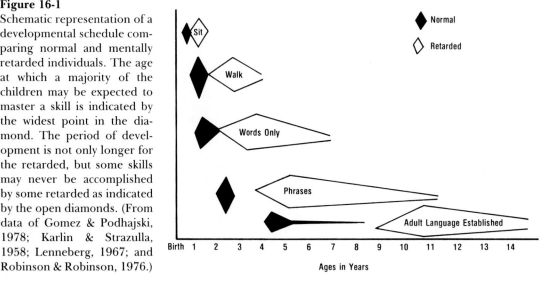

trainable group in particular had difficulty with simple declarative sentences and questions. The authors theorized that this may reflect a particular problem in the use of the subject form by children with deviant language.

Another study (Naremore & Dever, 1975) explored whether there were quantitative or qualitative differences in the language of 30 educable mentally retarded who were matched with normals on the basis of mental age. The authors explored both syntactic and fluency variables, and found that the fluency variables proved more interesting than did the syntactic complexity results. While the normals used filled pauses to signal that they were not yet finished speaking, and used false starts to allow themselves to restate, the retarded simply repeated themselves. This repetition served only to stop the flow of speech and was viewed as a basic dysfunction. This study supported the observation of qualitative differences between the language of normals and the mentally retarded. In their discussion, the authors raised the question of whether a retarded individual ever reached the proficiency and overall language level of a normal child of 6 years, or of 10 years, for example.

Figure 16-1 illustrates a schedule of development of language, sitting, and walking with the expected range of variation for both the normal and the retarded. The importance of the quantitative delay does not negate the validity of specific qualitative differences that have been observed in the use of certain morphemes and inflectional forms or syntactic structures, which may reflect the specific cognitive complexity of these forms. Or perhaps, as Schiefelbusch (1972) has suggested, the differences may be due to a tendency of some retardates to use memorized or rote forms rather than generalizing rules. Differences in language knowledge and performance may be expected to be related to differences in the level of concept development.

Speech Performance

In addition to language impairments, speech disorders are common among the mentally retarded. These include phonological, voice, and stuttering defects. No single researcher has attempted to analyze the total prevalence of speech defects in the mentally retarded. However, by combining the results of four separate studies, some idea of the observed frequency can be suggested (Table 16-2). Impairment of articulation is the most common defect, particularly in children with neuromotor problems. Voice and fluency problems are also common.

No pattern of articulation defects can be considered "typical" of the retarded, except that speech sound errors are found in

Table 16–2
Observed Range of Frequency of Various Speech
Defects among the Mentally Retarded

Type of Defect	Level of Retardation			
	Mild	Moderate	Severe	Profound
Articulation	8–53%	72%	80%	95%
Voice		22%	58%	62%
Stuttering		10%	45%	

*Adapted from material reported by Yoder and Miller (1972, p. 90); Schlanger (1973, pp. 16–20); Robinson and Robinson (1976, p. 236); and Schielfelbush (1972, p. 215).

greater abundance than among normal children. Among the mildly retarded, the prevalence of phonological defects ranges from a reported low of 8 percent up to 53 percent, while in the more severely impaired it ranges from 72 to 95 percent. Analysis of error phonemes has been done, and, not surprisingly, retarded children, like normal children, have more difficulty perfecting the more complex consonant sounds such as /th/, /v/, /s/, /z/, and /ch/. J. L. Bangs (1942) found that the articulation errors of the retarded corresponded very closely to the errors made by normal children, with the exception that the retarded tended to omit many more consonants occurring in the final position in words.

Children with neurological impairment show obviously higher percentages of articulation problems, and Down's syndrome children appear to be at special risk. Although Down's and normal children seem to use the same basic phonologic rules, Down's children use these rules inconsistently. In Blager's study (1980), many of the errors of Down's children did not seem to follow any rules, whereas the other severely retarded children performed similarly to age-matched normal children in that their errors followed rules. Blanchard (1964) had previously observed this, and suggested that children with Down's may have an inability to maintain long-term psychomotor programming. The cerebellum, which is important in motor performance, is significantly smaller in Down's children, and this may account for their inconsistent production. In addition, the hypotonicity of tongue and lips may also interfere with articulation (Cromer, 1974).

Voice and phonation disorders have been particularly studied among the Down's population. Benda (1960) commented that a "low"-pitched voice in Down's children was attributable to thickened laryngeal mucosa. However, Weinberg and Zlatin (1970) studied 27 Down's children, and their results not only failed to support a lowered fundamental frequency for the Down's population but indicated that their subjects had higher-pitched voices. They noted that since the children were more like younger normal children in terms of weight and especially height, this finding was not surprising. An immature body build suggests an immature larynx. A study of adults with Down's syndrome (Moran & Gilbert, 1978) confirmed that their mean fundamental voice frequency was higher than that of nonretarded adults of the same age and sex. They also noted the smaller stature and retarded sexual development of the Down's individuals and suggested a possible relationship between retarded physical development (including the larynx) and a high, immature-sounding voice.

Stuttering has also been reported in prevalence studies. This problem is less often observed among the profoundly retarded (see Table 16-2), possibly because their speech may be too limited to easily observe this symptom. Other researchers suggested that the profoundly retarded do not stutter because they may lack self-observation and self-consciousness about their ability to communicate (Schlanger, 1973). The occurrence of symptoms of stuttering among the verbal retarded ranges from 10 to 45 percent, with a higher incidence among those with Down's syndrome.

THE INTEGRATIVE APPROACH

The integrative approach recognizes that concepts must be established prior to development of knowledge of the linguistic code and the performance of that code in the comprehension and expression of language. Once a concept is established, it must be associated with the verbal symbol, and only after that association is formed will the individual be able to comprehend and express the word or phrase symbolizing the concept. The integrative model (Figure 16-2) reflects this fundamental defect in conceptualization, which is subsequently reflected in the delay of other aspects of language development.

Mentally retarded individuals characteristically show uniform depression in all concepts of equal abstraction and complexity. In general, the retarded can comprehend words matching the concepts they possess, and unless they have a motor speech problem, they can usually say these same words. In contrast, the child with clinical language disorder demonstrates some concepts that are appropriate for his chronological age. His conceptual deficits are often specific to certain concepts such as space or time, for example. As has been noted in Chapter 13, children with clinical language disorders may demonstrate that they have concepts for which they lack the words. It is also possible for these children to have markedly greater ability to comprehend than to express language. This is seldom true of mentally retarded children.

As the mentally retarded child develops vocabulary, the content words tend to be highly correlated with the concepts the child possesses. Specific, or qualitative, problems may appear in the development of some of the closed class of words due in part to the abstract nature of such concepts as relative location (prepositions), changing time (tense), and shifting reference (pronouns such as *I* versus *you*).

The relationship of concept development, as measured by intelligence level, and verbal expression can be appreciated by comparing how Arthur and Robert, two retarded individuals seen by the authors of this volume, describe the same two pictures. Although the boys were seven years apart in chronological age, their levels of concept development were roughly comparable, as illustrated by the vocabulary and semantic relations they expressed (Table 16-3). Both boys expressed existence through their naming of items in the pictures. Both also expressed the relations of action + object, while Arthur also used agent + action. Their choice of vocabulary suggests the insights each boy had into the pictures. In picture 1, Arthur correctly noted the smoke resulting from something burning on the stove. When discussing picture 2, neither boy commented on the lighted birthday cake visible through the window of the house or the fact that children were bringing presents to the house.

Figure 16-2
The integrative model of language showing the effect of a conceptual problem on the other dimensions of language. Affected units of language are marked with an asterisk.

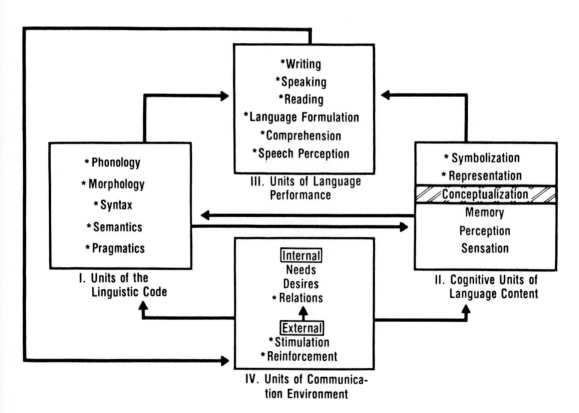

Table 16–3
Vocabulary and Semantic Relations of Two Retarded Boys*

Picture*	Arthur (Age 17, Moderately Retarded)	Robert (Age 10, Mildly Retarded)
1	The lady talking. Children. Fire. Smoke.	Grandmother. Trees and four children.
2	Ringing the doorbell.	Door knob. Girl buzzing.

*As recorded by the authors of this volume during the course of clinical research.

Although it has been stated that the language of the mentally retarded individual shows inevitable delay, this may not always be expressed in the same manner. Some mentally retarded individuals, with the same slow acquisition of concepts as Arthur and Robert, may sound fluent. Children diagnosed as hydrocephalic have been observed to produce fluent, well-articulated speech empty of real meaning (E. Schwartz, 1974; Swisher & Pinsker, 1971). Often, these children use language effectively as a greeting and to establish interpersonal contact. Clare, age 6, another child who was seen by the authors of this book, illustrates what Swisher and Pinsker (1971) have called "cocktail party talk." Clare had spinal bifida and hydrocephalus. When Clare saw the author in the hall she moved her wheelchair to meet her, and the following exchange took place:

Clare: Hi there.
Adult: Hi Clare. How are you?
Clare: I'm just fine, thank you. How are you feeling today? My goodness, you look nice. That is such a pretty dress. I really like your dress. . . .
Adult: (Begins to move away.)
Clare: Goodbye now. Have a good day.

Clare could be observed continuing down the hall repeating essentially the same conversation with others she met. Casual observers considered Clare to be "quite bright," yet objective testing indicated a significant delay in concept development. Very little of what Clare said signified anything beyond the empty content of social phrases. Like Arthur and Robert, Clare's language performance reflected her delayed concept development.

ASSESSMENT

The language specialist has several unique contributions to make to the assessment of the individual with confirmed or suspected diagnosis of mental retardation: (1) to assist in clarification of the distinction between other language problems and the language delay inherent in intellectual impairment; (2) to describe the linguistic system of the child; and (3) to assist in choosing the mode of language instruction appropriate for the child.

Despite current technology, children with undetected hearing loss and/or with little or no knowledge of English are still being labeled as mentally retarded. The language specialist has a primary responsibility to rule out these two possible factors in the diagnosis of mental retardation. Some retarded children, especially children with Down's syndrome, have better visual than auditory skills (Blager, 1980) and may express themselves better through gesture or sign language than through speech. The language specialist should clarify how such factors may have influenced the diagnosis of retardation and especially the assignment of a child to a particular degree of retardation. Also, the language specialist is in a unique position to observe how the child's environment has influenced the language he has learned and currently uses.

The description of the child's current linguistic functioning is the primary responsibility of the language specialist. Since the language code is standard, the same vocabulary, semantic intentions, semantic relations, mean length of utterance (MLU), grammatic forms, and sentence types need to be evaluated in the mentally retarded child as are analyzed in any other child. The functional use the mentally retarded child makes of his language is still infrequently analyzed, yet it is of vital concern. Many mentally retarded children have had negative testing experiences and require considerable patience and sometimes the use of unorthodox techniques in obtaining samples of spontaneous speech. Before concluding the evaluation, the language specialist should pursue selected tests of the cognitive skills essential to language performance. These include perception, memory, and attention, as well as some indication of the non-verbal concepts the child may have acquired.

An important diagnostic concern of the language specialist is determination of the mode of language instruction for each child, for example whether speech or non-oral communication should be the goal of intervention. Adler (1976) pointed out that oral communication skills in the retarded are a function of the following factors: (1) the clinical-genetic syndrome; (2) the severity of the retardation; (3) the psychosocial environment of the child; and (4) the structure and function of the auditory and oral system. Once the first three factors have been investigated, careful exploration of the oral structure can be completed.

McDonald (1980, p. 60), discussed children who are "at risk" for speech production. He indicated that he had not seen any children with grossly defective chewing, sucking, and swallowing who were able to speak intelligibly. If these vegetative functions, along with other support systems such as respiration, are seriously impaired, then this additional neuromotor defect, in con-

Table 16–4
Verbal Language Potential of Mentally Retarded*

Age (Years)	Degree of Retardation			
	Mild	Moderate	Severe	Profound
3	Names	4 to 6 Words	1 to 2 Words	None
6	300 Words	Names	4 to 6 Words	1 to 2 Words
9	Sentences	300 Words	Names and phrases	4 to 6 Words and gestures
12	Conversation	Sentences	300 Words	Phrases
15	Conversation	Conversation	Sentences	Up to 300 words

*Adapted from material in (1) Gomez and Podhajski (1978), which was adapted from Grossman H (Ed) (1973): *Manual of Terminology and Classification in Mental Retardation.* Washington, DC: American Association of Mental Defectives, and (2) Lillywhite and Bradley (1969).

junction with the clinical syndrome, the severity of the retardation, and the child's environment, may all be weighed to decide whether non-oral communication should be recommended.

Still further guidelines for deciding the mode of communication were offered by Chapman and Miller (1980). They suggested that children may be candidates for nonvocal communication if they meet certain criteria such as a failure to utter intelligible words and a defect of the speech mechanism, combined with evidence that the child's cognitive development is at a sensorimotor stage 6. These criteria indicate the importance of the child's level of conceptual development in the acquisition of either oral or non-oral language systems.

Whether cognitive potential is estimated using Piaget's stages of growth or through the use of intelligence tests, the relationship of cognitive levels to language performance retains its importance. An effort to relate tested intelligence and oral expressive language was made by the AAMD (Grossman, 1973) and was modified by Gomez and Podhajski (1978) (Table 16-4). This table does not imply that every retarded person will attain a particular level of verbal proficiency, nor does it imply that everyone will be limited to these levels. It does, however, offer evidence that even profoundly retarded individuals may achieve speech.

INTERVENTION

Society, medical and educational specialists, and even retarded individuals themselves are coming to realize that the retarded have potential and are entitled to live lives of dignity and fulfillment. The goals of language intervention should reflect a blending of the child's cognitive potential, his need to use language, and his current linguistic levels. For many retarded individuals, the goal is not normal, adult language but rather a limited or restricted verbal or non-oral system sufficient to meet their needs. With the emergence of this philosophy, considerable effort has been made to develop speech in children who have never exhibited expressive language. Programs such as that developed by Bricker & Bricker (1970) have been successful in fostering speech in some previously nonverbal children; however, they have not been totally successful. Consequently, non-oral programs have become increasingly popular for training severely and profoundly retarded children. These programs include sign language, gestural systems, total communication, Blissymbols, and communication boards, to name only some of the options.

Few efforts have been made to compare the effectiveness of the various intervention methods. Kahn (1981), however, has compared the success of signs versus verbal language training in profoundly retarded nonverbal children. His subjects were twelve hearing children with IQs below 20, who were between the ages of 4.5 years and 8.5 years at the beginning of the project. Each child was randomly assigned to one of three groups, and received instruction in either language, signing, or an area other than language. After three years of daily, individual training sessions lasting approximately 20 minutes, the results were reviewed. All four subjects in the sign group had learned some signed words, and all could produce at least one phrase in sign language. Only two children in the speech group had learned to say any words, and only one had learned to combine words into phrases. These findings were interpreted to mean that some nonverbal retarded children will benefit more from sign language than speech training. Significantly, both groups who received language training learned more language skills than did the placebo group, a finding that lends support to proponents of language training for even the profoundly mentally retarded.

Kahn's research (1981) also lends support to the importance of the child's level of cognitive development to the acquisition of either oral or non-oral language. Prior to initiating training, Kahn administered the Uzgiris and Hunt (1975) scales to all subjects, and found that achievement of object permanence and causality was significantly related to success in learning either mode of language.

The question has been raised as to whether conceptual levels deemed necessary for communication can be raised through direct training. There is still no consensus of opinion, but it appears that environmental and experiential "enrichment" programs are proving more promising than attempts to actually "teach" concepts. Programs of intervention should be chosen with the understanding that language reflects the individual's experience with the world. The mentally retarded must experience objects and people as they relate to each other in time and space. A curriculum limited to teaching the child to produce a series of words or grammatic forms using a behavioral modification paradigm may well succeed, but intervention is not complete until the child has been assisted in using those words spontaneously to express his own needs and ideas.

outline

language
disorders
among
children with
hearing loss

17

Hearing keeps people in touch with their surroundings. Beginning before birth and continuing throughout life, hearing constantly monitors the environment. Hearing impairment is a developmental tragedy because it deprives the child of the normal verbal input necessary for language development.

The first question parents of a hearing-impaired child usually ask is "Will my child learn to speak?" The answer depends upon a number of variables, including the parameters of the hearing loss and the method of training chosen for the child. Because it is difficult to understand or evaluate the language produced by hearing-impaired children without appreciation of these variables, this chapter begins with a discussion of hearing loss and the means so far devised to assist hearing-impaired children to learn language. Next the effects of impaired hearing on the various dimensions of language are presented. Finally, the integrative approach to the language of the hearing impaired is discussed, along with implications for assessment and intervention.

In a discussion of hearing loss, three variables are of significance to those responsible for the management of hearing-impaired children: (1) the degree and type of the hearing loss; (2) the etiology of the loss, and (3) the age of onset of the loss.

Degree and Type of Hearing Loss

Hearing loss is typically classified on a continuum from mild to profound. Figure 17-1 shows the differing degrees of hearing loss and the descriptive terms that refer to them. All of the studies reported in this chapter apply to children with mild, moderate, severe, or profound loss. The extent of this loss, especially in the speech frequencies (500, 1000, 2000 Hz), has a great influence on the individual's capacity to understand speech (Wiley, 1980). Individuals with mild loss of hearing can understand speech under most circumstances; persons with moderate loss have frequent difficulty; those with severe loss understand speech only if it is amplified; and those with a profound loss may not be able to understand even amplified speech.

The type of the hearing loss is also significant. Individuals with a loss of hearing only above 2000 Hz (a common high-frequency loss) have difficulty understanding words with such

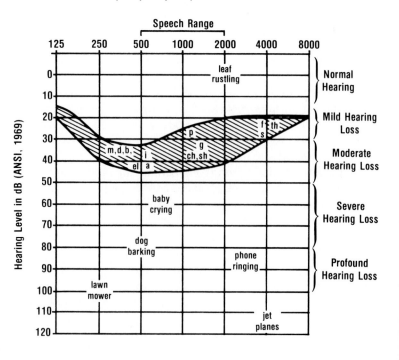

Figure 17-1
Degrees of hearing loss shown on the margin of a pure-tone audiogram. The shaded area indicates the range of loudness for conversation as well as the intensity of certain phonemes. The loudness levels of several environmental sounds are also shown. (From Northern and Downs [1978] and Weir [1980].)

high-frequency phonemes as /f/, /s/, and /th/ (Figure 17-1). However, they might be able to understand words containing low-frequency sounds very well. Currently, the ability to understand speech is tested using several standard lists of words. A number of audiological laboratories are devising more sophisticated sentence material and other innovative methods to analyze speech perception (Jerger, 1978).

Etiology

Hearing loss in children may be congenital or acquired. Congenital hearing loss may be hereditary or the result of prenatal toxic conditions or other causes. Acquired hearing loss may also result from various toxic illnesses or from specific ear infections such as otitis media.

A high percentage of congenital deafness is hereditary, according to Konigsmark (1972), G. R. Fraser (1976), Swisher (1976), and Northern and Downs (1978). A consensus of these studies suggests that almost 50 percent of congenital deafness is hereditary. However, some 40 percent of the inherited cases are the result of autosomal recessive inheritance, which means that both parents must be the carrier of the same gene. Most parents of hearing-impaired children have no family history of deafness and are not deaf themselves. This, of course, complicates the problem of proving hereditary deafness. According to Bergstrom, Hemenway, & Downs (1971), the marriage of two deaf persons gives only a slightly increased risk of deafness in their children. Identification of genetic deafness requires skilled evaluation by geneticists, yet only one school for the deaf (Clarke School) provides genetic counselling to its students.

In his review of the genetic basis for hearing loss, Konigsmark (1972) identified over sixty different types of hereditary hearing loss and gave criteria for distinguishing them. None of these sixty types were associated with observable physical anomalies; however, there are a wide number of obvious birth defects associated with hearing loss. Northern and Downs (1974, 1978) listed eighty-three distinct hereditary syndromes that have associated hearing loss, the most obvious of which are those affecting craniofacial structures (such as cleft palate), those affecting the central nervous system, endocrine and metabolic disorders, and chromosonal defects such as Trisomy 13, 18, and 21 (Down's syndrome). The high incidence of hearing loss among children with Down's syndrome was discussed in Chapter 16.

The most common nonhereditary causes of congenital hearing loss are maternal toxic diseases contracted during the early months of pregnancy. The most common are rubella and cyto-

megalovirus (Northern & Downs, 1978), and other causes include syphilis, toxemia, and diabetes. Clinical evaluation of
hearing should begin at birth or as soon as any high-risk factor
for hearing loss is noted. The high-risk factors determined by
the American Association of Otolaryngology and Ophthalmol-
ogy, the American Speech and Hearing Association, and the
American Association of Pediatrics are (1) history of hereditary
deafness in the family; (2) maternal rubella; (3) fetal infections;
(4) defects of ear, nose, or throat; (5) weight of less than 1500
grams at birth; (6) bilirubin more than 20 milligrams per 100
milliliters of serum; and (7) congenital cytomegalovirus (Lloyd
& Dahle, 1976).

Infants who display any of the above signs of high risk for
hearing loss should have their hearing tested immediately, and
at regular stages thereafter, until normal hearing, or the level of
the loss, is established. One study (F. B. Simmons, 1980) indicated that one in fifty-two infants in an intensive care nursery
has a hearing loss, as compared to only one in one thousand in a
well-baby nursery.

Children born with normal hearing may lose their hearing
during infancy or childhood due to various diseases, such as
measles, mumps, meningitis, encephalitis, or other infections requiring the use of ototoxic drugs, which may seriously affect
hearing. In addition, continuing or severe ear infections (acute,
chronic, or serious otitis media) may also affect hearing.

Age of Onset

In terms of language development, the time of onset of the
hearing loss is most significant. Children are commonly
grouped according to whether their hearing loss was prelin-
gual—prior to 3 years of age and before the acquisition of much
of the linguistic code—or prevocational—prior to 18 years of
age (Northern & Downs, 1978). The primary remediation task
for the prevocationally deaf is to preserve their language and
continue its growth. For the prelingually deaf, the major goal is
to establish language; it is this group that is the focus of this
chapter.

Other children in whom the time of hearing loss is considered
significant are those with minimal auditory deficiency (Northern
& Downs, 1978), children who sustained middle ear disease pri-
or to age 2. Holm and Kunze (1969) found that children with
hearing ranging from near normal to a loss of greater than 25
dB were lower in all language skills than were children in the
control group. Howie, Ploussard, and Sloyer (1976) found that
children with at least three recorded episodes of otitis media in

the first year of life showed significantly lower mean scores on the WISC-R than did the control group. Other researchers also linked minimal auditory deficiencies in early life with subsequent lowered achievement in school.

Northern and Downs (1978) summarized what they considered significant hearing loss in the first 2 years of life as (1) hearing loss over 15 dB; (2) serous otitis media in a child under 18 months more than half the time within a period of 6 months; and (3) fluctuating loss (0 to 15 dB) more than half the time for 1 year.

In a well-reasoned article, Ventry (1980) pointed out methodological problems in some of the research used to support the claim of minimal auditory deficiency. He noted, for example, that Holm and Kunze (1969) considered their work a "pilot study" and that they did not match their sixteen subjects on the basis of intelligence or environmental stimulation. Ventry (1980, p. 151) summarized his position by saying, "I do not take issue with the hypothesis that there may be a link between conductive hearing impairment and language, learning, and auditory dysfunction . . . but the research in this area is difficult and at present a definitive answer is impossible." A cause-effect relationship cannot be assumed simply because two conditions co-occur.

Children with unilateral hearing loss may also have language problems. Northern and Downs (1978) found that 30 percent of such children whom they studied were delayed in their academic program by an average of $1\frac{1}{2}$ years. Again, there is no way of proving that the unilateral hearing loss *caused* the academic lag. However, children with such a loss require at least yearly audiometric evaluation to make sure that they do not lose hearing in their good ear. They also require preferential seating, and the teachers should be told implications of unilateral hearing loss.

For any child with a hearing loss, whether mild or profound, routine audiometric rechecks are of vital importance. Northern and Downs (1978, p. 170) report that there is a high degree of middle ear disease among deaf children. Other types of hearing loss, such as that associated with congenital cytomegalovirus infections, may be progressive (Dahle et al., 1979). Children so affected require especially careful monitoring to make sure that they do not continue to lose hearing acuity.

METHODS OF TEACHING LANGUAGE TO THE HEARING IMPAIRED

Except for the deaf children of deaf parents, who learn sign language as their native language, severe and profoundly hearing-impaired children must be formally taught their first language.

Sign language was introduced into the United States in 1851 and adopted by Galludet for the American School for the Deaf.

Alexander Graham Bell

Alexander Graham Bell maintained that his deepest commitment in life was as a teacher of the deaf. It was his devotion to the search for better means of providing amplification and instruction for the deaf that led him to the invention of the telephone, which he patented when he was 29 years old. In addition, Bell also invented the first audiometer and the telegraph system. In 1877 he founded the Bell Telephone Company.

This deep attachment to the deaf undoubtedly resulted from his close personal relationship with the hearing impaired. His mother was severely hearing impaired, but her speech and language were reported to be good. His father was a phonetician who developed an instructional system called Visible Speech. When Bell moved to Boston from Edinburgh, Scotland, where he was born in 1847, he taught his father's system of visible speech at several schools, including the Clarke School for the Deaf. Bell subsequently married one of his deaf students, Mabel Hubbard. Prior to devoting his full time to research, Bell also taught at Boston University.

The Alexander Graham Bell Association for the Deaf was organized and named in Bell's honor in 1890 to promote the teaching of speech and lip reading for the deaf. This association publishes the *Volta Review* and its Volta Bureau prints and distributes various professional publications.

During the same period, the English and Germans were stressing oral education using parents to teach natural language to their children. These oral methods gained acceptance in the United States with the founding of Clarke School for the Deaf (1867) and the Lexington School for the Deaf (1879). Alexander Graham Bell urged a "natural approach" in teaching oral language to young deaf children, and the major thrust for oralism was established in this country.

Oralism

Oralism is the combined use of amplification, auditory training, speech, lip reading, and written language in the instructional approach. Within oralism, numerous techniques and methods have been introduced to make language learning easier. Fitzgerald (1949) combined six parts of speech, on a chart that the children memorized as a guide to generating their own sentences. d'Arc's approach (1958) stressed the learning of seven basic sentence patterns. During the 1960s, a number of programs using behavior modification were introduced.

In a letter to a director of a special shool, Anne Sullivan Macy, Helen Keller's teacher, wrote to explain something of her philosophy of teaching the deaf.

Helen learned language almost as unconsciously as a normal child. As I look back it seems as if Helen was always on the jump when I was teaching her. We were generally in the open air doing something. Words were learned as they were needed. She rarely forgot a word that was given to her when the action called it forth, and she learned a phrase or even a sentence as readily as a single word when it was needed to describe the action.*

*From Joseph Lash: *Helen and Teacher: The Story of Helen Keller and Anne Sullivan Macy.* New York: Delacorte Press, 1980. Reprinted with permission.

At the Lexington School for the Deaf in New York City, Groht (1958) devised and subsequently published her approach to teaching "natural language." This approach is based on concept development so that language becomes a means to an end rather than an end in itself. The oralists, of whom Groht is one, felt strongly that deaf children had to take their place in the hearing world and ideally should receive their education in the aural-oral mode.

Acoupedics—Aural Approach

The oral programs in Europe have traditionally placed an especially strong emphasis on listening skills. Initially, it was assumed that children with severe and profound hearing losses would rely heavily on lip reading to learn language. However, during the 1940s in Holland, Dr. Henk Huizing began a program of putting hearing aids on infants and working with the infants and parents at home, stressing auditory stimulation. The purpose was to teach language through the use of auditory training alone, placing special emphasis on the vibrotactile awareness of low-frequency sound (Asp, 1975). The program proved so successful (in the opinion of its advocates) that it was recommended that lip reading be avoided entirely until auditory orientation was established. Acoupedics was proposed by Dorren Pollack (1970, p. 13) as a "comprehensive habilitation program for the hearing-impaired infant and his family which includes an emphasis upon auditory training without formal lip reading instruction." In an acoupedic program, a child is not classified on the basis of his hearing loss but upon his ability to use residual hearing. The basic techniques of the program include a unisensory training approach to develop hearing perception and an auditory feedback mechanism to develop speech. Hearing is trained maximally and intensively, and the child is not allowed to attend to any visual cues.

Total Communication

Despite the energy put into oral education of deaf children, the Babbidge report (1965) submitted to the Department of Health, Education and Welfare stated that deaf education was almost exactly where it had been 150 years before. The deaf left high school with only a fourth- to sixth-grade reading level and a crude command of spoken English (Northern & Downs, 1974). Most teachers in oral schools did not know any system of sign language, and consequently students who were not functionally oral taught each other to sign in a kind of "underground." Oral

A popular novel of the 1970s told the poignant story of a deaf couple who had graduated from a school for the deaf that allowed only oral language to be used.* When this young man and woman left school their oral language was limited and their reading proficiency was only at the fourth-grade level. Once they married, they had to cope with the hearing world concerning employment, insurance, credit, mortgage payments, and the birth of their child. As they grappled with these problems, the husband met some deaf people who knew sign language. After he had achieved minimal proficiency with sign language he suggested to his wife that perhaps there were words for things not seen or touched and for thoughts more complex than 'go' and 'stay.' The young husband longed to share with his wife the feelings and pictures inside of himself for which he still had no words.

*Joanne Greenburg: *In This Sign.* New York: Avon Books, 1970.

schools did not hire deaf teachers, so students lacked role models.

Vernon and Koh (1970) compared the achievements of orally versus manually trained deaf. They found deaf children of deaf parents to be superior on almost all measures, despite the fact that the deaf parents had less education and performed more menial jobs than the hearing parents. A major difference was that the children of deaf parents learned signing as their native language, and even without preschool training they scored higher by 1.2 to 1.6 grades than did the orally trained deaf who had preschool training. The study revealed that 82 percent of the manual communicators passed college entrance exams, whereas only 51 percent of the orally trained students passed (Vernon & Koh, 1970).

When some of the above studies were undertaken, sign language was considered less than a language and more like a primitive gesture system lacking inflection and grammar. To sign was to acknowledge linguistic failure. Several linguists who began their careers studying the emerging language of normal children began to study sign language. Bellugi and Klima (1972) concluded that each sign contained the following three parameters: (1) a hand configuration; (2) a place of articulation in relation to the body; and (3) hand movement. These parameters may be combined in many ways, and the use of space, direction, and movement are all crucial. Space provides intonational-type cues of pause and questioning. Direction can signal semantic changes so that a simple reversal of direction can change *join* into *disconnect.* Movements have many meaning such as tense, number, and subject as opposed to object (Bellugi & Klima, 1972).

Further study by Bellugi and Klima (1978) showed that there are a number of different sign languages and they differ just as spoken languages do. American Sign Language (ASL) is used by most prelingually deaf Americans who sign. ASL is totally different from spoken English and is a fully complete language capable of expressing any level of abstraction (Bellugi & Klima,

LANGUAGE DISORDERS AMONG CHILDREN WITH HEARING LOSS

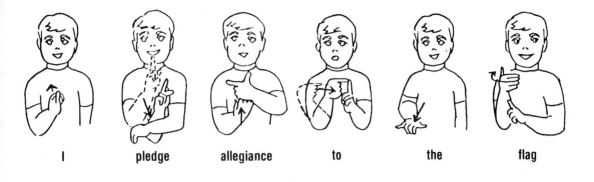

| I | pledge | allegiance | to | the | flag |

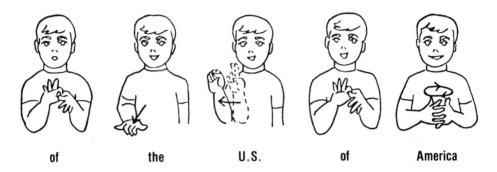

| of | the | U.S. | of | America |

1978). ASL appears to be even more highly inflected than English.

Total communication is the combination of amplification, speech, and lip reading with signing and written language in the educational process. Proponents of total communication feel that every deaf child has the right to learn language using all means available. If this program is to be successful the child's parents and siblings must also learn sign language and use this combined method at home.

Although American Sign Language is probably the most commonly used sign language, there are a number of other systems. Two systems designed for replicating spoken English as closely as possible are Seeing Essential English and Seeing Exact English (SEE_1 and SEE_2). These methods are taught in the hope of improving reading and writing skills among the hearing impaired (Moores, 1978, p. 186). In addition to the systems of sign language, there is a system of finger spelling with one sign for each letter of the alphabet. Figure 17-2 shows a portion of the Pledge of Allegiance in SEE_2 while Figure 17-3 illustrates the single word *flag* expressed in SEE_2 and in finger spelling. In the United States, no one learns finger spelling as a native language; it is used mainly to supplement communication by spelling unusual or difficult words.

Figure 17-2
The Pledge of Allegiance in the system of sign language known as SEE_2. (Redrawn with permission from Gustason G, Pfetzing D, Zawolkow E (1980): *Signing Exact English.* Silver Spring, Md.: Modern Signs Press.)

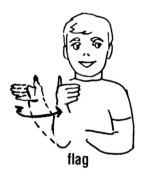

flag

The Sign in SEE₂

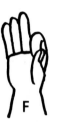 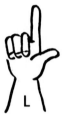 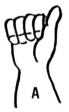 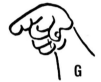

F   L   A   G

Finger Spelling

Figure 17-3
The difference between sign language (SEE₂) and finger spelling. (Redrawn with permission from Gustason G, Pfetzing D, Zawolkow E (1980): *Signing Exact English.* Silver Spring, Md.: Modern Signs Press.)

THE EFFECT OF HEARING LOSS ON THE DIMENSIONS OF LANGUAGE

The Cognitive Dimension

The cognitive abilities of sensation, perception, and conceptualization are all affected by hearing impairment.

Sensation and Perception

Perception of the speech signal is fundamental to matching auditory stimuli to concepts. Only after this association is made do words emerge. Consequently, the degree of hearing loss as measured by audiometric testing cannot be used to accurately predict a child's potential for acquiring oral language. The child's residual ability to perceive and discriminate speech sounds is of vital importance.

Vibrotactile input is thought by some to improve speech perception. Asp (1975) pointed out that most deaf children have measurable hearing, at least below 500 Hz. He felt that with proper training even the profoundly deaf child could use hearing to improve speech. Asp suggested that by utilizing the vibrotactile sense, a child could gain valuable information about the suprasegmental features of speech, including rhythm and stress. Such early training might be expected to improve the temporal aspects of speech, which are so often impaired. Asp recommended the use of vibrotactile input from bone oscillators in the training of young deaf children.

Some researchers believe that the profoundly hearing impaired perceive all sound vibrotactilely rather than auditorily. Erber (1979) found that thresholds of response to auditory stimuli obtained on the hand and from the ear were identical, especially for 250 and 500 Hz. Erber felt that the severely and profoundly hearing impaired could best be distinguished on the basis of their ability to perceive speech. The profoundly deaf cannot distinguish among consonants or among words, nor can they identify the number of syllables in words. However, even the profoundly deaf can distinguish some basic emotions, such as sadness versus happiness from voice quality.

Conceptualization

Because of the interrelationship of thought and language, the capacity of the deaf for sophisticated thought has been questioned by educators and the general public throughout the ages. The work of Furth has had great impact on the theory of the thought processes of the deaf. Furth's book, *Thinking Without Language* (1966), and a number of other publications by Furth have been influential in modifying educators' opinions about the language and thought of the deaf. Furth affirmed the independence of thinking from language. Furth, whose experiments were modeled upon the work of Piaget, emphasized the importance of experience for developing the mind. He advocated a reordering of priorities in the education of the deaf, in which education for thinking would take priority over instruction in language. Furth strongly affirmed that despite their typically poor instruction, prejudice, and discrimination, the majority of the deaf adequately adjust to the world. He interpreted this survival as a tribute to the deaf and a testimony to their basic intelligence.

A criticism of the work of Furth has been made by Moores (1978) who pointed out that Furth assumed in his work and in his choice of experimental subjects that the deaf did not know much language. He judged the deaf to be linguistically deficient, based upon their reading achievement scores and their oral language ability. Despite the fact that Moores quoted Furth as indicating that signing is the natural language of the deaf, Furth still judged the language of his subjects in terms of the oral language standard of the hearing community. (Moores, 1978). Moores concluded that Furth studied thought, not language, in the deaf.

Liben (1978) pointed out that the deaf probably have experiential deficiencies. Piaget's theories emphasized the importance of the child learning about the relationships of objects to each other and to people and the consequences of action on objects. The sense of hearing is functional from the seventh month of

Hans Furth

Although the intelligence of the deaf has been a topic of interest for centuries, no single researcher has become so associated with the exploration of this subject as Hans Furth. Using Piaget's theories as a basic premise, Furth has investigated the thinking processes of the deaf and drawn educational implications. His book, *Thinking Without Language* (1966), is considered a classic discussion of this subject.

Furth was born in Vienna, Austria, and obtained his first degree from the Royal Academy of Music in London as a pianist. In 1950 he received a B.A. in philosophy from Charterhouse in England, and subsequently obtained his Ph.D. in psychology from the University of Portland in 1960. Furth then joined the department of psychology at Catholic University in Washington, D.C., and became chairman of that department. Furth spent a year working with Piaget in Switzerland and subsequently interpreted the Swiss psychologist's work in *Piaget's Theory of Intelligence* and *Piaget for Teachers*.

gestation (Tomlinson-Keasey & Kelly, 1974) and is well developed at birth. The sensory limitations of the deaf child are operating significantly by the fourth month of life, as the child loses opportunities for feedback from himself and his environment in one significant modality. By 4 to 8 months, several modalities are lost: The child cannot coordinate vocalizations with any other sense. His cognitive structures lack auditory input. All of his information must be processed from vision, touch, taste, and smell (Liben, 1978; Tomlinson-Keasey & Kelly, 1974).

For the hearing child, spoken symbols are attached to mental images; for the deaf child learning sign language naturally from deaf parents, a gesture is attached to a mental image. The deaf infant who is not exposed to early auditory or visual language develops sensorimotor structures for organizing his environment that do not include language. The child has images with which to code his world but lacks the symbol system to communicate these images. Such a child also lacks the noncommunicative function of language, which the hearing child uses to name objects for the purpose of classifying them. This process facilitates concept development. Deaf children who learn to sign have been observed to engage in this monologue of sign (Tomlinson-Keasey & Kelly, 1974). There is evidence that while hearing subjects depend upon an auditory-oral coding system to assist in learning verbal material for short-term memory, the hearing impaired may code by either sign or semantic component (Moulton & Beasley, 1975). Collins-Ahlgren (1974) concurred that the manual deaf use manual-visual factors to code and store information. The deaf child is sometimes delayed in his ability to label objects that are unseen, and this may delay the deaf child's movement from concrete to abstract thinking.

The Communication Environment

The communication environment of the deaf infant differs from that of the normal child from the earliest months of life. While the deaf infant is limited to vision and touch as primary means of gaining information, his hearing parents attempt to reach him primarily through the auditory and visual channels. This leads to failed communication. Liben (1978) contended that 90 percent of the deaf children of hearing parents lack a system of communication and that these communication barriers extend through adolescence. These deaf children are also prevented from communicating easily with siblings and peers.

The normal infant pays attention to human speech very early; speech is soothing, and the infant localizes the sound of voice. Communication of affect occurs partially through the infant's interpretation of voice quality. Parent and child engage in vocal exchanges in coordinated and reciprocal patterns. For the hearing child of hearing parents, the child's first words are greeted by joy and the mutual sharing of this important milestone. Hearing parents of a deaf child often spend the child's early months in a state of uncertainty over the child's status of hearing. Once the diagnosis is made, the family undergoes shock and a period of mourning and depression. All of this modifies the parent's joy in interacting with the child. Hearing parents continue to place a high premium on first spoken words, which are anxiously awaited. The deaf child is aware that his parents value verbalization, and since verbalization tends to be delayed, speech too often becomes a part of a power struggle. The joy and reciprocity of communication are lost to both parent and child. One hearing mother of a deaf child indicated (H. S. Schlesinger & Meadow, 1972) that the reason she learned sign language and began total communication with her child was that she observed that the deaf mothers of deaf children communicated with joy and ease, and she too wanted to engage in playful and enjoyable exchanges with her daughter. The deaf child who remains mute may demonstrate negativism and fearfulness of adult disapproval and may become provocative to obtain adult attention. Deaf mutism is more often observed when words are anxiously and insistently forced by parents (H. S. Schlesinger, 1978).

H. S. Schlesinger and Meadow (1972) indicated a difference in the nature of parental communication for deaf parents and their deaf child. From birth, deaf parents introduced an abundance of tactile stimuli—running toys and fingers over the child's face and head, tickling, and tapping the child to gain attention. Signs were frequently made on the child's body, and the child would in turn make signs on the mother's body and face. The deaf parents engaged in frequent visual imitation of the child's actions, thus fostering reciprocal visual imitation.

Linguistic input from the environment is seriously modified for most deaf children during their early years. Maternal linguistic codes are different in the mother relating to a hearing child and the mother relating to a deaf child. Hearing parents of deaf children tend to use imperative control (Liben, 1978); 71 percent report spanking their deaf child, but only 25 percent use spanking with their hearing child. Explanations were given to hearing children, whereas the deaf children were simply told "no." In addition, there was a tendency for the hearing adults to control communication, and this carried over to a variety of school settings where communication was overwhelmingly dominated by teachers of deaf students; less than three percent of the classroom communication was initiated by the students (Liben, 1978).

Despite these barriers to communication, the needs and desires of deaf children to communicate appear just as great as those of normal children. This is supported by a study of the development of natural gesture in deaf children who lack any other means of communication. Goldin-Meadow and Feldman (1975) found that deaf children invented "names" for actions and objects, and syntactically coded semantic relations between actions and objects using a gestural system. These gestural skills developed in the same sequence as verbal skills in hearing children.

Oral Language Knowledge

Since it is generally agreed that the hearing impaired do not have problems in formulation or symbolization, the research literature appears to assume that the knowledge of the linguistic code is reflected in the performance. Consequently, the knowledge and performance of the code are studied simultaneously. The majority of studies of oral language investigated the performance of individuals with severe or profound losses. A survey of 16,000 children found that 75 percent of the hearing impaired actually had losses in these categories (Chasen & Zuckerman, 1976).

Cross-Sectional Studies*

In cross-sectional studies, subjects tended to be chosen from schools for the deaf and often numbered from 400 to 500 individuals (Quigley, Wilbur, & Montanelli, 1974, 1976; Wilbur, Quigley, & Montanelli, 1975), with 20 subjects ranking as a small number (Jarvella & Lubinsky, 1975; Power & Quigley, 1973). For many of the subjects, their method of language instruction was poorly defined. Silverman (1971) found that prior to 1968, some 85 percent of the prelingually deaf were exposed to an oral-aural method of instruction during their early years. Therefore, based upon the age of the subjects in the studies discussed here, it may be presumed that most of them were exposed to early oral training. Since the severely hearing impaired do not learn oral language without formal instruction, the method of

*The cross-sectional studies of oral language reported here focus on the severely and profoundly retarded.

instruction has a significant effect on the language produced. In some cases, problems in oral language observed in the studies may reflect bias or failure in instruction as much as they reflect the linguistic skill of the subjects.

Language was obtained from the subjects by asking them to describe pictures, to perform on a linguistic test, to repeat sentences, or, in a number of cases, to respond to written problems or questions. The responses on written language tests were presumed to reflect spoken language. In one older study, the normal controls were allowed to give their responses verbally while the deaf were required to write their responses (Templin, 1963). Swisher (1976) noted that there have been few studies of the spoken language of the deaf. This section focuses entirely on studies of oral language.

Vocabulary Development.   In 1963, Templin reported on the vocabulary of the deaf. Subjects between 11 and 14 years of age were asked to give definitions of words, synonyms, similarities, analogies and multiple meaning of words and to construct sentences. Responses matched with those provided by normal hearing children between 6 and 14 years of age. Templin (1963) found that by age 14, the hearing impaired were from 2 to 8 years below hearing children on all tests, with analogies, synonyms, and words with multiple meanings proving to be most difficult. This study supported the generally held opinion that the vocabulary of the deaf child was inferior to that of the hearing child.

Brannon and Murry (1966) concluded that the deaf (aged 12 to 13 years) tended to omit function words and to communicate using "telegraphic" speech. A. A. Simmons (1962) also found that the deaf (aged 12 to 15 years) used more nouns and verbs and fewer conjunctions and auxiliaries. Goda (1964) found that 75 percent of the verbal output of the deaf was composed of nouns and verbs in contrast to 60 percent for hearing individuals. Some researchers have suggested that the deaf chose these classes of words because this enabled them to maximize the information they conveyed (Elliot, Hirsh, & Simmons, 1967). MacGinitie (1964) suggested that the omission of function words may just be an economy of effort.

In a study of forty deaf 18-year-olds (Odom, Blanton, & Nunnally, 1967), using a procedure in which the subjects filled in missing words, it appeared that the deaf and normal controls used the same linguistic strategies in regard to semantic words, but not the same strategy, when attempting to predict syntactic words. Since the number of syntactic function words is low and forms a closed set, the difficulty the deaf had with these words may be associated with the possible idiomatic use of some syntactic words and a lack of appreciation of the semantic properties of these words.

Grammatic Structure. One of the marks of the mature speaker is the ability to conjoin sentences. Instead of saying, "The boy had lunch. The boy went home," it is more efficient to say, "The boy had lunch and went home," deleting the subject of the conjoined sentences. Wilbur et al. (1975) studied the capacity of deaf students (aged 10 to 18 years) to handle conjoined sentences. They found that it was most difficult for the deaf students to form relative clauses, though they had more success using conjunctions and forming questions. The deaf made some atypical errors of subject or object deletion in conjoining sentences that were never observed among normal controls. Swisher (1976) reported an unpublished study that found that the deaf produced more simple sentences using the same general vocabulary through the advancing age ranges. Studies (Goda, 1959) of the mean length of utterances showed that 12-year-old deaf children produced six-word sentences, and 16- to 18-year-old deaf students produced only seven-word sentences, on the average. In contrast to Goda, Swisher (1976) referred to an unpublished study of Simmons that found an average sentence length of almost ten words in 12-year-old subjects.

In other studies of grammatic structure, particular problems were identified with the comprehension and use of the passive (Power & Quigley, 1973); with the use of gerunds and infinitives (Quigley et al, 1976); with the use of relative pronouns (Wilbur, Montanelli, & Quigley, 1976), and especially with verb constructions (Presnall, 1973). It appears that syntactic development begins at a later age for deaf children and continues well into adolescence (Swisher, 1976).

Developmental Studies

H. S. Schlesinger and Meadow (1972) described the emergence of language in four deaf children. The parental styles of communication differed with these children in that one subject was the child of deaf parents while the other three were the children of hearing parents. All the parents chose to use total communication with their deaf child. The emergence of first signs actually seemed to precede the usual age of first spoken words. By age 15 months, one subject had a vocabulary of 19 signs, and at 18 months she used 117 signs. This is considerably in excess

---

The failure of many deaf individuals to learn to use various function forms, and especially the problems they have in using the verb system correctly, is illustrated by this exerpt from a letter written by a 19-year-old deaf college student to her mother.

Today the weather is lousy and coming down here by snow. I think this weather has a kind of weird for March. . . . Today my major will start, but I haven't have to go to the school today. . . . The major is Graphic Arts. I'll talk about my major when I'll get home. OK. I rather talk in person than write in the letter because it might cause the person to get misunderstood.*

*Reprinted with permission from Virginia Hewes: I Challenge the Profession. *The American Annals of the Deaf,* 122: 15–18, 1977.

of the expected number of spoken words among normal children of that age (see Chapter 7). Another subject was combining signs to form multiword utterances by 18 months. By age 2, it was observed that two of the subjects could switch from signing to spoken English, depending upon the ability of the listener. Another subject showed an increase in signs from 348 to 604 over a 4-month period during her third year (H. S. Schlesinger & Meadow, 1972).

The development of spoken English in 12 severely and profoundly deaf children who were being trained in an oral school was described by Curtis, Prutting, and Lowell (1979). These children, who were between 22 and 60 months of age, were placed in three groups: 2-year-olds, 3-year-olds, and 4-year-olds. Language samples were obtained in four different settings and recorded on videotape. The authors analyzed both oral language and nonverbal communicative acts to identify pragmatic and semantic intentions. The emergence of these intentions was then related to the subjects' chronological age. Results were analyzed so that both group and individual data could be retrieved and considered separately.

Group data indicated that 16 pragmatic categories and 13 semantic categories were used at least once in the study. As might be expected, based upon normal developmental data, the pragmatic category "labeling" was an important function for 2-year-olds. However, the finding that this category continued to be important for 4-year-olds was unexpected. "Acknowledgement" was very important for the 2-year-olds, but this category decreased in importance with age, as it does in normal hearing children. The category "description" increased in importance with age. The most common semantic category for all age groups was "performative" (an utterance occurring along with an action, e.g., "bye-bye"). There were marked individual differences between children in each age group, and Curtis et al. (1979) questioned whether these differences could be accounted for on the basis of hearing loss. While other studies (Brannon & Murry, 1966; Swisher, 1976) indicated a high correlation between hearing loss and language development, this study confirmed a relationship between the *aided* response level—not the unaided hearing level—and verbal and communicative abilities. Individual children used the same level of hearing very differently. Finally, this study confirmed that MLU was a good measure of strictly linguistic ability. The authors concluded that the young children in their study showed a compelling drive for communication. Even those who lacked a verbal means to "talk" attempted to encode meaning in some fashion.

Another study (Shafer & Lynch, 1981) followed the emerging language of six children enrolled in three different modes of training: oral instruction, aural instruction, and total communication. The subjects, who all had a severe or profound hearing loss, were videotaped interacting with their parents. The children were between 14 and 34 months of age and were just beginning to use single words when the study began. The development of substantives and function forms (as defined by Bloom) was observed. Regardless of the mode of instruction, all children developed function forms in the order reported by Bloom (1973) for her normal child. The size of the vocabularies at this early age varied according to the mode of instruction. The children trained in the oral or aural mode used a total of between seven and thirteen words at 2 years while the vocabularies for the children using total communication averaged fifty-seven signed and/or spoken words between 20 and 22 months of age. Only the children trained in total communication began to use a sufficient number of combined words to allow analysis of multiword utterances. Chaining was the most common means of combining words. Tiffany (27 to 33 months) produced chained utterances such as "up-up-hot-hurt" (describing a picture of smoke), and "bug-in-yellow" (showing a firefly in a bottle to teacher and classmates). These utterances differed from those usually reported for normal hearing children, because the deaf children were attempting to convey more complex concepts than the younger normal hearing child would encode in a chained utterance.

At all stages in this study (Shafer & Lynch, 1981), the children using total communication had larger vocabularies and a longer mean length of utterance. By 36 months of age, two of the three children using total communication were producing the majority of their utterances orally with no use of signing. This confirmed other studies showing that the early use of sign language tended to enhance rather than inhibit verbal expression. The third child had only vibrotactile response to sound and produced few oral-only utterances.

A further study of the acquisition of signed and spoken language was presented by H. S. Schlesinger (1978), who found that in deaf children exposed to sign language, the first sign appeared prior to the expected age of first spoken words. The semantic intentions expressed depended upon each child's cognitive development. The development of various morphologic forms has been charted in a number of studies (Crandall, 1978; Raffin, Davis, & Gilman, 1978; H. S. Schlesinger, 1978). These studies reaffirm the earlier claim of Bellugi and Klima (1972) that deaf children learning sign language express the full range of linguistic development, matching that of hearing children. The milestones of language seem to be the same.

These studies of emerging language in deaf children illustrate that despite sensory loss, deaf children develop concepts appropriately for their age. When learning sign language, concepts are linked to visual symbols at a somewhat earlier age than usually occurs with the auditory-oral symbols. With early diagnosis, amplification, and training, deaf children can learn to match concepts to verbal symbols at ages comparable to normal children. However, too much of the research focuses on the deaf child's lack of linguistic achievement rather than on the kind of detailed description of performance that could be used productively to influence programs of intervention.

Speech Problems of the Hearing Impaired

On the average, the naive listener can understand only 20 percent of the spoken words of the deaf (Ling, 1976). Ling (1976) reports studies showing that only 20 to 25 percent of the speech of deaf 12 to 15-year-olds is intelligible. Judgment of intelligibility was obviously related to the length of utterance (Monsen, 1978). Problems are observed with respiration, phonation, suprasegmental segments of rate, stress and juncture, the segmental elements of consonant and vowel production, and voice quality, which is characterized by excessive nasality. Forner and Hixon (1977) found abnormal respiratory function during speaking but not during normal resting breathing in the deaf. Monsen (1979) found the voices of deaf subjects excessively flat or abnormally changeable. The deviations showed that there was poor control of air supply, and the author indicated the need to avoid a tense vocal aperture. Deaf children need to be specifically taught to inhale prior to speaking.

In the opinion of Monsen (1976, 1979), there is something about the quality of the vowels that allows the listener to identify a deaf speaker. Although consonants are thought of as carrying the majority of information, vowels convey many cues about ad-

Helen Keller

Helen Keller was neither a scientist nor a researcher, yet she continues to represent high achievement for the communicatively handicapped. Keller was a great friend of Alexander Graham Bell, who wrote about her, "I feel that in this child I have seen more of the Divine than has been manifest in anyone I ever met before."*

Helen was a normal child when she was born in Tuxcumbia, Alabama; however, following an illness in her second year she lost both her sight and her hearing. Five years later her teacher, Anne Sullivan Macy, came to live with the family and to devote the remainder of her life to Helen. Helen was taught to communicate by spelling letters into the palm of the hand. She wrote in both Braille and in script, and she also learned to speak. Helen developed an early passion for poetry and corresponded with John Greenleaf Whittier when she was 9 years old. She felt that she could sense the flowing musical rhythm of poetry as it was communicated to her by her teacher's fingers moving in her hand.

Helen Keller graduated from Radcliffe College. She authored seven books, and supported herself and her household from her earnings as an internationally acclaimed lecturer. Several of her books told about her own life while others were religious and philosophical. In expressing her philosophy, Keller is quoted as saying, "I cannot understand why anyone should fear death. Life here is more cruel than death—life divides and estranges, while death, which at heart is life eternal, reunites and reconciles. I believe that when the eyes within my physical eyes shall open upon the world to come, I shall simply be consciously living in the country of my heart."*

*From Joseph Lash (1980): *Helen and Teacher: The Story of Helen Keller and Anne Sullivan Macy.* New York: Delacorte Press, 1980. Reprinted with permission.

jacent consonants. Monsen (1979) found that the deaf may reduce time and frequency of vowels, which contributes to reduced intelligibility. It is also possible that some unintelligibility in the deaf may be due to an aberrant glottal source. Stevens et al. (1976) reported on nasality, which is widely recognized as a problem in the speech of the deaf; he felt that this may be a result of articulatory error or velopharyngeal inefficiency. Certainly, lip reading provides no input regarding aspects of speech such as nasality or voicing. Black (1971) summed up the speech problems of the deaf by indicating that their speech differs from normal in all regards.

THE INTEGRATIVE APPROACH

The primary effect of severe hearing impairment is on language performance—especially auditory comprehension and speech production, which show delayed development. All other effects—those on the cognitive dimensions and on the knowledge of the linguistic code—occur indirectly as a result of not hearing spoken language at all or hearing it very imperfectly. In severe or profound hearing impairment, no type of auditory information, including that of language, enters the auditory system. Since the conceptual level of the cognitive dimension is intact in severe hearing loss (unless there is also a problem of mental retardation), percepts and concepts develop primarily from information received through the visual system. However, the refinement and rapid expansion of concepts ordinarily provided by language may not be available to the hearing-impaired child. Consequently, the linguistic code and its rules are not learned in the same manner in which the hearing child learns them; this is reflected in language performance. Since the conceptual system is intact, the severely hearing-impaired child can learn a symbol system. Figure 17-4 illustrates the dimensions of language affected by hearing loss and the alternative linguistic codes that may become a part of the linguistic knowledge and language performance of some hearing-impaired children.

Method A in Figure 17-4 represents the aural-oral method of instruction, employing amplified auditory input that may (in oral programs) or may not (in aural programs) be supplemented by lip reading cues. In both methods, the output is limited to speech. Since auditory input is restricted in the hearing impaired, auditory memory and perception are affected as are conceptualization and symbolization. These restrictions in the cognitive dimension influence the association of meaning with the linguistic code, and thus semantic learning is delayed. Since the child is limited in exposure to morphosyntactic and pragmatic rules, these language systems show corresponding delays in development. As previously noted, comprehension and speech performance may also be expected to be impaired. Method B of instruction is spoken English supplemented by visual

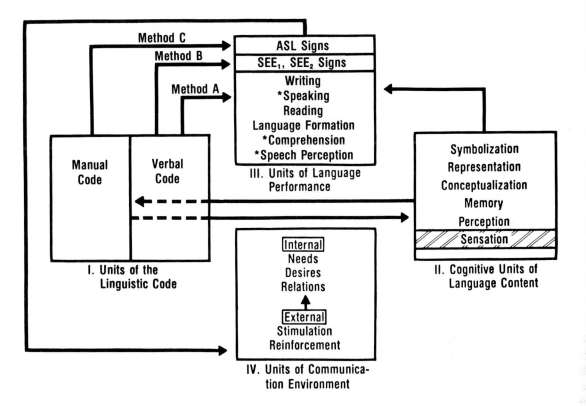

Figure 17-4
The integrative model of language showing the effect of a significant sensory loss on the dimensions of language. The particular impairment in oral language performance is identified with an asterisk.

signs that correspond exactly to the spoken words using a system of sign such as SEE₁ or SEE₂ combined with finger spelling. Method B utilizes the same procedure as Method A except that the auditory-oral code is augmented and clarified through the use of visual signs. Method C shows the substitution of another linguistic code, in this case ASL, for spoken English, thus bypassing speech perception and verbal expression. Although many children trained in total communication become proficient in both ASL and spoken English, method C illustrates that another linguistic code may be substituted without leading to deficits in the cognitive dimension of language or in the dimension of the communication environment.

The effect of varying degrees of hearing impairment on language performance may be illustrated by several children seen by the authors of this volume. The first boy was 4 years old before his severe high-frequency hearing loss was identified. Because his acuity in the low frequencies was completely normal, he always recognized the presence of speech, even very soft speech, but he frequently could not comprehend. Since he was an intelligent, observant boy, he realized that it was not acceptable to acknowledge that he did not understand what was said, so he guessed and often produced answers related to only one or two words in the question. When asked to describe pictures he was more fluent, but his descriptions were characterized by excessive naming. "A door and a tree and cake and a window and a girl and a girl and a window." "A doggy and a shirt and her hanging clothes and a window and a gate and bushes." Other problems in language development are also illustrated by these descriptions. He has the concept of plural, but is not always sure how to express it and so repeats "a girl and a girl." He names easily but still has not mastered the morphosyntactic systems. Consequently, he produces utterances such as "her hanging clothes."

The second child had a profound hearing loss and was fitted with a hearing aid that enabled him to identify the presence of speech at 40 dB. He was trained using an oral approach. At age 4 he described the same pictures as follows: "Present-party-birthday." "Dog-clothes-coat-running." These descriptions reflected his ability to identify key concepts, such as the children bringing presents to a birthday party, and he could use his limited vocabulary to express these concepts. At this time, he still related words only through the process of chaining. In this example, his vocabulary of substantive words appears better developed than his knowledge of function words.

Children with chronic mild or moderate hearing loss who have acute episodes of more severe impairment may have some conceptual impairment and a corresponding problem in vocabulary as a result of missing parts of the ongoing stream of speech in the environment. The difference between the moderately and severely hearing-impaired child and the retarded is the level of their concept development. Once remediation is provided, the hearing impaired have the potential of achieving a language level commensurate with their chronological age. In the opinion of the authors, the earlier a structured symbol system is introduced, the better chance the hearing-impaired child has of developing normal cognitive functions. The three methods indicated in Figure 17-4 illustrate the codes and modes of performance the deaf can use either as alternatives or supplements to the auditory-vocal code.

ASSESSMENT

The first responsibility of the language specialist is to participate in the confirmation of the hearing loss. At times, a language specialist may be the first professional to evaluate children who are "not talking." The responsibility to rule out hearing impairment in such children is obvious. Less obvious is the responsibility of the language specialist to act as an advocate for children in obtaining prompt audiometric evaluation and amplification if needed. One survey of parents of hearing-impaired children indicated that professionals, especially physicians, failed to listen to the concerns expressed by parents about their child's possible hearing problem. This failure resulted in delays of up to 24 months between the time the parents asked if their child could hear and a definitive diagnosis of deafness was made (Malkin, Freeman, & Hastings, 1976).

A more recent survey (F. B. Simmons, 1980) of newborns in a major medical center found that following initial screening, the average child was 9.8 months old when definitive rescreening was done; 13 months old when a hearing aid was recommended; and 22 months old before the hearing aid was actually acquired. Simmons stated that an obvious solution to this problem was to decrease the time interval between diagnostic recalls. He felt that "delayed auditory maturity" was seldom an adequate reason for postponing the decision on a child's hearing. (At the clinic with which Simmons was affiliated, appointments for audiological recall *must* be scheduled within 2 weeks of the first appointment, and a final opinion on hearing acuity must be offered within six weeks of the first appointment.) Whenever the audiologist is in doubt, brain stem evoked response (BSER) testing is requested, which must also be performed within 2 weeks of the date of the request. The justification for this rigid schedule is the short time available for maximum input to the child's rapidly developing brain.

With such guidelines in mind, the language specialist may become a more effective advocate in securing a final opinion on the child's hearing acuity, and also has an important role in urging proper reevaluation of the levels of hearing of children with diagnosed hearing loss. Language remediation may be expected to be gravely compromised without prompt, repeated, and reliable hearing testing, which should include aided thresholds and speech discrimination as early as possible. With careful training, a deaf child can be taught to identify certain toys, for example, so that speech discrimination can be tested by the audiologist even though standard tests of speech discrimination cannot be administered.

Another responsibility of the language specialist during assessment is to establish the child's level of linguistic functioning. The tests used with hearing impaired vary depending upon the purpose of the testing. If the language specialist has been asked to evaluate how a particular hearing-impaired child will do in a regular class, then the child should be tested using whatever tests are used for the normal children in the group in which he will compete. The consequence of failure to properly evaluate hearing-impaired children is suggested by research using the Boehm Test of Basic Concepts (Boehm, 1971). Davis (1974) tested twenty-four hearing-impaired children between the ages of 6 and 8 years old who were either enrolled in regular classes or who were being considered for enrollment in regular class. On this test of a child's ability to understand and follow basic directions commonly used in the lower primary grades, 75 percent of the hearing impaired scored below the tenth percentile in the concepts of quantity, space, and time, which are assumed to be important to early academic success. These scores raised serious questions about the advisability of transferring these children to regular classes until these concepts are mastered.

Sometimes it is important to know what concepts the hearing impaired child has acquired. In such instances, the use of tests that do not require the comprehension or use of spoken language, such as the Leiter International Performance Scale or the Hiskey-Nebraska Test of Learning Ability, would be appropriate.

For some hearing-impaired children, it is necessary to establish base line information about their ability to comprehend and use oral language and gestures. The Scales of Early Communication Skills for Hearing Impaired Children (Moog & Geers, 1975) is one such test. It can be completed by the child's teacher and is suggested as a first step in establishing realistic teaching objectives. The scales allow appraisal of receptive and expressive language skills as well as nonverbal receptive and expressive skills. The test was standardized on 371 hearing-impaired children between the ages of 2 years and 8 years, 11 months. (At present there are no commercial tests available for assessing competence in sign language.)

Analysis of spontaneous verbalization is as important for assessing the hearing impaired as for any other group of children. Although any of the methods previously discussed may be used, specific suggestions have been made for obtaining language samples with the hearing impaired (Kretschmer & Kretschmer, 1978). Because of the expected difficulty in understanding hearing-impaired children, a combination of visual and auditory records appears important. If videotaping is not practical, careful notes may be taken to supplement the audiotape. Kretschmer and Kretschmer also suggest standard eliciting procedures, and provide an analysis procedure that accounts for some of the unusual language performance of children whose techniques of syntactic, semantic, and pragmatic expression fall significantly below their cognitive awareness.

INTERVENTION

As discussed earlier in this chapter (pp. 373-377), there are three major methods for teaching children who have significant hearing impairment: oral, aural, and total communication methods. All modes of intervention require proper fitting and consistent use of hearing aids. Also, they are all dependent upon early identification and the participation of family members in the child's language learning process. The decision as to which children will enter which programs involves various professionals. The obvious goal is to choose the method of education that will be of most benefit to the particular deaf child. Downs (1974) proposed a deafness management quotient, which was designed to identify the language education program best suited to the child. This quotient provided a weighted scale for the following variables:

1. Residual hearing: 0–30 points
2. Central intactness: 0–30 points
3. Intellectual factors: 0–20 points
4. Family constellation: 0–10 points
5. Socioeconomic situation: 0–10 points

When the above formula awarded the child over 80 points, an auditory-oral approach was recommended. When the score was under 80 points, a total communication program was suggested.

Another approach to this decision-making process is the Feasibility Scale for Language Acquisition Routing (FSLAR) (Rupp et al., 1977). This scale analyzed seven prognostic factors including (1) amount and configuration of residual hearing; (2) age of the child; (3) parental interaction; (4) other possible handicaps; (5) child's behavior in testing; (6) "subjective" response to amplification; and (7) observed form of communication. According to the authors, the strength and practicality of the FSLAR is that it forces the professional to consider the many contributing variables and to reach a decision based upon all of them.

The speech of the deaf child also requires remediation. A program of speech instruction has been outlined in great detail by Ling (1976). This program specifies the steps that can be taken through brief daily practice to improve all parameters of speech, including respiration, phonation, rate, stress, juncture, vowel, and consonant production. The importance of low-frequency hearing (below 500 Hz) is stressed by Ling and is also put forward as a rationale for acoupedics.

The effectiveness of any intervention program for the deaf should be judged on the documented capability of that program to provide the children enrolled with language skills that are commensurate with their intellectual abilities. Whatever program of intervention is chosen, the goal of the program should be not only to develop language but also to foster the kind of communication that allows for good parenting and warm interpersonal exchanges between the hearing-impaired child and his family and peers. Also, although the hearing-impaired child has the right to learn articulate speech so that he may interact with the majority of people in the world, the attainment of intelligible speech in the absence of good language is an empty achievement.

outline

DEFINITIONS

Childhood Schizophrenia
Autism

CAUSES OF AUTISM

Psychogenic Causes
Organic Causes
Autism as a Genetic Disorder
Autism as a Neurological Abnormality

THE DIMENSIONS OF LANGUAGE AND AUTISM

The Communication Environment
Relationship Between Autism and the
Cognitive Dimension of Language
Splinter Abilities
Intelligence Testing
Effects of Autism on Knowledge and Performance of
the Linguistic Code
Mutism
Echolalia
Atypical Vocabulary Development
Pronoun Reversal
Morphosyntactic and Pragmatic Errors
Abnormalities of Voice and Articulation
Ability to Read by Rote

THE INTEGRATIVE APPROACH

ASSESSMENT

INTERVENTION

The Psychogenic Approach
The Behavior Modification Approach
Nonvocal Communication

language disorders among autistic children

18

AUTISM REMAINS AN enigmatic disorder and is one of the great tragedies that can confront a family. As one father said of his autistic son,"He is a tyranny you will never quite learn to live with; an obsession you will never learn to live without" (Greenfeld, 1978).

Although language deviation has always been considered characteristic of autism, earlier theories considered that the language disturbance was a reflection of an interpersonal disorder and that as interpersonal problems decreased, the language would spontaneously improve. Consequently, little direct attention was given to language intervention. More recently, language assessment and intervention have assumed pivotal significance in the management of autistic children (Ricks & Wing, 1976; Rutter, 1978b). It has been suggested that the most important factor in autism may be the associated language disorder.

DEFINITIONS

The term *autism* is sometimes used interchangeably with "emotional disorder" or "childhood schizophrenia." *Emotional disorder* is a generic term common in educational settings. It covers the severe behavioral problems discussed in this chapter and may also apply to the less serious adjustment problems often known as "behavioral disorders of childhood." These behavior disorders include numerous habit dysfunctions, which may be forerunners of later psychosomatic or neurotic problems, and disturbances of conduct, which may become character disorders (E. J. Anthony, 1970). A few of the behavioral disorders are handicapping enough that the children need enrollment in programs for the emotionally disturbed. Some of these children exhibit various speech and language problems, whereas others function adequately in school and exhibit no speech or language problems. This latter group is not discussed in this chapter.

Childhood Schizophrenia

Schizophrenic disorders in children have been recognized since the beginning of this century, but it was not until the 1940s that they began to arouse much interest (Bender, 1942; 1947; Bradley, 1941). Rutter (1972) believed that schizophrenia can begin in childhood and can be recognized by the same symptoms that characterize the adult disorder, including a fundamental disturbance of personality; a distortion of thinking (often including a sense of being controlled by alien forces); delusions, which may be bizarre; disturbed perception; and abnormal affect (Cooper et al., 1972). In most instances, the onset is insidious and the symptoms tend to occur during puberty. Over 80 percent of the thirty-three cases studied by Kolvin (1971) had auditory hallucinations and nearly half also had visual hallucinations. Mood was disturbed, affect was blunted, and mannerisms and grimacing were common. Of the parents, one in ten was schizophrenic. There was some tendency for the children to come from working class backgrounds. Most of the children tested were within the normal range of intelligence.

Autism

The disorder known as autism was identified by Kanner (1943) in a classic paper. He described a combination of factors as characteristic of the autistic child. These included extreme social isolation or "aloneness" from the very beginning of life, some flashes of purposeful behavior, and an obsessive desire to maintain "sameness" in all areas of life. In discussing the language of the autistic child, Kanner mentioned that verbal autistic children often focused on lists, slogans, or rhymes that had little communicative intention. Autistic children were noted to have a rather good rote memory and a tendency for echolalia and pronoun reversal.

Leo Kanner

Leo Kanner has been referred to as the "Dean of American child psychiatrists." While it is difficult to identify his single most significant contribution, his identification in 1943 of infantile autism has been of paramount importance. Kanner's publications number in the hundreds and include textbooks that are still classic. The effectiveness of his teaching has been demonstrated by the fact that his students are among the best known researchers in the area of autism and child psychiatry. Kanner was always a strong advocate for the care and welfare of mentally handicapped children, and his pioneering efforts continued into the 1970s when the *Journal of Autism and Childhood Schizophrenia* was founded under his editorial leadership.

Kanner was born in Austria and received his M.D. from the University of Berlin in 1919. He began his career working in electrocardiography at a Berlin Hospital. In 1924, he came to the United States and accepted an appointment in a psychiatric facility at Yankton, South Dakota. He joined the staff of the Johns Hopkins Hospital in 1928 and remained there until he became Professor Emeritus of Child Psychiatry in 1959.

Autism is still defined primarily by its behavioral manifestations: (1) impairment of interpersonal relationships; (2) impairment of language; (3) insistence on sameness; (4) disturbances of sensory input; and (5) disturbances of motility (Rutter, 1978a).

Impairment of Interpersonal Relationships. Although autism is generally accepted to mean withdrawal or aloneness, it is used in this instance to describe a failure to develop relationships with people. Kanner (1943) suggested that all the other symptoms occurred because of this profound social withdrawal, and although this position is no longer held, it continues to influence some approaches to autism. These disturbances in relating were summarized by Ornitz (1978, p. 118), who noted that 90 percent of the approximately seventy children reviewed by him and his colleagues appeared to be "in a shell" and "very hard to reach." Over 60 percent of them also (1) ignored people as if they did not exist; (2) avoided looking people in the eye; and (3) acquired objects by directing another's hand.

Impairment of Language. Language impairment is considered central to autism and will be discussed in detail later in this chapter. Those autistic children who develop speech tend to be echolalic and produce inappropriate (and therefore noncommunicative) utterances. Autistic individuals also have a tendency to reverse pronouns.

Insistence on Sameness and Aloneness. These two characteristics constitute the key symptoms of autism, according to Kanner and Eisenberg (1956). There are reports of some autistic children who refuse to have their clothes changed. Many will eat only a limited selection of food and may drink only from the same glass. Any change or upset in the child's established routine leads to violent temper tantrums that can be stilled only by the return to the routine.

Disturbances of Sensory Input. Many autistic children are first seen clinically because they are suspected of being deaf. Abnormalities of the visual modality are also common, and some autistic children are suspected of being blind. This neglect of the distance senses of hearing and vision appears to be related to the essential nature of "aloneness" of autism and is contrasted to the autistic child's attention to the proximal or more internalized senses of taste, touch, and smell.

Disturbances in Motility. In general, autistic children develop motor milestones at the expected ages (Wing, 1976a; DeLong, 1978, p. 209), and their families do not consider them motorically abnormal. However, there are physical symptoms that distinguish autistic children from others. The most prominent of these is flapping of the hands or arms in a repetitive manner, which was reported in 76 percent (Ornitz, 1978) and 62 percent of children surveyed (Coleman, 1978). Flapping tends to increase when the children are excited or when they are watching something, such as a spinning object, which they particularly enjoy. In addition, many of them engage in whirling, rocking, and prolonged head banging.

It is obvious that not all of these symptoms will be present in all children, but a majority of them are required to make a diagnosis of autism. The crucial distinction is that these symptoms *must* be present prior to 30 months of age in order for a child to be diagnosed as autistic (Rutter, 1978a).

The conditions of autism and schizophrenia in children have been distinguished as different disorders on the basis of their symptoms (Rutter, 1972; Wing, 1976b). Autism involves a failure of development while schizophrenia involves a loss of reality after it has already been established. Delusions and hallucinations are characteristic of schizophrenia, but are quite rare in autism. Marked remissions and regressions are expected in schizophrenia but are decidedly uncommon in autism, where a relatively steady course is much more usual. Mental retardation is a common accompaniment of autism but is less frequently associated with schizophrenia. The sex distribution is also different, with schizophrenia (especially in the adult form) occurring with about the same frequency in men and women, while autism is three to five times more common in boys than in girls (Ritvo et al., 1976). Family histories show that schizophrenia is rare in the families of autistic children, but occurs in about 10 percent of the parents of schizophrenic patients. Although these findings point to a clear distinction, not all researchers accept these distinctions; studies reported in this chapter follow the terminology used by each author, which means that there is some overlapping of terms.

Although the language specialist is not responsible for determining etiology, all assessment and intervention procedures may be affected to some degree by the language specialist's theory of etiology. Historically, the two major etiological theories are the psychogenic and the organic.

CAUSES OF AUTISM

Psychogenic Causes

In the first description of autism, Kanner (1943) pointed out that all eleven of his patients came from highly intelligent parents. Kanner emphasized the emotional coldness and obsessive qualities he saw in the parents of his autistic patients (Kanner & Eisenberg, 1955, 1956; Rutter, 1968), and he concluded that the disorder was partially due to lack of affection from the parents— a psychogenic disorder due to "emotional refrigeration." This view has been widely quoted despite Kanner's later (1971, p.141) caution that his clinical notes about the parents had been overstressed. He stated that the emergence of autistic symptoms from the beginning of life made it "difficult to attribute the whole picture . . . to parent–child relationship."

In his book, *The Empty Fortress* (1967), Bettelheim stressed the importance of introspection in understanding autism. It is therefore not surprising that he introduced his text by giving his own history, including his early program (between 1932 and 1938) of keeping autistic children in his own home. Later, Bettelheim headed a residential school for disturbed children and his book is based on his experience with forty autistic children. In Bettelheim's opinion, most institutions approach the psychotic child with the idea of assisting him to see the world as it really is. Bettelheim saw his task as creating for the child a world that was totally different from the one he abandoned in despair—a world that he could enter just as he was. Bettelheim believed that autism was psychogenic in nature and felt that it could be cured on a psychological basis. He said that he did not accept the hypothesis that autism was due to an organic defect and that he intended to continue treating it psychologically until such time as it became curable through pharmacology (Bettelheim, 1967, p. 403). Bettelheim also said, "Throughout this book I state my belief that the precipitating factor in infant autism is the parent's wish that his child should not exist" (p. 125).

There have been a number of objections raised to Bettelheim's hypothesis. The first objection concerns the early age (less than 30 months) at which the disorder must be manifested. It would seem that only the most severe parental abnormality could so quickly cause such a gross disorder as autism. With the exception of Bettelheim, most authors describe only subtle parental abnormalities. The second objection is that the parental abnormalities could be the *result* rather than the *cause* of the child's abnormal behavior. Rutter and Bartak (1971, p. 24) conclude that "autism is almost certainly not due solely to psychogenic influences."

Organic Causes

There have been increasingly strong claims that autism is due to organic brain disease. Several organic causes have been studied, including genetic disorder and neurological abnormality.

Autism as a Genetic Disorder

Several genetic possibilities have been investigated. Researchers have looked for possible chromosome abnormalities, but so far none have been found. Enough studies have been conducted that researchers like Wing (1976b) reject the proposal that a single gene is responsible for the disorder; however, the possibility that autism may be a polygenic or multifactoral inherited tendency is still to be explored, and there is a slightly raised occurrence (approximately 2 percent) of autism in the siblings of autistic children (Wing, 1976b). In a study of 21 same-sex twins in which at least one twin showed the symptoms of autism, Folstein and Rutter (1978) concluded that genetic factors are probably important, as did other researchers (Spence, 1976). The importance of biological hazards in the perinatal period, which may operate in combination with a genetic predisposition, are also mentioned. However, the mode of inheritance and exactly what is inherited remain uncertain.

Autism as a Neurological Abnormality

Follow-up studies done by Kanner (1971) suggested that there was no organic brain dysfunction among the autistic children he studied. All but one of Kanner's eleven patients had normal EEGs. However, other studies have shown a somewhat different picture. A follow-up of sixty-four children in England showed that eighteen of the sixty-four (28 percent) developed epileptic fits during adolescence (Rutter & Bartak, 1971). In another follow-up study (DeLong, 1978, p. 210) of seventeen autistic children, abnormal EEGs were found in eight cases. Other EEG records were marginal but only five of the seventeen were considered completely normal. Of these seventeen children, eight were left handed and three had no established hand preference. Others have suggested an abnormality of the function of the dominant hemisphere in autistic children (Ricks & Wing, 1976, p. 127). The most consistent abnormality was on pneumoencephalograms (where air is injected into the spinal cord cavity allowing visualization of the ventricals or openings in the brain). In this examination, fifteen of the seventeen cases demonstrated some brain abnormality, mainly on the left side, leading the author to hypothesize some type of temporal lobe lesion. The theory is that some damage to the left hemisphere is uncompensated for by transfer of function to the right hemisphere, and the overall consequence is that in autism one finds the most profound differences between the left and right hemisphere (DeLong, 1978). This theory makes no effort to account for the interpersonal abnormalities of autism.

Other rather extensive neurophysiologic studies have been carried out by Ornitz (1978), who did EEG studies and checked autonomic and vestibular responses. His findings, together with clinical observations of the strange sensorimotor behavior of autistic children, point toward a dysfunction of some system that modulates the interaction of sensory and motor process. He suggested that the vestibular system may be involved. In another report, edited by Coleman (1978, p. 185), seventy-eight autistic children from all over the United States were studied to search for chemical toxins in their blood. While some minor and unexplained antibodies were found, no metabolic problems were discovered. The author stated that this study provided no final answers but raised sufficient questions to justify further research.

Recently there has been a strong move away from viewing autism as an emotional problem caused by inadequate parenting, toward viewing it as a developmental disorder of organic origin. With this shift, the parents have been transferred from the

---

The following exerpts are from an essay written by the brother of an autistic boy.

I have a brain damaged brother. His name is Noah. My brother is a ten year old boy who can't talk, write and can't do most things a boy his age can do, such as throw or catch a ball. He goes to a special school and a special day care center in the afternoon.

In the morning, Noah usually gets up early and chants a low humming noise. Then in about fifteen minutes, he will walk down the hall to the living room where he sits on a certain love seat which he has made his.

If nobody teaches him he wanders from bedroom to bedroom, from living room to den. He knocks over pillows and blankets and chews on anything soft. . . . While doing this he is emitting the same noise as when he got up—or he is giggling or laughing or screaming. . . . After lunch he does the same thing he did before breakfast which accomplishes nothing—unless he studies.

I really don't know what my feelings about Noah are. Because I don't like thinking about the future for him. Once in a while I get mad at him for what he is because we can't take trips and do things a normal family does. But I shouldn't get mad at him. It's not his fault that he is the way he is.

Reprinted from Greenfeld J: *A Place for Noah*, pp. 308–309. Copyright 1978 by Holt, Rinehart, & Winston, Publishers.

---

cause of the problem to an integral part of the solution of the problem.

THE DIMENSIONS OF LANGUAGE AND AUTISM

When autism was first identified, behavioral characteristics such as aloneness and insistence on sameness received the greatest emphasis. These characteristics indicated a failure to establish a communicative relationship. The next dimension of language to be investigated was the extent of cognitive impairment among autistic children. Most recently, the particular linguistic symptoms of autistic children have been investigated.

The Communication Environment

Autism is essentially a disorder in interpersonal communication. From earliest life, the autistic child appears unable to establish a communicative partnership.

Kanner (1943) pointed out that normal children develop their first relationships through the exchange of a social smile at about 2 months of age. The parents of the autistic children he studied often reported that this social smile was missing in their children. The avoidance of gaze persists in older autistic children, who tend to respond to attempts to establish eye contact by moving away, turning away, averting their own gaze, or putting their head down. On the rare occasions when they make a social approach, older autistic children express much ambivalence, so that they approach timidly with their heads down. Autistic children may approach adults from the back or the side. Often, a positive response from the adult, such as a direct gaze or a smile, will immediately cause autistic children to withdraw once more. Wing (1978) suggested that eye contact may produce overarousal.

A study (Richer, 1978) of an 18-month-old autistic boy showed that he strongly avoided his mother, and that the mother's approaches to the child intensified his avoidance. Other mothers of autistic children report that their children rarely smiled or cried in distress, and appeared happiest when left entirely alone.

Developmentally, the normal child progresses from the exchange of mutual gaze to recognition of tones of voice and use of tone of voice to communicate. Turn-taking in vocal interaction between infants and their caretakers often occurs by several months of age. In addition, the normal infant is sensitive to the acoustic features that identify speakers and signal emotion and thereby communicate the intent of the utterance (Menyuk, 1978a). These same features are used by infants to mark their own utterances, and parents of normal children are quick to identify the basic intent of their child's cries. Experiments with parents of normal, autistic, and retarded children indicate that the parents of normal babies (both English and non-English speaking) could not pick out the voice of their own baby but could identify whether the cry represented want, frustration, greeting, or pleasant surprise. The results were comparable when repeated with retarded children. Parents of autistic children, however, could not interpret the sounds made by other autistic children, yet they could easily identify the voice of their own child and the intent of his cry. These studies suggest that from their earliest months, autistic children do not use voice quality to communicate the way other children do (Ricks, 1975).

During the first several months of life, normal infants begin to respond cooperatively to their caretakers by attempting to accommodate their bodies to the person holding them. Subsequently, they begin to raise their arms in anticipation of being picked up. Once again, parents of autistic children report that their children lacked any anticipatory response to being picked up, and, when they were picked up, they either held themselves stiffly or else seemed to "melt into" the adult's body (Rimland, 1964).

Other social behaviors that fail to develop in autistic children are vocal or gesture greetings such as "bye-bye" (Rutter, 1978a). Unlike normal toddlers, autistic children do not follow their parents about the house, run to greet them, or go to them for comfort. They also fail to develop bedtime routines. In short, they appear unacquainted with their caretakers, and, when being examined, may walk off with the examiner without seeming to recongize that person as a stranger. In fact, the only interpersonal contacts autistic children seem to enjoy are tickling and rough-house play. At such times, the child may laugh and express pleasure while seeming unaware of the adult who is providing the stimulation.

As autistic children become older, they fail to use gestures, head nods, facial expression, etc., to communicate (Ricks & Wing, 1975). They also fail to make any effort to reinforce the speaker, and seem unable to "read" the faces of others, just as they fail to use facial expressions themselves to communicate. Also, they pay no attention to clear-cut signs of disapproval at their socially inappropriate behaviors, such as hand flapping, rocking, and twirling.

As Chapter 9 discussed, in the normal child communication precedes the acquisition of words. This nonverbal communication consists of regulatory functions, the exchange of information as evidenced by pointing and mutual gaze, and greetings as expressed by attention and vocalization. Curcio (1978) studied twelve mute autistic children and concluded that protodeclarative acts such as pointing were absent. If pointing occurred at all, it served a requesting function. Eleven of twenty-seven autistic children studied by Wing (1971, p. 103) never pointed out anything for their parents to look at. Five of the twelve children studied by Curcio (1978) would guide the adult's hand to what they wanted. Imperatives were expressed primarily by screaming.

Another study, (Schuler, Fletcher & Davis-Welch, 1977) followed one 9-year-old autistic boy who had been mute until he was past 5 years of age. His first words expressed the function of *want*, usually food. A second function was also regulatory and was expressed by the use of *no*. This boy did not establish eye contact or otherwise attempt to secure the attention of his listeners. If ignored, he screamed or had a tantrum. Schuler (1980a) concluded that the nonverbal communicative behaviors of autistic children consist primarily of instrumental and regulatory functions.

The inability of autistic children to establish a communicative relationship appears to result in part from the following problems: (1) avoidance of gaze; (2) failure to smile or express any emotion except strong fear or frustration resulting in screaming or tantrums; (3) failure to engage in cooperative behavior such as infant play routines (i.e., bye-bye, patty-cake, etc.); and (4) failure to develop and use gestures such as pointing. This pervasive failure of autistic children to establish communication is characteristically expressed by their parents, who say such things as, "I can't reach him," "My child seems to be in a shell all of the time," or "It seems as if he can't see or hear us." Professionals describe the "vacuous distant stare" of the autistic child and the child's manner of "looking through you as if you were made of glass."

Relationship Between Autism and the Cognitive Dimension of Language

Autistic children are often first seen because it is suspected that they are hearing impaired. Bartak and Rutter (1976) found that approximately 80 percent of the autistic children they followed were believed to be deaf at some time during their developmental years. It has been observed that some autistic children do not exhibit a startle response. This has led some investigators to suggest that the reticular formation in the brain (where normal states of alertness are maintained) may be defective (Rimland, 1964, p. 96). In one study (Ornitz, 1978, p. 118), the sensory input in over seventy autistic children was investigated. It was found that 71 percent of them failed to respond normally to sounds. However in direct contrast to deaf children, some 42 percent of these autistic children were unusually agitated by loud noises. There are case reports of children who became frantically disturbed by sounds such as lawn mowers or vacuum cleaners. One little girl was so frightened by the vacuum cleaner that she would not even pass the closet where it was kept. This fear of loud sounds is in direct contrast to autistic children's willingness to produce loud sounds themselves. Another typical auditory symptom of autistic children is fascination with very faint sounds (Ornitz, 1978). None of these behaviors are characteristic of deaf children.

Abnormalities of the visual modality are also commonly reported (Wing, 1976a). Because autistic children are likely to stare into space or to excessively watch the flicking motions of their own fingers (characteristics of visually impaired children), they may be suspected of being blind or partially sighted. When they do take note of objects, they tend to be preoccupied with things that spin or with minor details of an object having nothing to do with its essential purpose. At any moment, they may let these objects fall from their hands as if they had never existed. Many autistic children seem preoccupied with the feel of things and may rub materials like fur or nylon hose for as long as they are permitted to do so.

Because of these frequently observed abnormalities of sensory response, a series of experiments was undertaken (G. Hermelin, 1976, p. 163) to explore the relationship between a specific sensory input and the devices used to interpret this input. It was Hermelin's conclusion that autism is not the result of abnormal functioning of a particular sensory channel; instead, autistic children seem unable both to organize stimuli and to generalize them into rules to make sense of their environment. DeMyer (1976) also concluded that autistic children's disabilities were in their failure to form abstractions about relationships, not in their sensations or perceptions of sensory stimuli.

Splinter Abilities

Despite their significant problems in most areas of development, some autistic children display one or two skills that appear normal or near normal for their age. These are often referred to as "splinter" abilities. A particular "splinter" ability of autistic children is their generally good rote memory. Hermelin and O'Connor (1970) found the immediate (short-term) memory of autistic children to be as good as or better than that of normal children of the same age. It has also been observed that autistic children, unlike both normal and mentally retarded children, can recall meaningless material equally as well as meaningful material. In another experiment, Hermelin and Frith (1971) had autistic children and normal controls repeat sentences ("We went to town") and nonsentences ("light what leaf we"). It is accepted that in normal children memory for sentences is superior to memory for random word strings. Not surprisingly, the normal children recalled the sentence material better, while the autistic children recalled the last words of *all* utterances better than the first words, regardless of meaningfulness. Since echolalia is a prominent symptom of the verbal autistic children, it is difficult to separate this apparent memory skill from the linguistic symptom of echolalia.

Autistic children may display other splinter abilities, which are often displayed in the fitting and assembly of objects and of block designs. Some degree of nonverbal understanding may also be inferred from the way these children learn to turn keys, unfasten latches, and climb fences. Proficiency on these tasks appears to be poorly related to language skills. However, in children as seriously impaired as autistics, any display of verbal or nonverbal skills might seem impressive. Evidence of splinter skills may have led Kanner (1943) to his original hypothesis that autistic children had "normal intelligence" that was somehow "locked in" and that would emerge following appropriate treatment. This theory persisted for many years, perpetuated in part because autistic children were so difficult to test. In formal testing situations, the responses of many autistic children were so atypical that no IQs could be established. This made it more difficult to challenge the theory that many autistics have relatively normal, albeit "locked-in," intelligence.

Intelligence Testing

It has now been determined that autistic children can undergo intelligence testing if careful techniques are used. Rutter and Lockyer (1967) found that 50 percent of a group of sixty-three autistic children functioned at a severely retarded level (IQs below 50). In another study, Lotter (1967) reported that 56 percent of a group of autistic children functioned in the severely retarded level. Hermelin and Frith (1971) found that 75 percent of the autistic children they studied were retarded. In a series of follow-up projects conducted at the Indiana University Medical Center, DeMyer (1976) concluded that most autistic children do not have normal intelligence. She divided autistic children into high, middle, and low groups based on their intelligence scores. Among her 155 subjects, who had a mean age of 5 years, she found that 75 percent of them had IQ scores below 51, and 94 percent had IQs below 67. When these same children were retested 6 years later, it was found that the initial IQ scores were predictive of how much the children would learn during a program of treatment. In addition, there was good correlation between initial IQs and those obtained 6 years later.

These studies suggest that the cognitive functioning of the autistic child is significantly impaired. Some investigators such as

Churchill (1972), Wing (1975), and Wing et al (1977) view autism primarily as a deficit of "central language" or cognition.

Effects of Autism on Knowledge and Performance of the Linguistic Code

Because of the profound interpersonal problems that characterize autism, it has been difficult to evaluate the various units of language performance and determine levels of speech perception and verbal comprehension. Among verbal autistics, it appears that verbal production often exceeds the level of auditory comprehension. Likewise, the reports of autistic children who read by rote suggest that the ability to "read" exceeds their ability to comprehend the meaning of the words they pronounce.

Mutism

Almost half of all autistic children never speak, and most who do speak show abnormal speech patterns (Rimland, 1964; Rutter, 1965). The incidence of mutism varies in the reported studies from approximately 28 percent (Lotter, 1967; Wolff & Chess, 1965) to 50 percent (Baltaxe & Simmons, 1975; Richer, 1978) to a high of 61 percent (Fish, Shapiro, & Campbell, 1966). The mutism seen in these children is unlike that of deaf children, for example, who maintain good interpersonal relationships and even work out their own gesture system. It is also unlike children with clinical language disorders, who are often very clever at expressing themselves nonverbally. Autistic children may be totally mute or may occasionally utter a word or a phrase. Some of the variability in the reported incidence of mutism may result from vague definitions of this term.

The period of mutism may be extended. Lotter's survey (1967) of thirty-two children showed that 19 percent were totally mute at 10 years of age, and another 31 percent were mute except for an occassional word or phrase. Some children reportedly remain mute all their lives. About 65 percent of the children in the DeMyer et al. study (1973) who were mute at age 5 years were still mute when retested several years later. Continued mutism has prognostic significance; several investigators have reported that the prognosis is more guarded for children who fail to speak by age 5 than for those who do speak by that age (DeMyer et al., 1973; Eisenberg, 1956; Rutter & Lockyer, 1967).

When the mute child produces an occasional word or phrase, it may be bizarre or atypical. Fay (1980a) gave examples of some of these rare utterances, which included "American flag," "chocolate," and "put the foot in the bed." These are totally unlike the first words of the normal child. Isolated utterances such as these sometimes suggest to the parents that their child has consciously chosen to refuse to speak. This tends to reinforce the hope that this is a capable child who is storing up information and knowledge that will suddenly be revealed. Actually, such utterances appear more likely to be delayed echolalia.

Among verbal autistic children, there are several characteristic abnormalities of speech and language. These include echolalia, atypical vocabulary development, pronoun reversal, and morphosyntactic and pragmatic errors. Abnormalities of articulation and voice are also common.

Echolalia

Immediate echolalia is the meaningless repetition of a word or group of words (Fay, 1980a, p. 25). This audiovocal behavior carries no meaning and has no apparent communicative function. Fraser, Bellugi, and Brown (1963), in their work on elicited imitation, contended that imitation was a perceptual-motor skill that did not work through the meaning system. Studies of imitation in normal children suggest that some children often echo spontaneously, whereas others do so very infrequently, if at all (Bloom, Hood, & Lightbown, 1974). In general, spontaneous echoing tends to disappear by age 3. Echolalia remains characteristic of autistic children and, to a lesser extent, of mentally retarded persons and those with various types of brain injury. In studies of disordered populations, it has been found that echolalia rarely occurs when the message is comprehended (Myklebust, 1957; Rutter, 1968). When the child fails to comprehend, he tends to produce an immediate echo. Fay (1969) indicated that when his subject comprehended an utterance, he would comply, not echo.

The first speech reported in at least 75 percent of the speaking autistic children was meaningless echoing of words spoken to them (Rutter, 1965; L. Wing, 1971). This echolalia may persist for several years or more (Baltaxe & Simmons, 1975) and appears to reflect a particular linguistic deviance. Autistic children may repeat just the last words of the phrase or an entire sentence, often with the inflection of the original speaker.

Many autistic children (and only autistic children) display delayed echolalia, which is the repetition of stored, usually echoic, utterances in a new and often inappropriate context (Fay, 1980b, p. 56). These utterances are sometimes considered "irrelevant responses," because the speech can be understood only by knowing the circumstances in which the phrase was first used. Delayed echolalia sometimes appears to have a communicative function and accounts for many of the bizarre-sounding utterances autistic children produce. Kanner (1946) described one boy who said "Peter eater" whenever he saw a stove or a sauce pan. His mother recalled that she was telling the nursery rhyme "Peter, Peter, Pumpkin Eater" when she dropped a sauce pan from the stove. He then adopted this highly individual and non-communicative referent. A child described by Kanner said "Rabbits don't cry. Dogs don't cry" whenever he was fearful. His mother reported that whenever he cried, she would point out that the toy animals were not crying. The child came to use the names of all of his animals in a kind of litany that he recited whenever he was upset. Another example, often repeated in the literature, is that of the boy who said the phrase "Don't throw the dog off the balcony" whenever he was tempted to throw something. Apparently his mother had told him at one time that he must stop throwing his toy dog off the balcony. A further characteristic of delayed echolalia is the tendency to echo not only the words but also the tone of voice and even dialectal characteristics (Ricks & Wing, 1976). A child seen by the authors of this book remarked during testing, "Tomorrow we go down here." This remark was made with the exact inflection and foreign accent of his mother. The utterance apparently had been made by his mother to indicate where he would go to be tested, and this boy repeated it upon arriving in the test room. The private reference autistic children make of speech is illustrated by these examples of delayed echolalia. Unless the origin of the phrase is known, it makes the verbalization appear even more bizarre.

Atypical Vocabulary Development

Once the autistic child has begun to talk, spontaneous vocabulary tends to convey little information and often lacks communicative function. The most readily acquired language skill is object naming (Fay, 1980b). Numbers of autistic children have been reported who show particular skill, and apparent pleasure, in learning the names of large collections of objects or pictures. Parents who have waited so long for the emergence of words often take this as a sign of underlying normal intelligence and begin to "stuff" the child with memorized lists. Kanner (1943) noted that many parents reported, usually with much pride, that their children had learned lists such as the alphabet, presidents, capitols, zoological or botanical terms, and prayers, at early ages. One child could recite an entire catechism at age 2 (Rimland, 1964).

Autistic children also tend to develop vocabularies that focus on a single topic. A 6-year-old boy seen by the authors of this book was fascinated by dates. His primary concern was always the day, the date, and the time of day. When he was asked during testing to describe a picture showing some children arriving for a birthday party, he said, "They sing happy birthday. What month? Maybe in June. My birthday is January 8" (which was correct). A 3-year-old also seen by the authors was interested in numbers and in letters of the alphabet. He had begun to speak by reciting the alphabet. When asked to describe a picture of several children listening to a lady telling a story, he responded by saying "That girl. That girl. That girl. Oh boy, a girl. Three. Three girls." When he was asked if that was all he had to say about the picture he spelled out, "Y—E—S."

The autistic child who uses words or sentences within a single context or to apply to a single topic lacks the ability to use this speech to communicate in any functional manner. Fay (1980b, p. 77) talks of this as "semantic binding" and aptly describes the words learned by autistic children as "cast in concrete." Autistic children appear unable to generalize the meaning of words. Each word or phrase continues to be used only as it was used in its original connotation.

Pronoun Reversal

A pathognomonic sign of the verbal expression of autistic children is pronoun reversal (substitution of *I* for *you*, etc.). Some theorists, like Bettelheim (1967), felt that this sign represented a lack of self-identification. It is now more generally recognized to be a function of echolalia (Rutter, 1968). Fay (1980b) concurred that autistic children were not actually reversing pronouns but simply repeating what they had heard. This problem may go beyond echolalia, reflecting an inability to cope with the shifting reference involved in learning deixis of person. Autistic children appear unable to grasp the changing roles of speaker and listener and fail to understand that *I* and *my* always refer to the speaker and *you* and *yours* always refer to the listener. As further linguistic studies are undertaken, there is increasing evidence that autistic children have equal trouble with other words that have "shifting" boundaries, such as *here/there, come/go,* and *bring/take.*

Morphosyntactic and Pragmatic Errors

Various morphosyntactic errors have been reported as common among autistic children. The most likely errors are omission of prepositions and conjunctions from phrases, resulting in a kind of telegraphic speech (Rutter, 1972; L. Wing, 1969).

Those autistic persons who have been most successful in developing verbal skills may still display what Schuler (1980, p. 107) called "conversational clumsiness." This inappropriate speech appears to result from the inability of autistic children to learn the rules of conversation. They fail to make initial judgments as to the appropriateness of their comments to the situation, and also fail to reinforce their listeners or to be guided by listener response to their own verbalizations. Ricks and Wing (1976) found that autistic children talked endlessly about topics of interest only to themselves. For example, one young man, when asked about his interest in music, would unfailingly respond with a recitation of all the records he had at home. Another young man described by Ricks and Wing (1976) talked to his aunt frequently on the phone. He always began each conversation with the words, "This is Charles Smith, your nephew, speaking."

Even the highest functioning autistic individuals have persisting problems with indirect questions and polite requests. An autistic person might well respond "yes" to the question, "Do you know what time it is?" Baltaxe (1977) found that politeness principles were frequently violated; humor and sarcasm continually baffled autistic individuals. Fay (1980b) presented the case of a high-functioning autistic adult who shared some of his experiences at a panel held at the 1975 conference of the National Society for Autistic Children. He said that he had difficulty in deciding what to say to different people, and that he once told a bank teller to her face that she was "sexy." He justified the remark by saying he had heard other men describing women using that term. He appeared not to understand that while the term might be used in personal conversations between men, it was not appropriate to use to a strange woman. He finally decided that this probably was not "the right thing to do."

Abnormalities of Voice and Articulation

Several researchers (Goldfarb et al., 1972; Ricks & Wing, 1976, p. 106) noted that the voices of autistic children tend to be jerky, with poor control of pitch and volume, and showing "odd" intonation patterns. Their voices seem to lack variation, being high-pitched and having a "parrot-like" monotony (Rimland, 1964, p. 14). Other vocal idiosyncrasies that have been noted include hoarseness, harshness, and hypernasality (Pronovost, Wakstein, & Wakstein, 1966). However, the autistic voice is most often described as monotonous. The literature often speaks of the voices of autistic individuals as sounding "mechanical," "hollow," "dull," or "wooden." Intonational peculiarities, particularly monotony, have often been explained on the basis of presumed emotional disorders. Articulation skills have been studied in both spontaneous speech and echolalia. Baltaxe and Simmons (1975) reviewed studies of phonology, which reported that autistic children followed the normal developmental sequence but at a delayed rate. This observation is confirmed by others (Cunningham, 1966; Goldfarb et al., 1972; Ricks & Wing, 1976).

Ability to Read by Rote

According to Kanner (1943), reading skill is acquired "quickly" by autistic children; he found that his subjects could read by 6 to 8 years of age, but they tended to read monotonously, without the capacity to appreciate the content of what they read. A number of children may also become preoccupied with the spelling of words. Some children learn to read signs and slogans on television or to read road signs. Rimland (1964) surveyed these reports of autistic children who learned to read with little comprehension, and reports on one child who wrote but did not speak. There have been a few reported instances of autistic children who demonstrated unusual rote reading ability (Cobrinik, 1974). Cobrinik (1974) suggested that this skill is due to preservation of a rote ability in the absence of adequate conceptual ability.

THE INTEGRATIVE APPROACH

In the integrative approach, the dimension of the communication environment is considered integral to language development. As Chapter 5 suggested, the infant's interaction with his social world is as crucial to language development as cognitive knowledge. Failure to establish social relationships influences the entire dimension of the communication environment. Whatever needs the autistic child may have to communicate, they are not expressed, and the child fails to engage in reciprocal behaviors with others, which eventually affects the amount and type of stimulation and reinforcement he receives from others. The dimensional model of language illustrates a primary failure at the level of the communication environment (Fig. 18-1).

A contributory factor in the failure of the autistic child to establish interpersonal relationships may be the atypical perceptual functioning that tends to foster social isolation. Neglect of the distance senses of hearing and vision leads to increased focus on the proximal senses of taste, smell, and touch. The suspected inability of the autistic child to integrate sensory input and categorize perceptual information results in significant reduction of higher cognitive functioning. The dual problems of establishing interpersonal relationships and interpreting and integrating sensory input result in the impairment of the knowledge and performance of language. Autistic and mentally retarded children both display severe language disorders, and many autistic children are also mentally retarded. However, diagostically and in their response to training, the autistic and the mentally retarded differ. The autistic tend to develop motoric and splinter nonverbal skills at a chronological age closer to normal than their mental age (based on intelligence testing) would predict. Thus an autistic child may walk at a fairly normal age and be

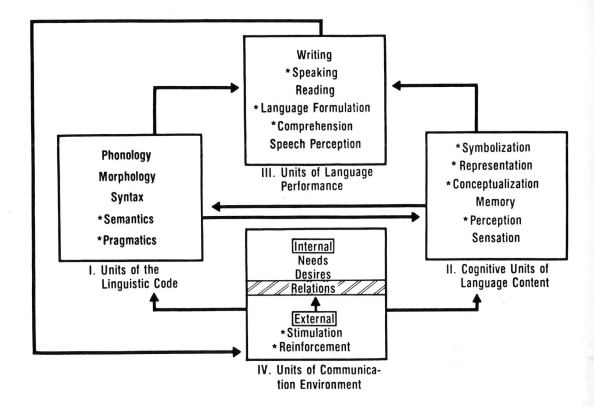

Writing
*Speaking
Reading
*Language Formulation
*Comprehension
Speech Perception

III. Units of Language
Performance

Phonology
Morphology
Syntax
*Semantics
*Pragmatics

I. Units of the
Linguistic Code

*Symbolization
*Representation
*Conceptualization
Memory
*Perception
Sensation

II. Cognitive Units of
Language Content

Internal
Needs
Desires
Relations
External
*Stimulation
*Reinforcement

IV. Units of Communica-
tion Environment

able to complete complicated puzzles—something mentally retarded children cannot do. But unlike autistic children, many mentally retarded children respond positively, and often warmly, to others. Personal attention is reinforcing to them, and they attempt to communicate. The verbal symptoms of autistic children are characterized by their basic lack of awareness of the listener.

Both the autistic child and the deaf child may fail to develop any verbal communication. Yet the deaf child is eager to communicate and will evolve his own gesture system if a language system is not provided for him.

Both the autistic child and the child with a clinical language disorder may fail to comprehend what is said to them. However, the problem of the child with a clinical language disorder is specific to the linguistic system, and such a child will perform willingly if the speaker's intentions can be conveyed through gesture or demonstration. Often, such a child will make good guesses of what is required based upon the context and his previous experiences. However, the autistic child fails to observe context and is no more able to respond to gestures than to verbal commands.

The severe and often dramatic communication problems of the autistic child illustrate the interactions between the various dimensions of language. He not only fails to develop the earliest

Figure 18-1
The integrative model of language showing the effects on the other dimensions of language of the autistic child's failure to establish communicative relations. Those units of language most likely to be impaired are marked with asterisks.

interpersonal communication but also fails to develop the concepts necessary to form the content of language. This leads to impairment in language performance, with particular abnormalities in the semantic and pragmatic systems (see Figure 18-1). Despite the problems presented by autistic children, professional interest in these individuals continues.

ASSESSMENT   Although the specific etiology of autism remains uncertain, research suggests that the symptoms are expressive of an underlying neurological, structural, chemical, or physiological disorder. Consequently, the differential diagnosis of autism requires a team effort involving medical specialists, language specialists, educators, and psychologists. At present, autism must still be diagnosed primarily by its behavioral components combined with a reported age of onset under 30 months. Behavioral observations and checklists are therefore important assessment tools. Criteria for these observations are contained in some texts on autism, such as the Ritvo et al. volume (1976). Behavioral checklists are also incorporated within various tests specifically designed to evaluate children suspected of being autistic. An example of one such test is the Autism Screening Instrument for Education Planning (Krug, Arick, & Almond, 1980). The items in this test are weighted for severity, so that an examiner can determine if a particular child behaves above or below the mean already established for the autistic population on which the checklist was normed. This instrument also includes an educational assessment of receptive and expressive language and speech imitation as well as estimates of attending behaviors and learning rates. Another recently published test, which has been used with large numbers of autistic individuals, is the Individualized Assessment and Treatment for Autistic and Developmentally Disabled Children: Psychoeducational Profile (Schopler & Reichler, 1979). The use of special tests designed for autistic individuals assists the evaluation team in separating the autistic from others with severe developmental disabilities.

The importance of establishing a level of intelligence is suggested by DeMyer (1976) who found that children with the highest intelligence scores made the greatest overall gains in treatment and education. Rimland (1964) found that the child's level of intelligence was linked with success in learning to speak. The degree and type of cognitive ability possessed by autistic children may be studied through the administration of nonverbal tests such as the Leiter International Performance Scale and the Hiskey Nebraska Test of Learning Ability, as well as the more common infant scales. In general, standardized administration procedures need to be modified. Often it will be necessary to reinforce each attempt by the child to perform in order to encourage continued participation in the testing procedure. Standardized testing must be supplemented by naturalistic observation of the child's ability to manipulate objects and engage in play.

Language evaluation has special relevance for overall prognosis in autistic children. Shapiro, Charandi, and Fish (1974) found that the potential for social and interpersonal recovery is greater among autistic children who begin to speak prior to their fifth year. Eisenberg (1957) concurred that if a child spoke by age 5, there was a 50 percent chance for some degree of social recovery. Based on an extensive review of the research relating speech to prognosis for recovery, Baltaxe and Simmons (1975) concluded that lack of language development was indicative of a guarded prognosis for improvement.

Because of the behavioral problems inherent in autism and the particularly personal referents developed by autistic children, no standardized language assessment could elicit the specialized vocabulary of some autistic children. Naturalistic observation of communicative behavior is therefore essential. Often it is necessary to ask a teacher or family member what the child can say, and then it is frequently necessary for that person to provide the appropriate stimuli. In this way the examiner can observe the child naming colors, saying the alphabet, or reciting television commercials, for example. The child's receptive language may also be specific to a few commands. Special attention should be paid to any attempts the child makes to relate to people or objects or to communicate spontaneously.

The principles underlying differential diagnosis of autism as opposed to other problems, such as clinical language disorders, have particular significance for the language specialist, and these have been discussed in the literature (Churchill, 1972; de-Hirsch, 1967). The autistic child displays certain prominent symptoms that affect language development, including a pervasive impairment in the ability to form relationships, as well as impairment in the intent to communicate and in the appropriate use of objects. These symptoms are not seen in such extreme form in children with other disabilities.

The language specialist should also assist in determining the mode of instruction that appears most appropriate for each child. Schuler (1980b) presented a series of issues that appear significant in the determination of the appropriate means of language instruction. These include characteristics of the child, learning characteristics, and practical opportunities for functional use of the language learned. Alpert (1980) also stressed the importance of careful assessment *prior* to choosing a mode of intervention. She suggested that assessment should include observation of the child's vocal and nonvocal communicative behaviors in a natural environment, as well as more formal language testing to assess vocal imitation, auditory discrimination, comprehension of vocabulary, and knowledge and use of syntax. It is also important to determine what is reinforcing for each particular child, since a system of reinforcement will be integral to whatever mode of instruction is finally chosen. Alpert (1980) cautioned that assessment, rather than a lengthy period of failure, should be used to choose the mode of instruction, because the longer a child remains without a means of communication, the less likely it is that he will acquire functional communication.

INTERVENTION Since emotional disturbance was first described by a psychiatrist (Kanner, 1943), it is not surprising that treatment originally began in psychiatry, with only the psychiatrist treating the child. Within the past ten years, there have been many new programs with a strong educational base, in which the main "interveners" are teachers (Sullivan, 1976, p. 293). In addition, parents are becoming increasingly involved in the treatment.

The Psychogenic Approach

Those who felt that the cause of autistic children's atypical behavior was parental treatment of the children "solved" this through complete and prolonged separation of the children from their home. Bettelheim (1967) removed the children he treated from their homes and placed them in an environment that was unstructured and completely accepting. This model was modified somewhat later by others (Mahler & Furer, 1972), who adapted it to include the children's mothers.

Play therapy is a less intensive, psychogenic approach to remediation (Axline, 1976). The child is allowed to set up his own play, and the therapist, by observing, gains insight into the child's problems, and so can help him work through these problems. Proponents of this method suggest that language development depends on the child's capacity to acquire an understanding of some level of symbolic representation, and that this capacity is most closely related to his ability to learn how to play. Others suggest that play may instead be based upon the same symbolic functioning as is speech (Shapiro, 1978). Environmental therapy presumes that the affective deficit is central to the impairment shown by the autistic child.

Objective testing of either the children treated or the methods of intervention is not usually a part of the psychogenic approach. Bettleheim's (1967) review of his patients illustrated some of the problems inherent in attempting to evaluate the success of this method. He described one of his patients, Laurie, as having made "good" progress, yet she was eventually institutionalized and regressed to the point where she responded to nothing. Based on this example, it is difficult to judge what Bettleheim meant when he indicated that 80 percent of those enrolled in his school had "fair to good" outcomes. Kanner and Eisenberg (1955) provided information on the status of the eleven individuals whom Kanner had diagnosed as autistic 30 years previously. Five were institutionalized, and only two were employed; one operated a duplicating machine, while the other, most successful of the group, worked as a bank teller but still lived with his parents.

The Behavior Modification Approach

This approach considers that the primary goal of therapy is not the fostering of a strong emotional bond between the adult and the child but rather the deliberate teaching of specific skills. Proponents of this method feel that firm external structure must be imposed because the handicap of autism has prevented the child from developing his own normal internal control of behavior. The goal of such therapy is not to emphasize a one-to-one relationship but rather to provide a highly structured, individualized learning program designed to help the child minimize his disabilities. Many programs currently use this approach (Sullivan, 1976).

Control of several types of behaviors is emphasized in the behavioral approach. Self-destruction and self-stimulation must be removed before language teaching can commence. Self-destructive behaviors include biting (which may become so severe that the child actually eats away part of his fingers or lips or creates severe sores on arms or shoulders) and banging (some children bang their heads until their corneas become detached). Attempts to increase the self-destructive child's positive feelings about himself through loving attention have apparently not met with much success (Lovaas, Schreikman, & Koege, 1973). However, when the self-destruction was seen as operant behavior

As remediation efforts for nonverbal children have increased, the programs designed by psychologists to teach language to apes have assumed added importance. Apparently, humans have always been intrigued by the possibility of "talking with" animals, and the most likely subjects for such experiments were the apes. Apes demonstrated not only the highest level of intelligence but also shared many physiological similarities with humans. According to the historical review by Hollis & Schiefelbusch,* a psychologist, Kellogg, proposed in the 1930s that an ape actually raised as a human might spontaneously learn to speak. So a chimpanzee, Gua, was raised with the Kelloggs' son. Although Gua learned many human behaviors, speech was not one of them. Two decades later, another chimpanzee, Vicki, was raised by the Hayses, a psychologist and his family. Unlike Gua, Vicki was given speech instructions. The Hayses kept Vicki for 6 years, but despite her rigorous training she only learned to say "papa," "mama," and "cup."

After this disappointment, it was suggested that a visual-kinesthetic approach to language might be more successful, and the Gardners began training a young chimpanzee named Washoe to use American Sign Language. At almost the same time, Premack taught another chimpanzee to use plastic chips as word units, and Rumbaugh utilized a computer system to provide a communication code. All of these animals have made good progress, and efforts continue with these and a second generation of apes. Adaptation of some of these techniques is now being made to improve nonspeech programs for handicapped children.

*Hollis JH, Schiefelbusch RL: A general system for language analysis: Ape and child. In Schiefelbusch RL, Hollis JH (Eds): *Language Intervention from Ape to Child.* Baltimore: University Park Press, pp. 5–42, 1979.

that could be extinguished through aversive stimuli (such as painful electric shock), there was an immediate termination of the behavior. Others have reported similar success.

Self-stimulatory behavior, which includes spinning, rocking, vacant gazing, and hand and finger twitching, makes a child much more difficult to teach and calls critical attention to him. Currently, researchers are exploring ways of using substitute self-stimulatory reinforcers to build more appropriate behavior. This research is still in its initial stages, and no judgment as to its effectiveness can yet be made.

Behaviorists like Lovaas (1977) admit that they know more about building behaviors than about acquiring language. Their language programs tend to be derived from the literature on discrimination learning. Most of their efforts have been directed toward severely impaired, often mute, autistic children. Lovaas' program commences by building first words and abstractions about relationships among objects and events, and progresses to installing social language used in conversation and information exchange (Lovaas, 1977).

The objective measurement of gains during treatment is fundamental to the behavioral approach. Various studies support the effectiveness of behavioral modification in changing the behaviors of autistic children (Wolf, Risley, & Mees, 1964; Wolf et al., 1967; Jones, Simmons, & Frankel, 1974). Using this technique, self-destructive behaviors can be decreased and attending behaviors increased. In mute children, it has been possible to successively shape vowel sounds into words and then increase the repertoire of words. Operant conditioning has also been used to teach an autistic child with immediate echolalia to answer questions appropriately (Freeman, Ritvo, & Miller, 1975).

A serious question concerning the use of behavior modification techniques to develop speech is whether the autistic child actually acquires a knowledge of language or is simply taught to produce a series of verbal responses. Researchers have not yet

Ivar O. Lovaas

Regardless of the method of intervention chosen for an autistic child, or for many children with developmental disabilities, the procedure used to teach the child may be based upon principles of behavior modification. Ivar Lovaas stated in *The Autistic Child* (1977, p. 1) that after all of the books on normal acquisition of language have been studied, the therapist was still faced with the problem of *how* to teach the child to speak. It is in the area of "how to teach" these difficult children that Lovaas has made the most significant contributions. As an advocate of behavioral modification, he influenced the training provided for large numbers of handicapped children.

Lovaas was born in Norway and educated in the United States. After receiving his B.A. degree from Luther College, he obtained a Ph.D. in psychology in 1958 from the University of Washington. His professional life has been devoted to teaching psychology at the University of Washington and currently at the University of California at Los Angeles. In addition, he has maintained an active interest in training facilities for autistic children, and has been actively involved in the study of the etiology and treatment of autism, especially in the aspects of language development and behavior modification.

determined whether linguistic rules can actually be taught. Completion of a speech program does not guarantee carryover of words into communication.

Nonvocal Communication

The failure of some autistic children to learn to speak is not surprising in view of their impaired intellectual and perceptual functioning (McLean & McLean, 1978). A number of nonspeech symbol systems exist, including various systems of signing, abstract plastic symbols, and printed words. All of these methods present certain advantages and disadvantages, which have been summarized by Alpert (1980).

Sign language is probably the most commonly used nonvocal means of communication, and its use with autistic children has steadily gained in popularity.

Results of preliminary studies on children who were trained to use sign language (Bonvillian & Nelson, 1976; A. Miller & Miller, 1973) show that even severely autistic children can learn to respond to signs, which contributes to their understanding of spoken language. Creedon (1973) reported on efforts to teach signs to autistic children. A superficial similarity was noted between signs and the hand movements that occur in the behavioral repertoire of some autistic children. Creedon felt that signs provided many opportunities for reinforcement and could be taught to children who display limited eye contact and an inability to play with objects or peers. Parents were included in this training program. All children were able to learn sufficient signs to express their immediate needs, and a few could sign on a more abstract level. A study by Konstantareas and Leibovitz (1977) indicated that simultaneous presentation of both speech and sign was preferable to use of sign alone because the use of signed speech has resulted in some autistic children progressing from spontaneous signed speech, to simultaneous sign and speech, and eventually to spontaneous verbal language (Schaeffer, 1980).

Regardless of the method of instruction chosen for autistic children, the close interaction between interpersonal communication, cognitive ability, and linguistic performance must be considered. It is still impossible to state whether the autistic child's inability to respond to the world accounts for the magnitude of his language problem, or whether his language problem accounts for his inability to respond to the world.

As J. K. Wing (1976, p. 14) noted, "Autistic children have a fascination which lies in the feeling that somewhere there must be a key which will unlock a hidden treasure.... In return for our attention, these children may give us the key to human language, which is the key to humanity itself."

outline

THE NATURE OF BILINGUALISM

The Bilingual Person
Diglossia and Bidialectism
Code-Switching, Borrowing, and Mixing

TYPES AND DEGREES OF BILINGUALISM

LANGUAGE ACQUISITION AND BILINGUALISM

Acquisition of First and Second Languages
Sequences of Acquisition
Age Differences in Second Language Learning
Processes and Strategies in Second Language Learning
Imitation in Second Language Learning
Simultaneous Acquisition of Two Languages
Sequential Learning of Two Languages
Social Aspects of Bilingualism
Educational Aspects of Bilingualism

BILINGUALISM AND THE DIMENSIONS OF LANGUAGE

LANGUAGE DISORDERS AND BILINGUALISM

Identification of the Language-Disordered Bilingual Child
Determination of Competency in Two Languages
Analysis of Language Differences
Linguistic and Social Environment
Contributing Cognitive Factors

ASSESSMENT

INTERVENTION

RESPONSIBILITIES OF THE LANGUAGE SPECIALIST

language disorders and bilingualism

19

IDENTIFYING, ASSESSING, AND providing intervention for a language-disordered child constitute a complex undertaking that requires considerable knowledge and skills. Providing these same functions for bilingual children requires even greater competency. Difficulties arise not only from a situation in which two languages must be analyzed instead of one, but also from other factors (1) the type and extent of bilingualism and how well is each language understood and spoken; (2) the bilingual models that have been used; (3) the age at which each language has been learned; (4) the social factors influencing the languages used; (5) the dialects of each language that are spoken; and (6) the degree of difference between the two languages.

Frequently, language specialists are asked to participate in activities other than the identification and assessment of and intervention for the language-disordered child. They may be asked to assist with determining language dominance for the purpose of appropriate classroom placement, or to participate in the development of educational policies for bilingual children.

The educational and clinical functions require knowledge about bilingualism in general and, specifically, its relationship to language acquisition. Additional information on the linguistic performance and needs of children learning a particular language in a specific cultural and social setting is essential. This knowledge will aid not only in the educational management of the bilingual child, but will also provide insights into the complexity of language acquisition for the monolingual child. This chapter provides current interpretations of the issues in bilingualism together with definitions of the terms used in the literature dealing with this topic. The effects of second language acquisition on linguistic performance and the factors influencing these effects are considered. Procedures in the assessment of the bilingual child are described, with special references to the identification and treatment of disordered language. Because the largest group of bilinguals in the United States are speakers of dialects of Spanish and English, this particular group is used to illustrate specific points regarding bilingualism; Spanish and English linguistic forms are selected to demonstrate points or principles that are discussed.

THE NATURE OF BILINGUALISM

The topic of bilingualism stimulates considerable controversy among educators. A factor that exacerbates the problem and causes poor communication is the failure to define and describe what is meant by bilingualism and other related terms.

The Bilingual Person

Although The Living Webster Encyclopedic Dictionary (1977) defines *bilingualism* as the capacity of using two languages often with equal facility, the term is commonly applied to individuals who are heterogeneous with respect to their linguistic abilities in two languages. As it is used currently, *bilingualism* reflects two language capabilities in a range of degrees. At one extreme is the complete symmetrical native control of two languages (Peñalosa, 1975). Very few persons, if any, possess such a degree of bilingualism. At the opposite extreme is a person who possesses at least one language skill (audition, speaking, reading, etc.) to a minimal degree in a second language (MacNamara, 1967). Cohen (1975) took this one step further by considering a person who possesses at least one language skill in each of two languages to be bilingual. He believed that this takes into account young children with some listening comprehension in each of two languages but no speaking ability. Bilingualism, thus broadly defined, describes a great number of individuals. The concerns these people present to language specialists are unique.

The disproportionate abilities in the two languages of a bilingual can take many forms. In some instances, performance in a second language (L2) may reach or approach performance in the first language (L1) in vocabulary and syntax but not in pronunciation, or in syntax and pronunciation but not in vocabulary. Cohen (1975) suggested that some linguistic areas, such as accent or pronunciation, influence listeners unduly about the degree of bilingualism. Thus, a speaker with a poor accent and less fluency but with greater knowledge of the language might not impress a listener as being as bilingual as one who pronounces the second language well but has marked deficiencies in its lexicon.

Diglossia and Bidialectism

Although Weinreich (1953) emphasized that linguistic diversity has its origins within each person as the languages he knows and speaks come in contact with one another, linguistic diversity also exists within and between communities or societies. As defined by Peñalosa (1975), diglossia refers to "situations" in which either two varieties of the same language or two different languages are used in the same society. Diglossia exists in communities where one variety of language is used for everyday affairs and another variety is used for formal communication, or in communities where one language may be the predominant language in the occupational area while a second language is used at home.

As stated in Chapter 5, unique modifications of a language, or a combination of two languages learned or shared by specified groups, are referred to as dialects. According to Sawyer (1975), to merit the term dialect a particular variety of language should have a stable structure, which can be taught to succeeding generations of a speech community. Sawyer did not consider a language that was in a fluid state from generation to generation to be a dialect, but rather an imperfect stage of the target language. Corder (1969a) referred to a language in a transitional state as interlanguage. (Some professionals label an individual bilingual if he speaks two dialects of the same language.)

Code-Switching, Borrowing, and Mixing

Alternation of dialects or languages with different groups of persons or between specific domains is known as code-switching. This occurs when speakers regularly use two or more languages or dialects; each is associated with specific activities, social situations, or speakers (Gumperz & Hernández-Chávez, 1975). For example, in a Mexican-American community, a change from English to Spanish may signal a change in the relationship (in the direction of greater personal warmth). The act of code-switching itself then conveys feelings and attitudes.

The concepts of borrowing and mixing are related to code-switching in that they all involve the alternation of two codes. In code-switching, the entire communication medium changes. In borrowing, words for new concepts not available in one language are borrowed from another (such as the French words *garage,* and *range,* and the Spanish words *lasso,* and *corral,* bor-

This is an example of language mixing in which both children speak and understand two languages (Lance, 1975, p. 152).

Carm: Cuentame del juego.
Tom: Primero they were leading diez pa' nada.
Carm: . . . . Diez a nada? Issah! Y luego?
Tom: Then there was our team to bat and we made . . . 'cimos dos carreras. And then ellos fueron a batear. Hicieron una and then nojotros 'cimos cinco. Depues 'ciron six.

rowed by English, or the English words *baseball* and *lunch* borrowed by Spanish (*beisbol, lonche*). Once a borrowed word is used frequently, it is incorporated into the lexicon of the borrowing language.

In mixing, the alternation involves only portions of the code; words from one language are interspersed into the other, but not consistently, nor is the direction of borrowing always the same (*from* the same language *to* the second). When the speaker is fluent in two languages, mixing occurs in conversation with others who are equally bilingual. Lance (1975) suggested that this does not imply that the speaker does not know a particular word in one language or the other, but rather that the word or phrase most readily available at the moment is the one uttered. In cohesive communities where mixing occurs consistently and systematically, there tends to be a fusion of two languages, with portions of both languages eventually becoming stabilized in a particular new form. This form is communicated to language learners within the society, thus the mixed language learned by a child is not modeled on monolingual representatives from the two languages but on the form of language used by the community (Cohen, 1975; Ervin-Tripp, 1978a).

In the Spanish-speaking areas of the United States, mixing of Spanish and English is common, the direction being ordinarily from English to Spanish but sometimes occurring in both directions. Borrowing exists primarily in the lexicon; English nouns, adjectives, and exclamatives are given the phonemic and syllabic patterns of Spanish, and, where appropriate, Spanish inflexional endings are added (Bowen, 1975).

TYPES AND DEGREES OF BILINGUALISM

There are probably as many different types of bilingualism as there are bilingual persons. Very few persons have exactly the same competence in two languages. The language in which an individual has greater competence is said to be the dominant language. For the purposes of assessment and education, it is well to use categories describing degrees of bilingualism. For Spanish and English, categories might be (1) mastery of Spanish (at age level) with minimal competency (the ability to understand or speak a few words) in English; (2) mastery of Spanish with moderate competency in English; (3) mastery of both languages more or less equally; (4) mastery of English with moderate competency in Spanish; and (5) mastery of English with minimal competency in Spanish. Actually, the above classification simplifies what is a much more complex situation in the United States, since there are many dialects of both Spanish and English, as well as differences from the core (standard) language.

When an individual's various linguistic environments (school, home, work, etc.) are considered along with the individual's language competencies and preferences, it becomes apparent that bilingualism is not a simple concept and should not be treated as such—particularly with regard to educational policies. With reference to the language of the Mexican-American community, Peñalosa (1975) stated that linguistic behavior is not simply a case of diglossia or bilingualism but rather multiglossia and multilingualism, with very complex relationships among the half-dozen codes in use. This view of the complexity of bilingualism is of particular importance in the identification and assessment of language disorders in the bilingual child.

LANGUAGE ACQUISITION AND BILINGUALISM

The methods of linguistic description and analysis that have been developed through the efforts of Brown and colleagues (1973) have led to a renewed interest in the acquisition of a second language (L2) by someone who has partially or completely acquired a first language (L1). The major issues related to the naturalistic acquisition of a second language were detailed by Wode (1978, p. 103):

1. Is there a developmental sequence for acquiring L2?
2. Is the sequence ordered in stages?
3. Do L1 and L2 have the same developmental sequence?
4. Is the sequence in L2 governed by any of the following variables?
   - Prior knowledge of L1
   - Structure of L2
   - Processes used in L2 acquisition
   - Similarity of processes in acquisition of L1 versus L2
   - Universality of processes and strategies for L2 learning

These questions have provided the content for studies of second-language learning. The conclusions are tentative, because only a limited number of children have been studied and the variables under which the studies have been conducted differ.

Acquisition of First and Second Languages

Traditional views have held that the acquisition of a second language is different from that of the first language. Current theory questions this conclusion. The evidence for this disagreement has been in studies of development in L2 (Ervin-Tripp, 1974; Carrow, 1971).

Sequences of Acquisition

A major question about second language acquisition is the sequence of development of specified linguistic forms; that is, do first and second language learners go through similar developmental stages? If the development of both languages is similar, studies will show a sequence of the development of linguistic forms in L2 similar to that found in L1.

In studying the language development of second-language learners, Ervin-Tripp (1974) found that the form and function of early sentences, their semantic redundancy, their reliance on short-term memory, their overgeneralization of lexical forms, and their use of simple order strategies were similar to processes seen in first-language acquisition. Carrow (1971) found that comprehension of vocabulary and selected syntactic forms in both Spanish and English followed a similar order in Mexican-American children.

Hakuta (1978) reported on the grammatic morpheme development of a Japanese girl aged 4 years, 11 months, and found that the acquisition of morphemes by the Japanese child was

Susan Moore Ervin-Tripp

After graduation from Vassar College, where she acquired a broad general education in art history, languages, and the social sciences, Susan Ervin-Tripp went to the University of Michigan where she completed her Ph.D. in Social Psychology. She has been a Professor of Rhetoric at the University of California since 1968.

Ervin-Tripp's earliest interest in languages was demonstrated by her having acquired French, German, Spanish, Latin, and Greek by the time she graduated from Vassar, because it was "such fun and seemed such a natural thing to do." Although her interest in language and psycholinguistics is broad, she developed interest in bilingualism because of dramatic personal experiences of bilingual friends who were troubled by a sort of multiple identity or multiple personality. In 1954, Ervin-Tripp contributed to the now classic report, *Psycholinguistics: A Survey of Theory and Research Problems,* edited by Osgood and Sebeok, which attempted to discover points of intersection between the linguists' conception of language as a structure of interrelated formal units, the psychologist's conception of language as a system of habits relating signs to behavior, and the communication specialist's conception of language as a means of transmitting information.

In the field of bilingualism, Ervin-Tripp's contributions have centered on the social variables involved in learning two languages. She stressed the need for identification with the native speakers and the assimilation of their values as prerequisites to acquisition of a second language. She described the effects of the social relationships as well as the emotional quality of the contexts in which a second language is learned on the meanings younger children associate with the language. Ervin-Tripp suggested that the differences between first and second language acquisition are in intent, motive, social milieu, and communicative choice—factors that are viewed as irrelevant to structure, and therefore left unexamined in first language acquisition.

Ervin-Tripp's scholarly works are considered significant contributions in the interdisciplinary studies on language. Of particular interest to the language scholar is her book, *Language Acquisition and Communicative Choice: Essays by Susan M. Ervin-Tripp.*

gradual and similar to that of the children reported by Brown (1973). However, the *order* or morpheme acquisition was different from that of Brown (1973) and de Villiers and de Villiers (1973a). This finding supported an earlier study by Dulay and Burt (1973), which investigated the sequence of development of a subset of Brown's 14 morphemes in 5- to 8-year-old children learning English as a second language. The correlation of the rank orders of acquisition of morphemes between the second-language learners of Dulay and Burt and those of de Villiers and de Villiers was not significant.

Ravem (1978), in a study of an adult Norwegian learning English, reported that although the subject did omit inflections and minor word classes (as do first-language learners), her English could not be classed as "telegraphic," because she transferred both content words and functors from her mother tongue. The difference in the details of acquisition order between learners of L1 and L2 was said by Dulay, Hernández-Chávez, and Burt (1978) to be due to cognitive sophistication, affective focus, acousticoarticulatory ability, and experience on the part of the L2 learner.

Although the sequence of development of linguistic forms in learning L2 has not been found similar to the sequence in L1, the order of development of forms in the same L2 is similar for its learners regardless of the first language spoken. Spanish and Chinese children studied by Dulay and Burt (1974) had virtually the same sequence of acquisition of eleven English functors, even though the grammar of the eleven equivalent functors is widely different in Chinese and Spanish. In studying adult learners of English as a second language, Bailey, Madden, and Krashen (1974) found that despite differences in adult learners with respect to the amount of instruction, exposure to English, and mother tongue, there was considerable agreement as to the relative difficulty of the set of grammatic morphemes studied. Wagner-Gough (1978) also noted similarity in developmental sequence regardless of previous experiences in a first language.

Age Differences in Second Language Learning

It has been the general belief that there is an optimum age for learning a second language, and that if children do not acquire language by this critical age, they will not be able to learn it with as much facility and accuracy. This belief has been supported by data presented by Penfield and Roberts (1959) on the age of completed lateralization of the brain, and by studies of relations between age and the ease of language restoration in aphasia. The hypothesis of optimum or critical age for learning a second language is currently under critical reexamination.

Snow and Hoefnagel-Höhle (1978) urged that in an investigation of age differences in L2 acquisition, the fact that language acquisition is not a monolithic process should be considered.

Language acquisition involves learning separate skills (vocabulary, stress, intonation, comprehension, expression, and reading). A complete test of the hypothesis that there are no age differences in L2 acquisition requires separate tests for these skills. Snow and Hoefnagel-Höhle reported that the adults they studied seemed to have an advantage over the children in acquiring the rule-governed aspects of langauge—morphology and syntax.

In general, the consensus seems to be that the greater ease with which a child learns a second language is more apparent than real, due to the expectations of accuracy in adult language, as well as the different communicative environment and needs of the adult. Ervin-Tripp (1974) stated that greater semantic demands are made on adults and that they attempt to communicate in a more complex form than do children; consequently, they appear to have greater difficulty than children. Additionally, the language input to an adult is quite different from the language input to a child (Butterworth & Hatch, 1978). The child is usually in a learning environment and guided in language learning for a longer period of time than the adult, and therefore may master the language better.

The primary difference between adults and children seems to be in the area of pronunciation. The attention of the adult is on vocabulary and syntax, and pronunciation is neglected. In fact, once an individual learns to read, his auditory processing system is not used to monitor his speech and the auditory system no longer functions effectively to learn new phonemic information. Ervin-Tripp (1974) suggested that for phonology, the optimum learning stage might be around 7 or 8 years of age.

Processes and Strategies in Second Language Learning

Imitation in Second Language Learning

Although current linguistic literature does not consider imitation to be a widely used strategy of children acquiring a first language, there is evidence to support the use of imitation in second-language learning. Huang and Hatch (1978), in studying acquisition of English by Paul, a Chinese child, described early imitation of words, phrases, and greetings. During Paul's first 3 weeks of exposure to English, he imitated frequently used imperatives such as "Get out of here!" "Let's go!" "Don't do that!" and "Don't touch!" Once Paul had "memorized" an utterance, he would use it in identical or similar situations, even though he was not aware of the units within the utterance. Gradually, he began using the forms in the manner in which they are used during acquisition by monolingual children. Huang and

Hatch interpreted Paul's initial second-language acquisition strategy to be different from that of learning a first language. His experience with one natural language system helped him in meaning, and his cognitive capacities made him capable of imitating complex sentences and attaching global meaning to them. This made it possible for Paul to learn English within a period of 4 months.

Wagner-Gough (1978) described the use of imitation by Homer, a Persian child. During the initial stages of acquisition of English, Homer imitated the speech and behavior of other children. When Homer successfully imitated a complete sentence of Mark, his best friend, Mark said, "Don't copy." Unintimidated, Homer shouted, "Don't copy," right back. According to Wagner-Gough, this imitative behavior in the second-language learner may be a way to commit to memory an unanalyzed linguistic pattern for future analysis and later application to a similar context. An analysis of portions of dialogue between Homer and native speakers of English revealed that the patterns addressed to Homer shaped his utterances. For example, in response to the command "Don't do that," Homer responded "Okay. Don't do that," meaning "Okay, I won't do that." In response to "Where are you going?" Homer replied "Where are you going is house," meaning "I'm going home." It may be that not only are the capacities of the second-language learner different from those of a child just beginning to acquire a first language, but the level of syntax used in the environment is also different. Since the L2 learner's cognitive behavior is obviously developed, there is no attempt to modify the input in the direction of simplification, as is often done with the L1 learner.

Simultaneous Acquisition of Two Languages

The process of learning two languages simultaneously is somewhat different from learning first one language and then a second. The common viewpoint has been that if two languages are learned at the same time, they should be learned from two distinct sources; otherwise children may have difficulties in language learning. This means that one language should be spoken to the child by one person and the other language by another person. Although there is some evidence supporting this point of view, it is not conclusive.

Studies have shown that children who are exposed to two languages (even from distinct sources) from infancy may use words from both languages without apparent awareness that they are speaking two distinct languages (Imedadze, 1978). However, as they begin making linguistic contrasts, they also begin to recognize separate patterns for two languages. Leopold (1954) considered bilingualism to be the separate learning of two sets of patterns. In the case of bilingualism, the patterns are both auditory-vocal codes. A child can, however, learn one code that is

Werner F. Leopold

Werner Leopold, a linguist, was an early innovator in the field of psycholinguistics in general and child language in particular. By his scientific studies and observations, he convinced American linguists that child language is a worthwhile and respectable field for research. His first volume of a four-volume landmark study, *Speech Development of a Bilingual Child,* appeared in 1939. This work was a precise and comprehensive description of the language learning process and of the emergence of two languages in his own child. His description included lexical, phonetic, syntactic, and semantic aspects of language. Leopold's diary method of reporting was later adopted by psycholinguists for studying child language. Although Leopold has published many scientific and theoretical papers, a second contribution that is of particular interest to the language specialist is his *Bibliography of Child Language,* published in 1952, which provides a comprehensive coverage of all published information on the topic. Leopold is Professor Emeritus of Linguistics and German, Northwestern University.

auditory-vocal and another that is manual. Learning two codes in itself should not normally present difficulty. In the simultaneous learning of two languages, Slobin (1973) found that forms in the two languages that symbolize the same meaning do not always appear at the same time, suggesting that the form for expression may be more complex in one language than in the other and therefore appears first in the less complex form (see Chapter 6).

Hatch (1978) observed that children acquiring two languages simultaneously separate them when communicating with different people during the second year of life. Imedadze (1978) reported similar results; phrases of mixed composition began to occur less and less often after the age of twenty months in the language of children exposed to two languages simultaneously. Dulay, Hernández-Chávez, and Burt (1978) concluded from a review of research that in all essential respects early simultaneous acquisition of two languages does not differ from acquisition of a single language. Imedadze (1978), however, rejected the idea that children consciously select a language for a specific listener. She explained the alternative autonomous functioning of two languages by the concept of *set,* which stipulates that the occurrence of a specific speech act (in either language) requires a need for communication and a situation in which it may be gratified, as well as the availability of means or instruments of communication. The bilingual child evolves two distinctive sets, which are functionally autonomous and alternatively actualized. Gumperz and Hernández-Chávez (1975) suggested that code selection is related to learned associations between particular speech varieties and the social environment. This may account for the child's ability to consistently address one person in one language and another person in another language.

It appears that simultaneous learning of two languages does not in itself pose problems for a child. If, however, the models and the time of exposure for one or both languages are inadequate, or if the child has a language disorder, a child may not reach optimum competence in either or both languages.

This anecdote illustrates the wisdom of young Mario, a Spanish-speaking child who knew little English. When he met a small English-speaking girl his own age, he selected the appropriate code—however meaningless—to establish communication with her.

After trying to get her attention with facial expressions, Mario spoke to her in his limited English. He was able to say only "Hey! Look! Watch! Here! Come!" and "Water!" (pointing to a nearby fountain). He judiciously avoided Spanish, limiting himself to only those linguistic items appropriate for use with the little girl (Fantini, 1974, p. 66).

Sequential Learning of Two Languages

Processes involved in learning two languages are different when one language is learned prior to the second one. In this situation, the data studied concern the effects of the first language on learning the second and the interference of the linguistic forms of the first on the second.

Influence of L1 on L2.   There is no unanimity of opinion regarding the effect of prior knowledge of one language on the acquisition of a second language. Wode (1978) proposed that L2 children do rely on prior knowledge of L1. He stated that both languages are acquired using the same set of principles but different surface forms. Furthermore, prior cognitive development leads to different strategies. Corder (1969b) stated that the cognitive development needed for learning a second language is quite different from that needed for the first.

Ravem (1978) not only concurred, but also indicated that there is active use of L1 knowledge in the acquisition of L2, and that this knowledge transfer is one of the learning processing strategies. He concluded that the more similar the linguistic means of expressing semantic notions in the two languages, the more directly will competency in the first language facilitate learning the second. For instance, in learning a second lan-

The listener who knows only one language finds all foreign languages equally strange sounding, yet linguists have discovered that languages may be grouped into "families" that are related to each other in basic ways. The largest and most completely studied language family is called Indo-European. Indo-European languages are spoken in most of Europe, North and South America, northern India, and Russia. Exceptions to this are Basque, Finnish, and Hungarian in Europe and the Native Indian languages in the Americas. The Indo-European languages are further divided into the Slavic languages (such as Russian and Bulgarian), the Romance languages (such as Spanish and French), and the Germanic languages (such as English). A comparison of the names assigned to the digits 1, 2, and 3 suggests some of the similarities and differences in vocabulary between Indo-European and Non-Indo-European languages (Fromkin & Rodman, 1974, pp. 236–240).

Indo-European				Non-Indo-European
Germanic		Romance		
English	German	Spanish	French	Pima (American Indian)
one	eins	uno	un	hermako
two	zwei	dos	deux	gohk
three	drei	tres	trois	waik

guage, the child he studied did not use telegraphese in the same way as do first-language learners. As this child began using English, she transferred both content words and functors from Norwegian, giving them an English stress and rhythm pattern.

Examples: Du skal have this one (You shall . . .) Vil du have coffee (Will you . . .)

As stated previously, the opposite view stipulates that the L2 learner uses the same strategies as used in learning L1 and will make the same transitional errors. Similarities between the sentence forms produced and understood by monolingual children and children learning a second language (Ervin-Tripp, 1974) provide evidence that second-language learners not only use the same strategies but also make the same transitional errors as in learning the first language. This implies that having learned one language neither helps or hinders second-language acquisition.

Interference. The issue of interference concerns intrusion of the semantic and syntactic forms of the first language on the second. The question of the presence of interference in second-language learning has not been definitively resolved in either direction. Dulay and Burt (1974) claimed that interference is virtually nonexistent in second-language learning by children. Supporters of the interference theory claimed that not only is there language interference from L1 to L2, but that it also is possible to predict the errors that the speakers of a specific second language will make after having learned a specific first language, by analyzing and contrasting the forms of both languages. This issue cannot be resolved by accepting either extreme. There is evidence to support the position that some errors of second-language learners are patterned on forms in the first language. Examples of errors made by French and Spanish subjects acquiring English were given by Chamot (1978) to illustrate transference of French and Spanish forms into English: *in* bed for *to* bed, *in* the school for *at* school, *in* TV for *on* TV. Chamot explained this incorrect preposition usage on the basis that semantic areas covered by English prepositions do not correspond entirely to their Spanish or French equivalents. Examples of other "errors" that are not found in the developmental stages of monolingual children, and that were similar to the L1 Spanish forms, were the relative clause word order "I don't know what is it" for "it is" and the omission of the pronoun *it* in "it is here."

In a study of English expressive language functions of Mexican-American children whose primary language was English, Carrow (1972a) found that their performance on expressive language tasks, although somewhat delayed with respect to age of mastery, was grossly similar to that followed by native speakers of English. Within the samples of language obtained, however,

LANGUAGE DISORDERS AND BILINGUALISM

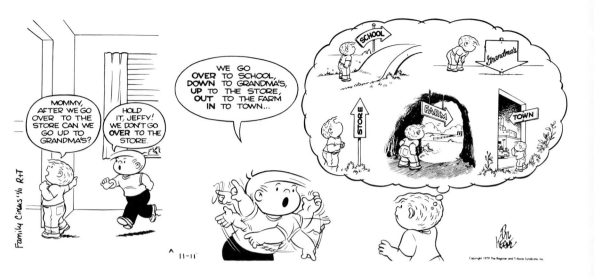

there were specific areas in both phonemic and structural aspects of language in which the development seemed atypical, suggesting the presence of linguistic intrusion from Spanish to English. The "interference" tended to decrease with age and was totally absent in some of the children. None of the subjects exhibited the full-blown system of variations often found in the English of adult native speakers of Spanish who are learning English.

It has been verified by research and observation that certain patterns in the phonology, syntax, and lexicon of L2 learners are reminiscent of L1. Are these 'errors' due to interference? The term interference implies that the first language keeps the individual from learning the second language accurately. There are, however, other explanations for this phenomenon, one of which suggests that the second-language learner has more to say than his abilities in the second language allow him to express. The learner may then employ L1 syntax or construction rules for utterances in L2, or he may overgeneralize the semantic aspect of forms in L2 that are similar to those in L1. In many instances, this procedure is part of the L2 developmental process, and the borrowed patterns disappear when the appropriate second-language patterns are acquired.

Since the environment in which the second-language learner functions on a day-to-day basis is not that of the second language, the learning contexts may be aberrant in both function and frequency of structure (Ervin-Tripp, 1974). Therefore, some of the borrowed patterns become "fossilized" and remain in the second language.

These fossilized language patterns, which are often referred to as residual foreign dialect, may influence language in a histor-

Prepositions are complicated even for the native speaker of a language. (The Family Circus by Bil Keane, reprinted courtesy of The Register and Tribune Syndicate, Inc.)

ic sense. Once a mixed pattern becomes fossilized, it becomes a model for future learners in that community. When all or parts of the mixed patterns are passed on from generation to generation, the resulting language spoken becomes a dialect. Psychological and social community cohesiveness contributes to the perpetuation of dialect. If the social community is large and the minority language therefore strong, fossilization is more likely. Children within such a community will be less likely to learn the second language without also learning such fossilized errors of transition.

Social Aspects of Bilingualism

Specific dialects used by speakers of second languages (e.g., the English of Mexican-Americans) may be preserved for other reasons. A dialect may serve to separate ethnic groups from one another—the insiders from the outsiders. Frequently, bilinguals living in a cohesive ethnic community will use the community dialect to speak to the insiders and the language of the outsiders to speak with those not in the community. The dialect becomes the symbol of the ethnic group and its culture, and thus produces and preserves group cohesiveness (Barker, 1975a). There is understandable resistance to changing the dialect to conform to the larger society. Criticism of the dialect becomes criticism of the ethnic group and its values.

Schumann (1969, 1976) stated that the difficulty experienced by a member of an ethnic group in acquiring the language of a larger group is related proportionately to the social distance between the groups. The social distance is defined by (1) the political, cultural, technical, and economic superiority of the dominant group; (2) the size of the ethnic group; (3) the attitudes of the groups toward each other—ethnic stereotypes, etc.; (4) the degree to which the cultures are similar; and (5) the intended length of residence of the member of the ethnic group. Schuman believes that social and psychological forces cause persistence of what he calls "pidginization" (simplified and reduced forms of speech used for communication between people with different languages).

Educational Aspects of Bilingualism

For decades there has been strong feeling in educational circles regarding the detrimental effects of being bilingual. Detrimental effects have been imputed in the areas of intelligence, language, emotional adjustment, and economic and social well-being. Current viewpoints explain the seemingly detrimental effects of bilingualism in a manner that removes the blame for these effects from the bilingualism itself and places it instead on the methods and interpretations used to study behavior of the bilingual child.

In general, bilingual children, as compared with monolingual children of the same age and social status using nonlanguage tests of intelligence, have not been found to be retarded *or* accelerated in their mental development. When verbal tests of intelligence are used for comparison, studies have shown that the bilinguals generally do not reach the level of monolinguals; this discrepancy decreases with age. Few studies have taken into consideration the degree and type of bilingualism.

Some bilinguals have been found to be less proficient in certain aspects of language than monolingual children of the same age, most frequently in understanding and speaking vocabulary and in articulation. This has been blamed on the type of bilingual environment and models as well as socioeconomic factors that have affected the milieu for learning. Young learners of a second language usually begin L2 before L1 has been completely mastered. Development of both languages may then be delayed with respect to monolinguals of the same age, the first language because learning may slow down when the second language is introduced. The differences in proficiency decrease with age as the subject's ability in the second language improves (Carrow, 1971, 1972a).

It is important, then, not to make generalizations about bilingualism or the bilingual child for the purposes of educational placement and intervention. Each child must be viewed independently, and his ability and language skills studied from the framework of his social community, linguistic environment, and level of competence in both languages. He cannot be compared with others unless they are similar in these aspects. In this way, it is possible to identify bilingual children who have language disorders.

BILINGUALISM AND THE DIMENSIONS OF LANGUAGE

A look at bilingualism in terms of the four dimensional approach illustrates the differences between the bilingual and monolingual speaker. As is shown in Figure 19-1, the cognitive and performance areas are essentially the same for bilingual and monolingual speakers. However, the linguistic structure and the communications environment dimensions differ for the bilingual individual, who must learn two sets of rules in each of the oral linguistic structure categories as well as two sets of relations between the phonemic and graphemic systems, for although many of the letters are common to numerous languages, the association between the sounds and letters is not. The communication system of the bilingual may also be different from that of the monolingual, because the bilingual interacts not only with two codes but also (often) with two cultural and social groups. The functions of language may differ in different cultural and social groups, and the response and feedback to the language of a bilingual may not be the same as for a monolingual speaker, particularly if the bilingual has not mastered the dialect being spoken.

In addition to the problems inherent in bilingualism alone, the bilingual language-disordered child must attempt to master two codes with a language-learning system that is ineffective even for one. The patterns of language disorder are the same for the bilingual child as for a monolingual child, with the exception that the semantic/syntactic units may exhibit a confusion arising from attempts to associate concepts with two codes.

The reciprocal relationship between cognition and the elements of the linguistic code is somewhat modified in bilingualism. On one hand, a second lexicon and a second grammar may convey different nuances of meaning, which in turn communicate images and concepts that may not be available in the first

Figure 19-1
Model illustrating two codes in the dimension of language knowledge, the dimension that distinguishes the bilingual from the monolingual speaker.

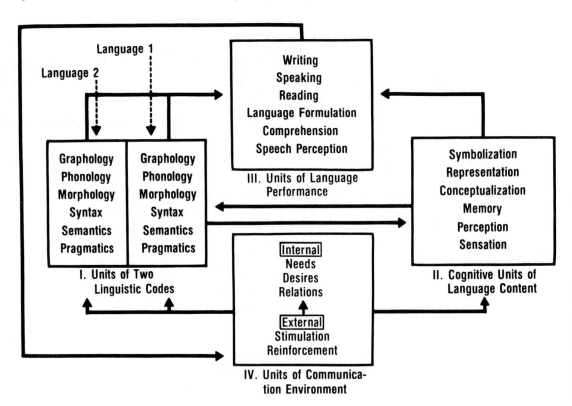

Zimbardo and Ruch (1977, p. 142) provided a transcript of an experimental session in hypnosis research with a student who could neither speak nor understand Spanish but who spent several years in Mexico as a child. Consider the implications of this report for language learning, memory, and bilingualism:

Hypnotist: You are going back in time, getting younger and younger until once again you are five years old. . . . you are at your own birthday party.

Chuck: Que linda! Que torta mas grande y tantas velas! Hay uno, dos, tres, cuatro, cinco, y uno mas para darme mi deseo especial.

language. The bilingual person has the richness of meaning of both languages, but must learn two codes for the same meanings. Although this may appear to be a difficult task, learning a second or even third code does not usually present problems for the typical child who has adequate bilingual models.

LANGUAGE DISORDERS AND BILINGUALISM

There are bilingual children who have disorders of language not because of their bilingualism but because they are subject to the same factors that cause language disorders in the monolingual child. The language differences may be part of an overall developmental delay, or may be a specific disorder of the language acquisition or language behavioral processes. The procedure whereby one sorts out the nature of the problem so that appropriate educational management steps can be taken is complicated by the presence of bilingualism. As has been discussed, bilingualism is not a simple, unitary phenomenon; it is complex and variable, and the type and degree of bilingualism of a child is as unique as the child.

Identification of the Language-Disordered Bilingual Child

In educational settings where there are many bilingual children, it is relatively easy to select those having special difficulty in learning language, particularly a second language, because they will learn language differently than the other bilingual children. Where there are few bilingual children, it is harder to identify factors that may be functions of learning two languages and those that are due to language disorders. The identification of a language disorder in a bilingual child must take into account the following: (1) competencies of the child in both languages; (2) the semantic, grammatic, and pragmatic differences between the two languages under consideration; (3) the linguistic and social environments; and (4) contributing cognitive factors.

Determination of Competency in Two Languages

In making judgments about the presence or absence of a language disorder in a bilingual child, the language specialist needs to evaluate the child's competency in both languages. In the case of a Mexican-American child, for example, both Spanish and English abilities in comprehension and production must be assessed. Spanish may be the child's native language but not the dominant language. There are Mexican-American children who neither speak nor understand Spanish. On the other hand, the child may have considerable proficiency in Spanish when he begins to learn English and, consequently, the development of English seems to be, and in fact is, delayed when compared to monolingual English speakers. This delay, however, may only indicate that the child is progressing through the normal developmental stages at a later age than the monolingual child.

Analysis of Language Differences

The sampling procedures used for determining whether the language of a bilingual child is disordered are similar to procedures used to study monolingual children except that for the bilingual child, both languages must be tested. The interpretation of the findings of the procedures are different, however. The various sources of linguistic error must be determined so that areas of disorder may be identified. If language difference alone is used as a criterion for language disorder, then a large proportion of bilingual children would be inappropriately labeled language-disordered. The differences in the phonology, morphology, syntax, and semantics from the adult form of both languages must be viewed in part from the standpoint of the typical differences related to normal developmental stages of language and in part to those differences that are typical of the development of a second language. The errors may be developmental, transitional, dialectal, due to language interference, or in the case of the language-disordered child, specific to the disorder.

The developmental stages of first-language learners are relatively uniform with respect to linguistic behavior. Linguistic structures at the various developmental stages are similar among children but differ from the adult models. These developmental characteristics are found in the language of bilingual children also, and comprise the bulk of their identified "errors." The most important factors causing developmental differences from the adult language are (1) omission of major constituents; (2) omission of morphemes; (3) overgeneralization; and (4) misordering. While these errors reflect incomplete language acquisition, it is important to remember that the child learns quickly, and therefore approximations to adult forms become closer and closer to the target, reaching it in a relatively short period of time.

Certain characteristics in the acquisition of language are atypical of the L1 learner but typical of the L2 learner. During the learning stages, the L2 learner may use forms, structures, or lexicons from the first language to "substitute" for forms in the second language that he has not yet learned. He does this because of the inadequacy of his L2 forms for expressing complex ideas. If the learning process is continuous, these errors are transitional and will disappear from the language as the learner masters L2. For the same reason, an L2 learner may overgeneralize the semantic features identified with a word; this is particularly noticeable with prepositions. When prepositions are phonemically similar, the semantic confusion is magnified. Until a L2 learner learns which semantic features are associated with the specific lexicon and which are not, he will overgeneralize from L1 and use features of L1 in L2. Overgeneralization is often a transitional error and, if the learning is continuous, forms will gradually be associated with the correct semantic features.

Other than the common forms that are part of a regional or local dialect, there is usually no consistent pattern of errors found in bilingual children—even those who have a common first language. Child A may have one type of residual pattern or single error, child B may have another, and child C may have no residual at all, although they may all come from the same environment.

Prior to the determination of a language disorder in a bilingual child, the language specialist must identify and rule out (1) the developmental linguistic patterns that are typical of the language development; (2) the transitional linguistic patterns that are typical of the L2 learners—those patterns that are characteristic of individuals of one particular language acquiring a particular second language; (3) the dialectal patterns that have been fossilized in a community; (4) the patterns that are individually fossilized by the child; and (5) the linguistic patterns or errors that arise from emotional stress or fatigue. Once the above factors are identified, the language specialist is in a position to examine other factors that may be due to the disorder.

Linguistic and Social Environment

The adult form of the language against which the child's structure is judged must be that of the particular dialect of the language spoken in the community to which the child belongs. The language specialist must be conversant with the dialectal forms of the target language spoken in the child's community.

The judgment of the linguistic competence of a bilingual child must also be evaluated against the language models—of both the first and second languages. If the language models contain many fossilized errors, the child's language will reflect these. It is also important to ascertain the child's attitudes toward both L1 and L2. Frequently, a child is reluctant to demonstrate knowledge of either the first or the second language due to the social forces in his environment that penalize the use of one or the other.

Contributing Cognitive Factors

Since intelligence correlates so highly with language, it is also necessary to assess cognitive functioning in the bilingual child. As with the language-disordered monolingual child, the most valid method of evaluating intellectual ability in the bilingual is nonverbal. Once cognitive levels are established, language levels in both L1 and L2 can be evaluated with reference to intelligence.

ASSESSMENT   The procedures for evaluating the language of a bilingual child based on spontaneous speech samples are similar to those used with a monolingual speaker. The factors involved in the evaluation of the results of the linguistic analysis of the child have already been reviewed. However, because of the complexity of identifying language disorders in the bilingual child, it is frequently necessary to obtain additional information about his linguistic performance as compared to his peers. It may therefore be helpful to use standardized tests in addition to the more naturalistic approaches. If the examiner does not know both languages of the bilingual child, she may find test administration a better means of language analysis than spontaneous speech samples. Some tests require minimal knowledge of the language for administration and scoring, particularly if a native speaker of the language is used to provide the test stimuli. However, the use of the norms of standardized tests with bilingual children may present validity problems.

Collecting normative data for language tests of monolingual children is a difficult procedure—one that limits the applicability of the results obtained. Norming an instrument for use with bilingual children is considerably more complex, considering the complexity of bilingualism. Norms should reflect the population to which they will be applied. How is a linguistically homogenous population of bilinguals identified for use in norming a language test? If the norms are not obtained from a linguistically homogeneous population or stratified according to degrees and types of bilingualism, what information will they provide? Take, for example, a test of English or Spanish syntax standardized on a representative sample of Hispanics—Cubans, Puerto Ricans, and Mexican-Americans—at various levels of proficiency in English. This population may include children who are just beginning to learn English as well as those who speak it exclusively, and their Spanish proficiency may encompass the same distribution of ability. The combinations of abilities in both languages are infinite. In this population, what does a "mean" performance in either language at any age indicate? The standard deviation would be so large as to make meaningful comparisons impossible. Thus, the only valid method of standardizing such instruments is to provide norms for speakers who have reached a relatively homogeneous level of proficiency for their age.

Another problem in standardizing measures of language concerns the differences in the semantics of forms, particularly of vocabulary, among the dialects. This problem exists with any test of language but is magnified in populations with a variety of heterogeneous and semi-isolated dialects of the same language. It is difficult to select words for test instruments that are commonly used by children and that are universally acceptable by speakers of all dialects of a language. The choice of specific words might penalize speakers of one dialect. If the words in a test are changed to conform to local dialectal usage, the relative difficulty of the test instrument is changed also, making comparison with norms invalid.

A method suggested by Carrow-Woolfolk (1978) to provide valid data for the comparison of the language status of bilingual children is to develop local norms. This can be done easily by selecting about fifty children at specific age levels who represent the language of the community and the range of linguistic abilities within the age group. (Children whose parents have recently entered the community should not be used.) Mean scores and standard deviations computed at each age level will provide a base for comparing children from the same linguistic and community background. A child can then be evaluated against the framework of children of his own linguistic community.

INTERVENTION

Procedures used in language intervention with bilingual children are similar to those used with monolingual children. With a bilingual child, however, it is necessary to decide what language or languages to use in intervention. If a child has a severe language disorder or is developmentally slow in general, being taught in two languages will exacerbate the confusion. The severely disordered child should be taught one language only, and the language of the home and school should be the same whenever possible. For children with moderate language disorders, a single language should be used for instruction, but the language of the home may differ. Usually, the language chosen for instruction should be that of the majority in the locality, the language in which the child will ultimately work. Use of a single language for instruction eliminates the complexity of acquiring two codes for learning and expressing the concepts of the school. For instance, children would speak Spanish in the home, but would be taught only English in school.

Children who have no language disorder and who are within normal intellectual levels can learn and be taught in two languages in schools that have sufficient numbers of children of the same first language to warrant bilingual education. The decision to be made in this situation is which of the many dialects of the two languages should be taught in the school. The answer to this question is not simple. On one hand, the dialect of the local community is a bona fide language and should be treated as such. Dialectical usage should be acceptable in oral communication for discussing problems related to subject matter in, e.g., history and math. Children should not be "corrected" for these dialectal differences. At the same time, these children need to know the language of the majority because it is possibly in the larger community that they will earn a living. Therefore, the language of the majority should be taught in speech, English, and Spanish classes, with the condition that it is considered an alternate way of communicating—not necessarily a better way. The Hispanic children may need to learn, then, four codes or dialects: two in Spanish and two in English.

The above approach is defended by Gonzalez (1973, pp. 224): "While I accept the position that one dialect is just as linguistically valid as another, I submit that dialects do not operate in a social vacuum. Their effectiveness rests, not in that one is as valid as the other, but in using each dialect in its proper social context." He also said that while the child's Spanish should not be ridiculed, he should also be exposed to other varieties of language, including Standard Spanish.

RESPONSIBILITIES OF THE LANGUAGE SPECIALIST

Effective decisions relating to the linguistic aspects of bilingualism, particularly those made with the language-disordered bilingual, ideally should be made by a language specialist who speaks both languages and is familiar with dialect. If this is not possible, the clinician should try to utilize members in the community to assist in assessing the problems of the children. Misconceptions about bilingualism and the bilingual child have been prevalent in the schools of the United States, and consequently bilingual children have not always received the education that is best for them. The language pathologist can aid other specialists in the understanding of the linguistic issues in bilingualism and assist in making appropriate placement decisions.

appendices

appendix a: rules for calculating
MLU

An utterance is not always easy to define because it may, or may not, be a sentence in the grammatical sense. An utterance can be defined as a verbalization or a verbal string whose boundary is marked by inflection—either rising or falling. A sentence is an utterance with structured grammatical relationship between the elements.

$$\text{The mean length of utterance} = \frac{\text{Total number of morphemes or words}}{\text{Total number of utterances}}$$

Brown (1973) provided rules for calculating the MLU and his rules are based upon the use of morphemes not words. Brown's rules may be summarized as follows.

Rules for Calculating MLU (Morphemes)

1. Count as one morpheme all compound words *(pocketbook, choo-choo, night-night)*; all diminutives *(doggie, mommy)*; all irregular past tenses *(got, did, want, saw)*.
2. Count as separate morphemes all auxilliary verbs and *gonna, wanna,* and *hafta.* Also count as separate morphemes the plural, possessive, third person singular /s/, past, and progressive.
3. Do not count fillers (uh, umm).

Although they are less frequently used, there are also rules for calculating the MLU using words (McLean & McLean, 1978).

Rules for Calculating MLU (Words)

1. Count all single words. Include in this count all inflected and compound words. Count as single words connected words such as "Winnie the Pooh."
2. Do not count fillers (umm, uh).

appendix b: suggestions for interpreting semantic intentions

The following devices have been gathered from various longitudinal studies of language development.

1. Encourage expansion by the adult. If the child says "ice/mommy" and the parent expands "Is that mommy's ice?" the semantic relation is clarified.
2. Observe the child's acceptance or nonacceptance of the adult's expansion.
3. Give great credence to the interpretation made by an adult familiar with child.
4. Assume that the child's gesture indicates an important element of the communication. Always record gestures.
5. Observe the child's vocal stress because stress may clarify the intended meaning. New and important information in an utterance tends to be stressed.
6. Observe the child's word order; there is a tendency for the child to follow adult word order even in two-word utterances.
7. Consider that the productivity of forms may contribute to establishing correct reference. If a child consistently uses *hat* to indicate something worn on the head and then says *daddy* while pointing to his father's hat, it may be presumed that since *hat* has been used productively this occurrence of *daddy* suggests possession.

references

Adler, S (1976): The influence of genetic syndromes upon oral communication skills. *J Speech Hear Disord* 41:136–138

Alajouanine T, Lhermitte F (1965): Acquired aphasia in children. *Brain* 88:654–662

Alpert C (1980): Procedures for determining the optimal nonspeech mode with the autistic child. In Schiefelbusch (Ed): *Nonspeech Language and Communication: Analysis and Intervention.* Baltimore: University Park Press, pp 391–420

American College Dictionary (1963). New York: Random House

Annett M (1973): Laterality of childhood hemiplegia and growth of speech and intelligence. *Cortex* 9:4–33

Anthony EJ (1970): The behavior disorders of childhood. In Mussen P (Ed): *Manual of Child Psychology* (ed 3). New York: John Wiley & Sons, pp 667–764

Apgar V, Beck J (1972): *Is My Baby All Right? A Guide to Birth Defects.* New York: Trident Press

Aram DM, Nation JE (1975): Patterns of language behavior in children with developmental language disorders. *J Speech Hear Res* 18:229–241, 1975

Argyle M, Cook M (1976): *Gaze and Mutual Gaze.* Cambridge: Cambridge University Press

Asch SE (1968): The doctrinal tyranny of associationism: Or what is wrong with rote learning. In Dixon TR, Horton DL (Eds): *Verbal Behavior and General Behavior Theory.* Englewood Cliffs: Prentice-Hall, pp 214–228

Asher J (1972): Children's first language as a model for second language-learning. *Mod Lang J* 56:133–138

Asp CW (1975): Measurement of aural speech perception and oral speech production of the hearing impaired. In Singh S (Ed): *Measurement Procedures in Speech, Hearing and Language.* Baltimore: University Park Press, pp 191–218

Aten J, Davis J (1968): Disturbances in the perception of auditory sequences in children with minimal cerebral dysfunction. *J Speech Hear Res* 11:236–245

Austin JL (1962): *How to Do Things with Words.* Cambridge: Harvard University Press

Axline V (1976): Play therapy procedures and results. In Schaefer CE (Ed): *Therapeutic Use of Child's Play.* New York: Jason Aronson

Babbidge HS (1965): Education of the deaf. A Report to the Secretary of HEW by his Advisory Committee on Education of the Deaf. U.S. Government Printing Office 0–765–119

Bailey N, Madden C, Krashen SD (1974): Is there a "natural sequence" in adult second language learning? *Language Learning* 24:235–243

Baltaxe C (1977): Pragmatic deficits in the language of autistic adolescents. *Pediatr Psychol* 2(4):176–180

Baltaxe, C, Simmons J (1975): Language in childhood psychosis: A review. *J Speech Hear Disord* 40:439–458

Bandura A (1971): *Psychological Modeling.* Chicago: Aldine-Atherton

Bangs JL (1942): A clinical analysis of the articulatory defects of the feebleminded. *J Speech Hear Disord* 7:343–356

Bangs TE (1961): Evaluating children with language delay. *J Speech Hear Disord* 26:16–18

Bangs TE (1968): *Language and Learning Disorders of the Pre-Academic Child.* New York: Appleton-Century-Crofts

Bangs TE (1979): *Birth–Three Developmental Scale.* Hingham, Mass.: Teaching Resources

Bankson N (1977): *Bankson Language Screening Test.* Baltimore: University Park Press

Barker GC (1975): Social functions of language in a Mexican-American community. In Hernandez-Chavez E, Cohen AD, Beltramo AF (Eds): *El Lenguaje de los Chicanos.* Arlington, Va: Center for Applied Linguistics, pp 170–182

Barry H (1962): *The Young Aphasic Child.* Washington, DC: Alexander Graham Bell Assoc for the Deaf

Bartak L, Rutter M (1975): Language and cognition in autistic and "dysphasic" children. In O'Connor N (Ed): *Language Cognitive Deficits and Retardation.* Wolburn, Mass: Buttersworth, pp 193–202

Bartak L, Rutter M (1976): Differences between mentally retarded and normally intelligent autistic children. *J Aut Child Schizo* 6:109–120

Basser, LS (1962): Hemiplegia of early onset and the faculty of speech with special reference to the effect of hemispherectomy. *Brain* 85:427–460

Bates E (1975): Peer relations and the acquisition of language. In Lewis M, Rosenblum LA (Eds): *Friendship and Peer Relations: The Origins of Behavior,* vol 4. New York: John Wiley & Sons

Bates E (1976a): *Language and Context: The Acquisition of Pragmatics.* New York: Academic Press

Bates E (1976b): Pragmatics and sociolinguistics. In Morehead DM, Morehead AE (Eds): *Normal and Deficient Child Language.* Baltimore: University Park Press, pp 411–463

Bates E, Benigni L, Bretherton I, Camaioni L, Volterra V (1977): From gesture to the first word: On cognitive and social prerequisites. In Lewis M, Rosenblum L (Eds): *Interaction, Conversation, and the Development of Language.* New York: John Wiley & Sons, pp 247–308

Bates E, Camaioni L, Volterra V (1975): The acquisition of performatives prior to speech. *Merrill-Palmer Quarterly,* pp 205–226

Bateson MC (1975): Mother–infant exchanges: The epigenesis of conversational interaction. In Aaronson D, Rieber RW (Eds): *Developmental Psycholinguistics and Communication Disorders.* New York: New York Academy of Sciences, Annals of the New York Academy of Sciences, vol 263, pp 101–113

Bayley N (1968): *Bayley Scales of Infant Development.* New York: Psychological Corporation

Bedrosian JL, Prutting C (1978): Communication performance of mentally retarded adults in four conversational settings. *J Speech Hear Res* 21:79–95

Bellugi U (1971): Simplification in children's language. In Huxley R, Ingram E (Eds): *Language Acquisition: Models and Methods.* New York: Academic Press, pp 95–119

Bellugi U, Klima ES (1972): The roots of language in the sign talk of the deaf. *Psychology Today* 6:59–64

Bellugi U, Klima ES (1978): Structural properties of American sign language. In Liben LS (Ed): *Deaf Children: Developmental Perspectives.* New York: Academic Press, pp 43–68

Bellugi-Klima U (1969): Language Acquisition. Paper prepared for symposium on "Cognitive Studies and Artificial Intelligence Research," University of Chicago Center for Continuing Education

Benda CE (1960): *Mongolism and Cretinism.* New York: Grune & Stratton

Bender L (1942): Childhood schizophrenia. *New Child I,* pp 138–140

Bender L (1947): Childhood schizophrenia: Clinical study of 100 schizophrenic children. *Am J Orthopsychiatry* 17:40–56

Benedict H (1978): Language comprehension in 9–15 month old children. In Campbell R, Smith P (Eds): *Recent Advances in the Psychology of Language: Language Development and Mother–Child Interaction.* The Hague: Mouton, pp 57–69

Bensberg G, Sigelman C (1976): Definitions and prevalence. In Lloyd L (Ed): *Communication Assessment and Intervention Strategies.* Baltimore: University Park Press, pp 33–72

Benton A (1978): The cognitive functioning of children with developmental dysphasia. In Wyke MA (Ed): *Developmental Dysphasia.* New York: Academic Press, pp 43–62

Bereiter C, Engelmann S (1966): *Teaching Disadvantaged Children in the Preschool.* Englewood Cliffs: Prentice-Hall

Bergstrom L, Hemenway WG, Downs MP (1971): A high risk registry to find congenital deafness. *Otolaryngol Clin North Am* 4:369–399

Berko J (1958): The child's learning of English morphology. *Word* 14:150–177

Berko Gleason J (1973): Code switching in children's language. In Moore TE (Ed): *Cognitive Development and the Acquisition of Language.* New York: Academic Press

Berko Gleason J, Weintraub S (1978): Input language and the acquisition of communicative competence. In Nelson KE (Ed): *Children's Language,* vol 1. New York: Gardner Press, pp 171–222

Bernstein B (1970): A sociolinguistic approach to socialization: with some reference to educability. In Williams F (Ed): *Language and Poverty: Perspectives on a Theme.* Chicago: Markham, pp 25–61

Berry P, Marshall B (1978): Social interaction and communication patterns in mentally retarded children. *Am J Ment Defic* 83:44–51

Bettelheim B (1967): *The Empty Fortress: Infantile Autism and the Birth of Self.* New York: Free Press

Bever TG (1968): Associations to stimulus–response theories of language. In Dixon TR, Horton DL (Eds): *Verbal Behavior and General Behavior Theory.* Englewood Cliffs: Prentice-Hall, pp 478–495

Bever TG (1970): The cognitive basis for linguistic structures. In Hayes JR (Ed): *Cognition and the Development of Language.* New York: John Wiley & Sons, pp 279–353

Birdwhistle RL (1970): *Kinesics and Context.* Philadelphia: University of Pennsylvania Press

Black JW (1971): Speech pathology for the deaf. In Connor LE (Ed): *Speech for the Deaf Child: Knowledge and Use.* Washington, DC: Alexander Graham Bell Assoc for the Deaf, pp 154–169

Black JW, Moore WE (1955): *Speech: Code, Meaning, and Communication.* New York: McGraw-Hill

Black P, Shepard R, Walker E (1975): Outcome of head trauma: Age and post traumatic seizures. In *Outcome of Severe Damage to the Central Nervous System.* New York: Ciba Foundation Symposium, pp 215–226

Blager FB (1980): Speech and language development of Down's syndrome children. *Seminars in Speech, Language, and Hearing* 1:63–72

Blanchard I (1964): Speech patterns and etiology in mental retardation. *Am J Ment Defic* 68:612–617

Blank M (1978): Review of "Toward an understanding of dyslexia: psychological factors in specific reading disability." In Benton AL, Pearl D (Eds): *Dyslexia, An Appraisal of Current Knowledge.* New York: Oxford University Press, pp 113–122

Blank-Greif E, Berko Gleason J (1980): Hi, thanks, and goodbye: More routine information. *Language in Society* 9:159–166

Bliss L, Allen D, Walker G (1978): Sentence structures of trainable and educable mentally retarded subjects. *J Speech Hear Res* 21:722–731

Bloom L (1970): *Language Development: Form and Function in Emerging Grammars.* Cambridge, Mass: MIT Press

Bloom L (1971): Why not pivot grammar? *J Speech Hear Disord* 36:40–50

Bloom L (1973): In *One Word at a Time: The Use of Single-word Utterances before Syntax.* The Hague: Mouton

Bloom L (1974): Talking, understanding, and thinking. In Schiefelbusch RL, Lloyd LL (Eds): *Language Perspectives—Acquisition, Retardation, and Intervention.* Baltimore: University Park Press, pp 285–313

Bloom L, Hood L, Lightbown P (1974): Imitation in language development: If, when and why. *Cognitive Psychology* 6:380–420

Bloom L, Lahey M (1978): *Language Development and Language Disorders.* New York: John Wiley & Sons

Bloom L, Lahey M, Hood L, Lifter K, Fiess K (1980): Complex sentences: Acquisition of syntactic connectives and the semantic relations they encode. *J Child Lang* 7:235–261

Bloom L, Lifter K, Hafitz J (1980): Semantics of verbs and the development of verb inflection in child language. *Language* 56:386–412

Bloom L, Lightbown P, Hood L (1975): Structure and variation in child language. *Monographs of the Society for Research in Child Development.* Chicago: University of Chicago Press, serial 160, 40:2

Bloom L, Miller P, Hood L (1975): Variation and reduction as aspects of competence in language development. In Pick A (Ed): *Minnesota Symposia on Child Psychology,* vol 9. Minneapolis: University of Minnesota Press

Bloom L, Rocissano L, Hood L (1976): Adult–child discourse: developmental interaction between information processing and linguistic knowledge. *Cognitive Psychology* 8:521–552

Bloomfield L (1933): *Language.* New York, Henry Holt

Bloomfield L (1964): Literate and illiterate speech. In Hymes D (Ed): *Language in Culture and Society.* New York: Harper & Row, pp 391–396

Bloor D (1977): The regulatory function of language. In Morton J, Marshall J (Eds): *Psycholinguistics: Developmental and Pathological.* Ithaca, New York: Cornell University Press, pp 73–97

Boas F (1911): *Handbook of American Indian Languages.* Washington, DC: Smithsonian Institution

Boehm AE (1971): *Boehm Test of Basic Concepts Manual.* New York: Psychological Corporation

Bonvillian JD, Nelson KE (1976): Sign language acquisition in a mute autistic boy. *J Speech Hear Disord* 41:339–347

Boomer DS, Laver JDM (1973): Slips of the tongue. In Fromkin V (Ed): *Speech Errors as Linguistic Evidence.* The Hague: Mouton, pp 120–131

Bowen JD (1975): Adaptation of English borrowing. In Hernandez-Chavez E, Cohen AD, Beltramo AF (Eds): *El Lenguaje de los Chicanos.* Arlington, Va: Center for Applied Linguistics, pp 115–122

Bowerman M (1973a): *Early syntactic development: A cross-linguistic study with special reference to Finnish.* Cambridge: Cambridge University Press

Bowerman M (1973b): Structural relationships in children's utterances: Syntactic or semantic? In Moore T (Ed): *Cognitive Development and the Acquisition of Language.* New York: Academic Press, pp 197–214

Bowerman M (1976): Semantic factors in the acquisition of rules for word use and sentence construction. In Morehead DM, Morehead AE (Eds): *Normal and Deficient Child Language.* Baltimore: University Park Press, pp 99–181

Bowerman M (1978a): Semantic and syntactic development: A review of what, when, and how in language acquisition. In Schiefelbusch RL (Ed): *Bases of Language Intervention.* Baltimore: University Park Press, pp 97–189

Bowerman M (1978b): Words and sentences: Uniformity, individual variation, and shifts over time in patterns of acquisition. In Minifie FD, Lloyd LL (Eds): *Communicative and Cognitive Abilities—Early Behavioral Assessment.* Baltimore: University Park Press, pp 349–397

Bowerman M (1978c): The acquisition of word meaning: An investigation into some current conflict. In Waterson N, Snow C (Eds): *The Development of Communication.* New York: John Wiley & Sons, pp 263–287

Bradley C (1941): *Schizophrenia in Childhood.* New York: Macmillan

Braine MDS (1963): The ontogeny of English phrase structure: The first phase. *Language* 39:1–13

Braine MDS (1971): On two types of models of the internalization of grammars. In Slobin DI (Ed): *The Ontogenesis of Grammar.* New York: Academic Press, pp 153–186

Braine MDS (1976): Children's First Word Combinations. *Monographs of the Society for Research in Child Development,* 41:1–97 (serial 164)

Brannon JB, Murry T (1966): The spoken syntax of normal, hearing impaired and deaf children. *J Speech Hear Res* 9:604–610

Brewer WF: Is reading a letter-by-letter process? A discussion of Gough's paper. In Kavanagh JF, Mattingly IG (Eds): *Language by Ear and by Eye.* Cambridge, Mass: MIT Press, pp 359–365

Bricker WA, Bricker DD (1970): A program for language training for the severely retarded handicapped child. *Exceptional Children* 37:101–111

Bricker WA, Bricker DD (1974): An early language training strategy. In Schiefelbusch RL, Lloyd LL (Eds): *Language Perspectives—Acquisition, Retardation, and Intervention.* Baltimore: University Park Press, pp 431–468

Brown R (1958): *Words and Things.* New York: Free Press

Brown R (1965): *Social Psychology.* New York: Free Press

Brown R (1968): The development of wh questions in child speech. *J Verbal Learn Verbal Behav* 7:279–290

Brown R (1973): *A First Language: The Early Stages.* Cambridge, Mass: Harvard University Press

Brown R, Bellugi U (1964): Three processes in the child's acquisition of syntax. *Harvard Education Rev* 34:133–151

Brown R, Cazden C, Bellugi U (1973): The child's grammar from I to III. In Ferguson CA, Slobin DI (Eds): *Studies of Child Language Development.* New York: Holt, Rinehart and Winston

Brown R, Fraser C, Bellugi U (1964): Explorations in grammar evaluation. In Bellugi U, Brown R (Eds): The acquisition of language. *Monographs of the Society for Research in Child Development* 92:79–92 (serial 29)

Brown R, Hanlon C (1970): Derivational complexity and order of acquisition in child's speech. In Hayes JR (Ed): *Cognition and the Development of Language.* New York: John Wiley & Sons, pp 11–55

Brown R, Lenneberg E (1954): A study in language and cognition. *J Abnorm Soc Psychol* 49:454–462

Bruner JS (1965): The course of cognitive growth. *Am Psychol* 19:1–15

Bruner JS (1974–1975): From communication to language—A psychological perspective. *Cognition* 3:255–287

Bruner JS (1975): The ontogenesis of speech acts. *J Child Lang,* 2:1–19

Bruner JS (1978): From communication to language—A psychological perspective. In Markova I (Ed): *The Social Context of Language.* New York: John Wiley & Sons, pp 17–48

Bruner JS, Goodnow JJ, Austin GA (1956): *A Study of Thinking.* New York: John Wiley & Sons

Burium N, Rynder J, Turnure J (1974): Early maternal linguistic environment of normal and Down's syndrome children. *Am J Ment Defic* 79:52–58

Butterworth G, Hatch E (1978): A Spanish-speaking adolescent's acquisition of English syntax. In Hatch EM (Ed): *Second Language Acquisition.* Rowley, Mass: Newburg House, pp 231–246

Byrne M (1978): Appraisal of child language acquisition. In Darley F, Spriesterbach DC (Eds): *Diagnostic Methods in Speech Pathology.* New York: Harper & Row, pp 102–177

Calvert K (1973): An investigation of the relationship between the syntactic maturity of oral language and reading comprehension scores. *Dissertations Abstract International,* 33B, pp 4838–4839. Ann Arbor: University Microfilm International

Cardenas DN (1975): Mexican Spanish. In Chavez-Hernandez E, Cohen AD, Beltramo AF (Eds): *El Lenguaje de los Chicanos.* Arlington, Va: Center for Applied Linguistics, pp 1–6

Carroll JB (1964): *Language and Thought.* Englewood Cliffs: Prentice-Hall

Carroll JB (1964): Words, meanings, and concepts: Part I, their nature. In De Cecco JP (Ed): *The Psychology of Language, Thought, and Instruction.* New York: Holt, Rinehart & Winston, pp 219–228

Carrow E (1971): Comprehension of English and Spanish by preschool Mexican-American children. *Mod Lang J* 55:299–305

Carrow E (1972a): Auditory comprehension of bilingual and monolingual preschool children. *J Speech Hear Res* 15:407–412

Carrow E (1972b): Assessment of speech and language in children. In McLean JE, Yoder DE, Schiefelbusch RL (Eds): *Language Intervention with the Retarded.* Baltimore: University Park Press, pp 52–58

Carrow E (1973): *Test of Auditory Comprehension of Language (TACL)* (ed 5). Hingham, Mass: Teaching Resources Corp

Carrow E (1974a): A test using elicited limitations in assessing grammatical structure in children. *J Speech Hear Disord* 39:437–444

Carrow E (1974b): *Carrow Elicited Language Inventory.* Boston: Teaching Resources Corp

Carrow E, Maulden M (1973): Children's recall of approximation to English. *J Speech Hear Res* 16:201–212

Carrow MA (1968): The development of auditory comprehension of language structure in children. *J Speech Hear Disord* 33:99–111

Carrow-Woolfolk E (1978): Letter: Reply to Rueda and Perozzi (letter). *J Speech Hear Disord* 43:555–558

Carrow-Woolfolk E (1980): *Teaching Reading Through an Auditory Method.* Houston: Communication Press

Carrow-Woolfolk E (1981): *The Carrow Auditory and Visual Abilities Test.* Hingham, Mass: Teaching Resources Corp

Carter CH (Ed) (1978): *Medical Aspects of Mental Retardation* (ed 2). Springfield, Ill: Charles C Thomas Publisher

Cassirer E (1953–1957): *Philosophy of Symbolic Forms* (3 vols). New Haven: Yale University Press

Cazden CB (1965): Environmental assistance to the child's acquisition of syntax. Unpublished dissertation, Harvard University

Cazden CB (1968): The acquisition of noun and verb inflections. *Child Development* 39:433–438

Cazden CB (1971): The psychology of language. In Travis L (Ed): *Handbook of Speech, Hearing, and Language Disorders.* New York: Appleton-Century-Crofts

Cazden CB (1973): Play with language and metalinguistic awareness: One dimension of language experience. Paper presented at the Second Lucy Sprague Mitchell Memorial Conference: Dimensions of Language Experience. New York: Bank Street College of Education

Cazden CB, Brown R (1975): The early development of the mother tongue. In Lenneberg EH, Lenneberg E (Eds): *Foundations of Language Development.* New York: Academic Press, pp 299–311

Chamot AV (1978): Grammatical problems in learning English as a third language. In Hatch EM (Ed): *Second Language Acquisition.* Rowley, Mass: Newburg House, pp 175–189

Chapman RS, Kohn LL (1978): Comprehension strategies in two and three year olds: Animate agents or probable events. *J Speech Hear Res* 21:746–761

Chapman RS, Miller JF (1975): Word order in early two and three word utterances: Does production precede comprehension? *J Speech Hear Res* 18:356–371

Chapman RS, Miller JF (1980): Analyzing language and communication in the child. In Schiefelbusch RL (Ed): *Nonspeech Language and Communication.* Baltimore: University Park Press, pp 160–196

Chappell GE (1973): Childhood verbal apraxia and its treatment. *J Speech Hear Disord* 38:362–368

Chappell GE, Johnson GA (1976): Evaluation of cognitive behavior in the young nonverbal child. *Lang Speech Hear Serv Sch* 7:17–27

Chase RA (1966): Evolutionary aspects of language development and function. In Smith F, Miller GA (Eds): *The Genesis of Language, A Psycholinguistic Approach.* Cambridge, Mass: MIT Press, pp 253–269

Chasen B, Zuckerman W (1976): The effects of total communication and oralism on deaf third-grade "rubella" students. *Am Ann Deaf* 121:394–404

Cherry C (1957): *On Human Communication.* New York: John Wiley & Sons

Chomsky C (1969): *The Acquisition of Syntax in Children from 5 to 10.* Cambridge, Mass: MIT Press

Chomsky N (1957): *Syntactic Structures.* The Hague: Mouton

Chomsky N (1965): *Aspects of the Theory of Syntax.* Cambridge, Mass: MIT Press

Chomsky N (1967): Review of Skinner's *Verbal Behavior.* In De Cecco JP (Ed): *The Psychology of Language, Thought, and Instruction.* New York: Holt, Rinehart & Winston, pp 325–339

Chomsky N (1970): Phonology and reading. In Levin H, Williams JP (Eds): *Basic Studies on Reading.* New York: Basic Books, pp 3–18

Church J (1961): *Language and the Discovery of Reality.* New York: Random House

Churchill D (1972): The relationship of infantile autism and early childhood schizophrenia to developmental laryngeal disorders of childhood. *J Aut Child Schizo* 2:182–197

Clark EV (1971): On the acquisition of the meaning of "before" and "after." *J Verbal Learn Verbal Behav* 10:266–275

Clark EV (1973): What's in a word? On the child's acquisition of semantics. In Moore TE (Ed): *Cognitive Development and the Acquisition of Language.* New York: Academic Press, pp 65–110

Clark EV (1974): Some aspects of the conceptual basis for first language acquisition. In Schiefelbusch RL (Ed): *Language Perspectives—Acquisition, Retardation, and Intervention.* Baltimore: University Park Press, pp 105–128

Clark EV (1977): Strategies and the mapping problem in first language acquisition. In MacNamara Jr (Ed): *Language Learning and Thought.* New York: Academic Press, pp 147–168

Clark HH (1970): The primitive nature of children's relational concepts. In Hayes JR (Ed): *Cognition and the Development of Language.* New York: John Wiley & Sons, pp 269–278

Clark HH (1973): Space, time, semantics and the child. In Moore TE (Ed): *Cognitive Development and the Acquisition of Language.* New York: Academic Press, pp 27–63

Clark R (1974): Performing without competence. *J Child Lang* 1:1–10

Cobrinik L (1974): Unusual reading ability in severely disturbed children. *J Aut Child Schizo* 4:163–175

Cofer CN (1961): *Verbal Learning and Verbal Behavior.* New York: McGraw-Hill

Coggins T (1979): Relational meaning encoded in the two-word utterance of stage I Down's syndrome children. *J Speech Hear Res* 22:166–178

Cohen A (1973): Errors of speech and their implication for understanding the strategy of language users. In Fromkin V (Ed): *Speech Errors as Linguistic Evidence.* The Hague: Mouton, pp 88–92

Cohen AD (1975): Assessing language maintenance in Spanish speaking. In Chavez-Hernandez E, Cohen AD, Beltramo AF (Eds): *El Lenguaje de los Chicanos.* Arlington, Va: Center for Applied Linguistics, pp 202–220

Coleman M (1978): A report on the autistic syndromes. In Rutter M, Schopler E (Eds): *Autism: A Reappraisal of Concepts and Treatment.* New York: Plenum Press, pp 185–199

Coleman M (1980): An overview of Down's syndrome. *Semin Speech Lang Hear* 1:1–8

Collins-Ahlgren M (1974): Teaching English as a second language to young deaf children: A case study. *J Speech Hear Disord* 39:486–499

Conrad R (1972): Speech and reading. In Kavanagh JF, Mattingly IG (Eds): *Language by Ear and by Eye.* Cambridge, Mass: MIT Press, pp 205–240

Cooper FS (1972): How is language conveyed by speech. In Kavanagh JF, Mattingly IG (Eds): *Language by Eye and by Ear.* Cambridge, Mass: MIT Press, pp 25–46

Cooper JE, Kendell RE, Gurland B, Sharpe L, Copeland J, Simon R (1972): *Psychiatric Diagnosis in New York and London,* Monograph No. 20. London: Oxford University Press

Corder SP (1969a): Idiosyncratic dialects and error analysis. In Schumann JH, Stenson N (Eds): *New Frontiers in Second Language Learning.* Rowley, Mass: Newbury House, pp 100–114

Corder SP (1969b): The significance of learner's errors. In Schumann JH, Stenson N (Eds): *New Frontiers in Second Language Learning.* Rowley, Mass: Newbury House, pp 90–100

Corrigan R (1978): Language development as related to stage B object performance development. *J Child Lang* 5:173–189

Cramblit NS, Siegel GM (1977): The verbal environment of a language-impaired child. *J Speech Hear Disord* 42:474–482

Crandall KE (1978): Inflectional morphemes in the manual English of young hearing impaired children and their mothers. *J Speech Hear Res* 21:372–386

Creedon MP (1973): Language development in non-verbal autistic children using a simultaneous communication system. Reprint ED-78624, Bethesda: EDRS Leasco Information Products

Cromer RF (1974): Receptive language in the mentally retarded: Processes and diagnostic distinctions. In Schiefelbusch RL, Lloyd LL (Eds): *Language Perspectives—Acquisition Retardation, and Intervention.* Baltimore: University Park Press, pp 237–268

Cromer RF (1976): The cognitive hypothesis of language acquisition and its implications for child language deficiency. In Morehead DM, and Morehead AE (Eds): *Normal and Deficient Child Language.* Baltimore: University Park Press, pp 283–335

Cromer RF (1978): The basis of childhood dysphasia: A linguistic approach. In Wyke MA (Ed): *Developmental Dysphasia.* New York: Academic Press, pp 85–134

Crook, WG (1975): *Can Your Child Read? Is He Hyperactive?* Jackson, Tenn: Pedicenter Press

Crosby F (1976): Early discourse agreement. *J Child Lang* 3:125–126

Crowder RG (1972): Visual and auditory memory. In Kavanagh JF, Mattingly IG (Eds): *Language by Ear and by Eye.* Cambridge, Mass: MIT Press, pp 251–276

Crystal D, Fletcher P, Garman M (1976): *The Grammatical Analysis of Language Disability: A Procedure for Assessment and Remediation.* London: Edward Arnold

Cunningham M (1976): A five year study of the language of an autistic child. *J Child Psychol Psychiatr* 7:143–154

Curcio F (1978): Sensorimotor functioning and communication in mute autistic children. *J Aut Child Schizo* 3:281–292

Curtiss S, Prutting CA, Lowell EL (1979): Pragmatic and semantic development in young children with impaired hearing. *J Speech Hear Res* 22:534–552

Cutting JE, Kavanagh JF (1975): On the relationship of speech to language. *ASHA* 17:8:500–506

Dahle AJ, McCollister FP, Stagno S, Reynolds DW, Hoffman HE (1979): Progressive hearing impairment in children with congenital cytomegalovirus. *J Speech Hear Disord* 44:220–229

Dale PS (1976): *Language Development: Structure and Function.* New York: Holt, Rinehart & Winston

Dales RJ (1969): Motor and language development of twins during the first 3 years. *J Genetic Psychol* 114:263–271

Damico J, Oller J (1980): Pragmatic versus morphological syntactic criterion for language referrals. *Lang Speech Hear Serv Sch* 11:85–94

Darley FL (1979): *Evaluation of Appraisal Techniques in Speech and Language Pathology.* Mass: Addison-Wesley

Darley FL, Aronson AE, Brown JR (1969): Differential diagnostic patterns of dysarthria. *J Speech Hear Res* 12:246–249

Darley FL, Spriestersbach DC (1978): *Diagnostic Methods in Speech Pathology.* New York: Harper & Row

Darley FL, Winitz H (1961): Age of first word: Review of research. *J Speech Hear Disord* 26:272–290

Davis J (1974): Performance of young hearing-impaired children on a test of basic concepts. *J Speech Hear Res* 17:342–351

deAjuriaguerra J, Jaeggi A, Guignard F, Koches F, Maguare M, Roth S, Schmid E (1976): The development and prognosis of aphasia in children. In Morehead D, Morehead AE (Eds): *Normal and Deficient Child Language.* Baltimore: University Park Press, pp 345–385

d'Arc J Sr (1958): The development of connected language skills with emphasis on a particular methodology. *Volta Review* 60:58–65

Deal JL, Darley FL (1972): The influence of linguistic and situational variables on phonemic accuracy in apraxia of speech. *J Speech Hear Res* 15:639–653 de Hirsch K (1967): Differential diagnosis between aphasic and schizophrenic language in children. *J Speech Hear Disord* 32:3–10

DeLong GR (1978): A neuropsychologic interpretation of infantile autism. In Rutter M, Schopler E (Eds): *Autism: A Reappraisal of Concepts and Treatment.* New York: Plenum Press, pp 207–217

DeMyer MK, Barton S, DeMyer E, Norton A, Allen J, Steele R (1973): Prognosis in autism: A follow-up study. *J Aut Child Schizo* 3:199–216

DeMyer MK (1976): Motor, perceptual motor and intellectual disabilities of autistic children. In Wing L (Ed): *Early Childhood Autism: Clinical, Educational and Social Aspects.* New York: Pergamon Press, pp 169–193

Denckla MB, Rudel R (1976): Naming of object-drawings by dyslexia and other learning disabled children. *Brain and Language* 3:1–15

Dennis M, Whitaker H (1977): Hemispheric equipotentiality and language acquisition. In Segalowitz S, Gruber F (Eds): *Language Development and Neurological Theory.* New York: Academic Press

deSaussure F (1959): *Course in General Linguistics.* New York: Philosophical Library

DesLauriers A, Carlson C: *Your child is asleep: Early infantile autism.* Homewood Ill: Dorsey Press, 1969

de Villiers JG, de Villiers PA (1973): A cross-sectional study of the acquisition of grammatical morphemes. *J Psycholinguistic Res* 2:261–278

de Villiers JG, de Villiers PA (1978a): Semantics and syntax in the first two years: The output of form and function and the form and function of the input. In Minifie FD, Lloyd LL (Eds): *Communicative and Cognitive Abilities: Early Behavioral Assessment.* Baltimore: University Park Press, pp 309–348

de Villiers JG, de Villiers PA (1978b): *Language Acquisition.* Cambridge, Mass: Harvard University Press

de Villiers PA, de Villiers JG (1972): Early judgments of semantic and syntactic acceptability in children. *J Psycholinguistic Res* 1:299–310

Dihoff RE, Chapman RS (1977): First words: Their origins in action. Stanford University, *Papers and Reports on Child Lang Dev* 13:1–7

Doll EA (1964): *The Vineland Social Maturity Scale.* Minneapolis: Educational Test Bureau

Donaldson M, Balfour G (1968): Less is more: A study of language comprehension in children. *Br J Psychol* 59:461–471

Donaldson M, Wales R (1970): On the acquisition of some relational terms. In Hayes JR (Ed): *Cognition and the Development of Language.* New York: John Wiley & Sons, pp 235–278

Dore J (1974): A pragmatic description of early language development. *J Psycholinguistic Res* 3:343–350

Dore J (1975): Holophrases, speech acts, and language universals. *J Child Lang* 2:21–40

Dore J (1977): Illocutionary acts. In Freedle RO (Ed): *Discourse Production and Comprehension.* Norwood, NJ: Ablex, pp 227–244

Dore J (1979): Conversational acts and the acquisition of language. In Ochs E, Schieffelin (Eds): *Developmental Pragmatics.* New York: Academic Press, pp 339–361

Dore J, Gearhart M, Newman D (1978): The structure of nursery school conversation. In Nelson K (Ed): *Children's Language,* vol 1. New York: Gardner Press, pp 337–395

Downs M (1974): The deafness management quotient. *Hear Speech News* 42:8–9, 26–28

Downs M (1980): The hearing of Down's individuals. *Semin Speech Lang Hear* 1:24–38

Dulay HC, Burt MK (1973): Should we teach children syntax? *Language Learning* 23:245–258

Dulay HC, Burt MK (1974): Natural sequences in child second language acquisition. *Language Learning* 24:37–53

Dulay HC, Hernandez-Chavez E, Burt MK (1978): The process of becoming bilingual. In Singh S, Lynch J (Eds): *Diagnostic Procedures in Hearing, Language and Speech.* Baltimore: University Park Press, pp 251–304

Eakin S, Douglas VI (1971): Automatization and oral reading problems in children. *J Learn Disord* 4:31–38

Edelsky C (1977): Acquisition of an aspect of communicative competence: Learning what it means to talk like a lady. In Ervin-Tripp S, Mitchell-Kernan C (Eds): *Child Discourse.* New York: Academic Press

Edwards JR (1979): *Language and Disadvantage.* New York: Elsevier North Holland

Eimas PD, Sequiland ER, Tusczytz P, Vigorito J (1971): Speech perception in infants. *Science* 171:303–306

Eisenberg L (1956): The autistic child in adolescence. *Am J Psychiatry* 112:607–612

Eisenberg L (1957): The course of childhood schizophrenia. *AMA Archives of Neurology and Psychiatry* 78:69–83

Eisenson J (1968): Developmental aphasia: A speculative view with therapeutic implications. *J Speech Hear Disord* 33:3–13

Eisenson J (1972): *Aphasia in Children.* New York: Harper & Row

Eisenson J, Auer JJ, Irwin JV (1963): *The Psychology of Communication.* New York: Meredith

Eisenson J, Ingram D (1972): Childhood aphasia: An updated concept based on recent research. *Acta Symbolica* 3:108–116

Ekman P (1975): Face muscles talk every language. *Psychology Today* 4:35–59

Elliott LL, Hirsh IJ, Simmons AA(1967): Language of young hearing-impaired children. *Language and Speech* 10:141–158

Emde RN, Katz EL, Thorpe JR (1978): Emotional expression in infancy II. Early deviations in Down's syndrome. In Lewis M, Rosenblum LA (Eds): *The Development of Affect,* vol 1: *Genesis of Behavior.* New York: Plenum Press, pp 351–360

Emerick L, Hatten JH (1974): *Diagnosis and Evaluation in Speech Pathology.* Englewood Cliffs: Prentice-Hall

Erber NP (1979): Speech perception by profoundly hearing-impaired children. *J Speech Hear Disord* 44:255–270

Ervin S (1964): Imitation and structure change in children's language. In Lenneberg EH (Ed): *New Directions in the Study of Language.* Cambridge, Mass: MIT Press, pp 163–189

Ervin-Tripp S (1970): Discourse agreement: How children answer questions. In Hayes JR (Ed): *Cognition and the Development of Language.* New York: John Wiley & Sons, pp 79–108

Ervin-Tripp S (1971): An overview of theories of grammatical development. In Slobin DI (Ed): *The Ontogenesis of Grammar: A Theoretical Symposium.* New York: Academic Press, pp 189–215

Ervin-Tripp S (1973): Some strategies for the first two years. In Moore TE (Ed): *Cognitive Development and the Acquisition of Language.* New York: Academic Press, pp 261–286

Ervin-Tripp S (1974): Is second language learning like the first? *TESOL Quarterly* 8:2, 111–127

Ervin-Tripp S (1978): Is second language learning like the first? In Hatch-Marcussen E (Ed): *Second Language Acquisition.* Rowley, Mass: Newbury House, pp 190–207

Ervin-Tripp S, Mitchell-Kernan C (1977): Introduction. In Ervin-Tripp S, Mitchell-Kernan C (Eds): *Child Discourse.* New York: Academic Press

Ewing A (1930): *Aphasia in Children.* New York: Oxford University Press

Fantini AE (1974): Language acquisition of a bilingual child: A sociolinguistics perspective. Ph.D. Dissertation, University of Texas

Fay WH (1969): On the basis of autistic echolalia. *J Comm Dis* 2:38–47

Fay WH (1980a): Aspects of speech. In Fay WH, Schuler AL (Eds): *Emerging Language in Autistic Children.* Baltimore: University Park Press, pp 21–50

Fay WH (1980b): Aspects of language. In Fay WH, Schuler AL (Eds): *Emerging Language in Autistic Children.* Baltimore: University Park Press, pp 53–85

Fay WH, Butler BV (1968): Echolalia, IQ and the developmental dichotomy of speech and language systems. *J Speech Hear Disord* 11:365–371

Ferguson CA (1964): Diglossia. In Hymes D (Ed): *Language in Culture and Society.* New York: Harper & Row, pp 429–439

Ferguson CA, Slobin DI (1973): *Studies of Child Language Development.* New York: Holt, Rinehart & Winston

Ferrier LJ (1978): Some observations of error in context. In Waterson N, Snow C (Eds): *Development of Communication.* New York: John Wiley & Sons

Fillmore CJ (1968): The case for case. In Bach E, Harms RT (Eds): *Universals in Linguistic Theory.* New York: Holt, Rinehart & Winston, pp 1–90

Fish B, Shapiro T, Campbell M (1966): Long-term prognosis and the response of schizophrenic children to drug therapy: A controlled study of Trifluoperazine. *Am J Psychiatry* 123:32–39

Fitzgerald E (1949): *Straight Language for the Deaf.* Washington, DC: Alexander Graham Bell Assoc for the Deaf

Flavell JH (1963): *The Developmental Psychology of Jean Piaget.* Princeton: Van Nostrand

Flavell JH, Wellman HM (1980): Metamemory. In Kail RV, Hagen JW (Eds): *Memory in Cognitive Development.* Hillsdale, NJ: Lawrence Erlbaum Assoc, pp 3–33

Fletcher JM (1980): Linguistic factors in reading acquisition: Evidence for developmental change. In Pirozzolo FJ, Wittrock MC (Eds): *Neuropsychological and Cognitive Processes in Reading.* New York: Academic Press

Fodor JA (1966): How to learn to talk: Some simple ways. In Smith F, Miller GA (Eds): *The Genesis of Language.* Cambridge, Mass: MIT Press, pp 105–123

Folstein S, Rutter M (1978): A twin study of individuals with infantile autism. In Rutter M, Schopler E (Eds): *Autism: A Reappraisal of Concepts and Treatment.* New York: Plenum Press, pp 219–241

Ford F (1973): *Diseases of the Nervous System,* vol III. Springfield, Ill: Charles C Thomas

Forner LL, Hixon TJ (1977): Respiratory kinematics in profoundly hearing-impaired speakers. *J Speech Hear Disord* 20:373–408

Foss DJ, Hakes DT (1978): *Psycholinguistics: An Introduction to the Psychology of Language.* Englewood Cliffs: Prentice-Hall, p 307

Foster R, Giddan J, Stark J (1973): *Assessment of Children's Language Comprehension.* Palo Alto: Consulting Psychologists Press

Frankenburg WK, Dodds JB, Fandal A (1967): *Denver Developmental Screening Test.* Denver: Ladoca Project and Publications Foundation

Fraser C, Bellugi U, Brown R (1963): Control of grammar in imitation, comprehension, and production. *J Verbal Learn Verbal Behav* 2:121–135

Fraser GR (1976): *The Causes of Profound Deafness in Childhood.* Baltimore: Johns Hopkins University Press

Freedle R, Lewis M (1977): Prelinguistic conversations. In Lewis M, Rosenblum LA (Eds): *Interaction, Conversation, and Development of Language.* New York: John Wiley & Sons, pp 157–186

Freedman PP, Carpenter RL (1976): Semantic relations used by normal and language impaired children at Stage I. *J Speech Hear Res* 19:784–795

Freeman BJ, Ritvo E, Miller R (1975): An operant procedure to teach an echolalic, autistic child to answer questions appropriately. *J Aut Child Schizo* 5:169–176

Fristoe M (1976): Communication assessment in the mentally retarded. In Mittler P (Ed): *Research to Practice in Mental Retardation, Vol 11: Education and Training.* Baltimore: University Park Press

Fromkin V (1972): Discussion paper on speech physiology. In Gilbert JH (Ed): *Speech and Cortical Functioning.* New York: Academic Press, pp 73–106

Fromkin V, Krashen S, Curtiss S, Rigler D, Rigler M (1974): The development of language in Genie: A case of language acquisition beyond the "critical period." *Brain and Language* 1:81–107

Fromkin V, Rodman R (1974): *An Introduction to Language.* New York: Holt, Rinehart & Winston

Fry E (1968): Do it yourself terminology generator. *J Reading* 11:428–430

Fry MA, Johnson CS, Muehl S (1970): Oral language production in relation to reading achievement among select second graders. In Bakker DJ, Satz P (Eds): *Specific Reading Disability: Advances in Theory and Method.* Rotterdam: Rotterdam University Press, pp 123–146

Furth H (1966): *Thinking Without Language.* New York: Free Press

Gall F (1825): *On the Function of the Brain and Each of Its Parts,* vol 1–6. Boston: Phrenology Library, March, Capen & Lyon

Gallagher TM (1977): Revision behaviors in the speech of normal children developing language. *J Speech Hear Res* 20:303–318

Gallagher TM, Darnton BA (1978): Conversational aspects of the speech of language-disordered children: Revision behaviors. *J Speech Hear Res* 21:118–135

Gardner H (1978): The development and breakdown of symbolic capacities: A search for general principles. In Caramozza A, Zuril E (Eds): *Language Acquisition and Language Breakdown.* Baltimore: Johns Hopkins University Press, pp 291–308

Gardner H, Winner E, Bechhofer R, Wolf D (1978): The development of figurative language. In Nelson K (Ed): *Children's Language,* vol 1. New York: Gardner Press, pp 1–38

Garrett M, Fodor JA (1968): Psychological theories and linguistic constructs. In Dixon TR, Horton DL (Eds): *Verbal Behavior and General Behavior Theory.* Englewood Cliffs: Prentice Hall, pp 451–478

Garvey C (1977): Play with language and speech. In Ervin-Tripp S, Mitchell-Kernan C (Eds): *Child Discourse.* New York: Academic Press

Gazzaniga MS (1974): Cerebral dominance viewed as a decision system. In Dimond SJ, Beaumont J (Eds): *Hemisphere Function in the Human Brain.* New York: John Wiley & Sons, pp 367–382

Geschwind N (1974): The anatomic basis of hemispheric differentiation. In Dimond SJ, Beaumont JG (Eds): *Hemispheric Function in the Human Brain.* New York: John Wiley & Sons, pp 121–183

Geyer JJ, Kolers PA (1976): Some aspects of the first stage of reading. In Singer H, Ruddell

RB (Eds): *Theoretical Models and Processes of Reading.* Newark, Del: International Reading Assoc, pp 217–241

Gibson EJ (1966): *The Senses Considered as Perceptual Systems.* Boston: Houghton, Mifflin

Gibson EJ (1971): Perceptual learning and the theory of word perception. *Cognitive Psychology* 2:351–368

Gibson EJ (1972): Reading for some purpose: keynote address. In Kavanagh JF, Mattingly IG (Eds): *Language by Ear and by Eye.* Cambridge, Mass: MIT Press, pp 3–19

Gibson EJ, Levin H (1975): *The Psychology of Reading.* Cambridge, Mass: MIT Press

Gilbert LC (1976): Speech of processing visual stimuli and its relation to reading. In Singer H, Ruddell RB (Eds): *Theoretical Models and Processes of Reading.* Newark, Del: International Reading Assoc, pp 176–185

Glucksberg S, Danks JH (1975): *Experimental Psycholinguistics: An Introduction.* Hillsdale, NJ: Lawrence Erlbaum Assoc

Goda S (1959): Language skills of profoundly deaf adolescent children. *J Speech Hear Res* 2:369–376

Goda S (1964): Spoken syntax of normal, deaf, and retarded adolescents. *J Verbal Learn Verbal Behav* 3:401–405

Goldfarb W, Goldfarb N, Braunstein P, Scholl, H (1972): Speech and language faults of schizophrenic children. *J Aut Child Schizo* 2:219–233

Goldin-Meadow S, Feldman H (1975): The creation of a communication system: A study of deaf children of hearing parents. *Sign Lang Studies* 8:225–236

Goldstein K (1948): *Language and Language Disturbances.* New York: Grune & Stratton

Gomez A, Podhajski B (1978): Language and mental retardation. In Carter CH (Ed): *Medical Aspects of Mental Retardation.* Springfield, Ill: Charles C Thomas, pp 51–65

Gonzalez G (1973): The analysis of Chicano Spanish and the "problem" of usage: A critique of Chicano Spanish dialects and education. *Aztlan* 2 (3):223–231

Goodman KS (1967): Reading: A psycholinguistic guessing game. In Singer H, Ruddel R (Eds): *Theoretical Models and Processes of Reading.* Newark: International Reading Association

Goodman KS (1970): Behind the eye: What happens in reading. In Goodman KS, Niles OS (Eds): *Reading Process and Program.* Urbana, Ill: National Council of Teachers of English, pp 3–38

Gordon D, Lakoff G (1976): Conversational postulates. In Cole P, Morgan J (Eds): *Syntax and Semantics, Vol 3: Speech Acts.* New York: Academic Press, pp 83–104

Gordon WL, Panagos JM (1976): Developmental transformational capacity of children with Down's syndrome. *Perceptual-Motor Skills* 43:967–973

Gott P (1973): Language after dominant hemispherectomy. *J Neurol Neurosurg Psychiatry* 36:1082–1088

Gough PB (1972): One second of reading. In Kavanagh JF, Mattingly IG (Eds): *Language by Eye and by Ear.* Cambridge, Mass: MIT Press, pp 331–358

Graham LW (1976): Language programming and intervention. In Lloyd LL (Ed): *Communication Assessment and Intervention Strategies.* Baltimore: University Park Press, pp 371–422

Gratch G (1975): Recent studies based on Piaget's view of object concept development. In Cohen L, Salapatck P (Eds): *Infant Perception: From Sensation to Cognition, vol II. Perception of Space, Speech and Sound.* New York: Academic Press, pp 51–96

Gray B, Ryan B (1973): *A Language Program for the Non-language Child.* Champaign, Ill: Research Press

Greenfield PM, Smith JH (1976): *The Structure of Communication in Early Language Development.* New York: Academic Press

Greenfield PM, Zukow PG (1978): Why do children say what they say when they say it?: An experimental approach to the psychogenesis of presupposition. In Nelson K (Ed): *Children's Language,* vol 1. New York: Gardner Press, pp 287–336

Greenwald C, Leonard LB (1979): Communication and sensorimotor development of Down's syndrome children. *Am J Ment Defic* 84:296–303

Groht M (1958): *Natural Language for the Deaf.* Washington, DC: Alexander Graham Bell Assoc for the Deaf

Grossman H (1973) (Ed): *Manual on Terminology and Classification in Mental Retardation.* (1973 Revision) Washington, DC: Am Assoc Ment Def

Grunwell P (1980): Developmental language problems at the phonological problems. In Jones FM (Ed): *Language Disability in Children.* Baltimore: University Park Press, pp 129–158

Guess D, Sailor W, Baer DM (1978): Children with limited languages. In Schiefelbusch RL (Ed): *Language Intervention Strategies.* Baltimore: University Park Press, pp 101–144

Guess D, Sailor W, Baer DM (1974): To teach language to retarded children. In Schiefelbusch RL, Lloyd L (Eds): *Language Perspectives—Acquisition, Retardation, and Intervention.* Baltimore: University Park Press, pp 529–563

Guess D, Keogh W, Sailor W(1978): Generalization of speech and language behavior. In Schiefelbusch RL (Ed): *Bases of Language Intervention.* Baltimore: University Park Press, pp 374–395

Gumperz JJ, Hernández-Chávez E(1975): Cognitive aspects of bilingual communication. In Hernández-Chávez E, Cohen AD, Beltramo AF (Eds): *El Lenguaje de los Chicanos.* Arlington, Va: Center for Applied Linguistics, pp 154–164

Gustason G, Pfetzing D, Zawolkow E(1972): *Signing Exact English.* Silver Spring, Md: Modern Signs Press

Gutmann AJ, Rondal JA(1979): Verbal operants in mother's speech to nonretarded and Down's syndrome children matched for linguistic level. *Am J Ment Def* 83:446–452

Guttman E(1942): Aphasia in children. *Brain* 65:205–219

Hagen JW, Jongeward RH, Kail RV(1975): Cognitive perspectives on the development of memory. In Reese HW (Ed): *Advances in Child Development and Behavior.* New York: Academic Press, pp 57–101

Hakes DT(1972): Effects of reducing complement constructions on sentence comprehension. *J. Verb Learn Verb Behav* 11:278–286

Hakuta K(1978): A report on the development of grammatical morphemes in a Japanese girl learning English as a second language. In Hatch EM (Ed):*Second Language Acquisition.* Rowley, Mass: Newbury House Publishing, pp 132–147

Hall ET(1959): *The Silent Language.* Garden City, NY: Doubleday

Hall ET(1969): *The Hidden Dimension.* Garden City, NY: Doubleday

Hall PR, Tomblin JB(1978): A followup study of children with articulation and language disorders. *J Speech Hear Dis* 42:227–241

Halliday MAK(1975): Learning how to mean. In Lenneberg, EH, Lenneberg E (Eds):*Foundations of Language Development,* vol 1. New York: Academic Press, pp 239–265

Halliday MAK(1978): *Language As Social Semiotic: The Social Interpretation of Language and Meaning.* Baltimore: University Park Press

Hammill D, Larsen S:(1974): The effectiveness of psycholinguistic training. *Except Child* 9:5–13

Hannah E (1977): *Applied Linguistic Analysis II.* Pacific Palisades, Calif: Sincom Associates

Hatch EM (1978): Introduction. In Hatch EM (Ed): *Second Language Acquisition, A Book of Readings.* Rowley, Mass: Newbury House, pp 1–22

Hayes JR (1970): *Cognition and the Development of Language.* New York: John Wiley & Sons

Head H (1926): *Aphasia and Kindred Disorders of Speech.* New York: Macmillan

Hebb DO (1949): *Organization of Behavior.* New York: John Wiley & Sons

Hécaen H (1976): Acquired aphasia in children and the ontogenesis of hemispheric functional specialization. *Brain and Language* 3:114–134

Hermelin B (1976): Coding and the sense modality. In Wing L (Ed): *Early Childhood Autism: Clinical, Education, and Social Aspects.* New York: Pergamon Press, pp 135–168

Hermelin B, Frith V (1971): Can autistic children make sense of what they see and hear? *J Spec Educ* 5:105–117

Hermelin B, O'Connor N (1970): *Psychological Experiments with Autistic Children.* London: Pergamon Press

Hewes V (1977): I challenge the profession. *Am Ann Deaf* 122:15–18

Hill A (1958): *An Introduction to Linguistic Structure.* New York: Harcourt Brace

Hollis JH, Schiefelbusch RL (1979): A general system for language analysis: Ape and child. In Schiefelbusch RL, Hollis JH, (Eds): *Language Intervention from Ape to Child.* Baltimore: University Park Press, pp 5–42

Holm VA, Kunze LH (1969): Effect of chronic otitis media on language and speech development. *Pediatrics* 43:833–839

Hopper R, Naremore RC (1978): *Children's Speech: A Practical Introduction to Communication Development.* New York: Harper & Row

Horton KB (1974): Infant intervention and language learning. In Schiefelbusch RL, Lloyd LL (Eds): *Language Perspectives—Acquisition, Retardation, and Intervention.* Baltimore: University Park Press, pp 469–492

Howie VM, Ploussard JH, Sloyer JL (1976): Natural history of otitis media. *Ann Otol Rhinol Laryngol (suppl)* 25, 85:18

Huang J, Hatch EM (1978): A Chinese child's acquisition of English. In Hatch EM (Ed): *Second Language Acquisition.* Rowley, Mass: Newbury House, pp 118–131

Hubbell RD (1977): On facilitating spontaneous talking in young children. *J Speech Hear Disord* 42:216–231

Hughes JP (1962): *The Science of Language.* New York: Random House

Hurtig R (1977): Toward a functional theory of discourse. In Freedle RO (Ed): *Discourse Production and Comprehension.* Norwood, NJ: Ablex Publishing, pp 89–106

Hutt ML, Gibby RG (1976): *The Mentally Retarded Child: Development, Education, and Treatment* (ed 3). Boston: Allyn and Bacon

Huttenlocher J (1974): The origins of language comprehension. In Solso RL (Ed): *Theories of Cognitive Psychology.* Hillsdale, NJ: Lawrence Erlbaum Assoc, pp 331–368

Huxley R (1970): The development of correct use of subject personal pronouns in two children. In Flores d'Asscais GB, Levett WJM (Eds): *Advances in Psycholinguistics.* London: North Holland, pp 141–165

Hymes DH (1967): The functions of speech. In De Cecco JP (Ed): *The Psychology of Language, Thought and Instruction.* New York: Holt, Rinehart & Winston, pp 78–88

Imedadze N (1978): On the psychological nature of child speech formation under condition of exposure to two languages. In Hatch EM (Ed): *Second Language Acquisition.* Rowley, Mass: Newbury House, pp 33–38

Ingram D (1974a): The relationship between comprehension and production. In Schiefelbusch RL, Lloyd LL (Eds): *Language Perspectives—Acquisition, Retardation and Intervention.* Baltimore: University Park Press, pp 313–335

Ingram D (1974b): Phonological rules in young children. *J Child Lang* 1:49–64

Ingram D (1975): If and when transformations are acquired by children. Paper presented to the Georgetown University Round Table, Washington, DC, March 1975

Ingram D (1976): *Phonological Disability in Children.* London: Edward Arnold

Ingram D (1978): Sensorimotor intelligence and language development. In Lock A (Ed): *Action, Gesture, and Symbol: The Emergence of Language.* New York: Academic Press, pp 261–290

Ingram TTS, Mason AW, Blackburn I (1970): A retrospective study of 82 children with reading disability. *Dev Med Child Neurol* 12:271–281

Inhelder B (1976): Observations on the operational and figurative aspects of thought in dysphasic children. In Morehead DM, Morehead AE (Eds): *Normal and Deficient Child Language.* Baltimore: University Park Press, pp 335–344

Inhelder B, Piaget J (1958): *The Growth of Logical Thinking from Childhood to Adolescence.* New York: Basic Books

Isakson RL, Miller JW (1976): Sensitivity to syntactic and semantic cues in good and poor comprehenders. *J Educ Psychiatry* 68:787–792

Jarvella RJ, Lubinsky J (1975): Deaf and hearing children's use of language describing temporal order among events. *J Speech Hear Res* 18:58–73

Jenkins JJ (1969): Language and thought. In Voss JF (Ed): *Approaches to Thought.* Columbus, Ohio: Charles E Merrill, pp 211–237

Jerger J (1978): Introduction: Hearing. In Singh S, Lynch J (Eds): *Diagnostic Procedures in Hearing, Speech and Language.* Baltimore: University Park Press, pp 25–28

Johnson DJ, Myklebust HR (1967): *Learning Disabilities: Educational Principles and Practices.* New York: Grune & Stratton

Johnston JR (1978): Language disorders: What are they and who has them? Miniseminar: Presented at ASHA Convention, San Francisco, 1978

Johnston JR, Schery TK (1976): The use of grammatical morphemes by children with communication disorders. In Morehead DM, Morehead AE (Eds): *Normal and Deficient Child Language.* Baltimore: University Park Press, pp 239–258

Jones FH, Simmons JQ, Frankel F (1974): An extinction procedure for eliminating self-destructive behavior in a 9-year-old autistic girl. *J Aut Child Schizo* 4:241–250

Kahn JV (1981): A comparison of sign and verbal language training with nonverbal retarded children. *J Speech Hear Res* 24:113–119

Kanner L (1943): Autistic disturbances of affective contact. *Nervous Child* 2:217–250

Kanner L (1946): Irrelevant and metaphorical language in early infantile autism. *Am J Psychiatry* 103:242–245

Kanner L (1971): Follow-up study of eleven autistic children originally reported in 1943. *J Aut Child Schizo* 1:119–145

Kanner L, Eisenberg L (1955): Notes on the follow-up studies of autistic children. In Hoch PH, Zubin J (Eds): *Psychopathology of Childhood.* New York: Grune & Stratton

Kanner L, Eisenberg L (1956): Early infantile autism 1943–1955. *Am J Orthopsychiatry* 26:556–566

Karlin IW, Strazzulla M (1952): Speech and language problems of mentally deficient children. *J Speech Hear Disord* 17:286–294

Katz JJ (1980): Chomsky on meaning. *Language* 56:1–14

Katz JJ, Fodor JA (1967): The structure of a semantic theory. In De Cecco JP (Ed): *The Psychology of Language, Thought and Instruction.* New York: Holt, Rinehart & Winston, pp 164–176

Keeney TJ, Smith ND (1971): Young children's imitation and comprehension of sentential singularity and plurality. *Language and Speech* 14:372–382

Keir EH (1977): Auditory information processing and learning disabilities. In Tarnopol L, Tarnopol M (Eds): *Brain Function and Reading Disability.* Baltimore: University Park Press, pp 147–176

Kennett KF (1967): Adaptive behavior and its assessments. In Mittler P (Ed): *Research and Practice in Mental Retardation, vol II: Education and Training.* Baltimore: University Park Press

Kimura D (1961): Cerebral dominance and the perception of verbal stimuli. *Can J Psychol* 15:166–171

Kimura D (1975): Cerebral dominance for speech. In Tower DB (Ed): *The Nervous System, vol 3: Human Communication and Its Disorders.* New York: Raven Press, pp 365–372

Kinsbourne M (1975): The ontogeny of cerebral dominance. In Aaronson D, Rieber RW (Eds): *Developmental and Communication Disorders.* Annals of New York Academy of Science, vol 263, pp 244–250

Kinsbourne M (1976): Minor hemisphere language and cerebral maturation. In Lenneberg EH, Lenneberg E (Eds): *Foundations of Language Development,* vol 2, pp 107–116

Kinsbourne M, Caplan PJ (1979): *Children's learning and attention problems.* Boston: Little Brown

Kirk SA, McCarthy JJ, Kirk WD (1968): *Illinois Test of Psycholinguistic Abilities,* revised ed. Urbana: University of Illinois Press

Klima ES, Bellugi U (1973): Syntactic regularities in the speech of children. In Ferguson CA, Slobin DI (Eds): *Studies of Child Language Development.* New York: Holt, Rinehart & Winston, pp 333–354

Kolvin S (1971): Psychoses in children—a comparative study. In Rutter M (Ed): *Infantile Autism: Concepts, Characteristics and Treatment.* London: Churchill Livingston, pp 7–26

Konigsmark, B (1972): Genetic hearing loss with no associated abnormality: A review. *J Speech Hear Disord* 37:89–99

Konstantareas MM, Leibovitz SF (1980): Auditory-visual vs. visual communication training with autistic children. Paper presented at ASHA Meeting, November. Cited in Fay W, Schuler AL: *Emerging Language in Autistic Children.* Baltimore: University Park Press, 1980

Kramer C, James S, Saxman J (1979): A comparison of language samples elicited at home and in the clinic. *J Speech Hear Disord* 44:321–330

Krashen S (1975): The critical period for language acquisition and its possible bases. In Aaronson D, Rieber R (Eds): *Developmental Psycholinguistics and Communication Disorders.* Annals of the New York Academy of Science, vol 263, pp 211–244

Krashen S (1976): Cerebral asymmetry. In Whitaker H, Whitaker H (Eds): *Studies in Neurolinguistics, vol 2.* New York: Academic Press, pp 158–192

Kretschmer RR, Kretschmer LW (1978): *Language Development and Intervention with the Hearing Impaired.* Baltimore: University Park Press

Krug DA, Arick JR, Almond PJ (1980): *Autism Screening Instrument for Education Planning.* Portland, Oregon: ASIEP Educational Co

Kubler-Ross E (1975): *On Death and Dying.* New York: Macmillan

LaBerge D (1972): Beyond auditory coding. In Kavanagh JF, Mattingly IG (Eds): *Language by Ear and by Eye.* Cambridge, Mass: MIT Press, pp 241–248

LaBerge D, Samuels SJ (1974): Toward a theory of automatic information processing in reading. *Cognitive Psychol* 6:293–323

Labov W (1970): The logic of nonstandard English. In Williams F (Ed): *Language and Poverty: Perspectives on a Theme.* Chicago: Markham, pp 153–189

Labov W (1972): *Language in the Inner City.* Philadelphia: University of Penn Press

Lackner JR (1968): A developmental study of language behavior in retarded children. *Neuropsychologia* 6:301–320

Lakoff R (1973): Language and woman's place. *Lang Soc* 2:45–80

Lance DM (1975): Spanish-English code switching. In Hernandez-Chavez E, Cohen AD, Beltramo AF (Eds): *El Lenguaje de los Chicanos.* Arlington, Va: Center for Applied Linguistics, pp 138–154

Langer SK (1942): *Philosophy in a New Key.* Cambridge, Mass: Harvard University Press

Latif I (1941): The physiological basis of linguistic development and the ontogeny of meaning. *Psychological Review* 41:55–85, 153–176, 246–264

Lee L (1966): Developmental sentence types: A method for comparing normal and deviant syntactic development. *J Speech Hear Disord* 31:311–330

Lee L (1971): *Northwestern Syntax Screening Test (NSST).* Evanston: Northwestern University Press

Lee L (1974): *Developmental Sentence Analyses.* Evanston: Northwestern University Press

Leiter RG (1969): *Leiter International Performance Scale.* Los Angeles: Western Psychological Services

Lenneberg EH (1967): *Biological Foundations of Language.* New York: John Wiley & Sons

Lenneberg EH (1969): On explaining language. *Science* 164:635–643

Lenneberg EH (1973): What is meant by knowing a language? In Pliner P, Krames I, Alloway T (Eds): *Communication and Affect: Language and Thought.* New York: Academic Press, pp 1–8

Leonard L (1972): What is deviant language? *J Speech Hear Disord* 37:427–446

Leonard L (1976): *Meaning in Child Language.* New York: Grune & Stratton

Leonard L (1978): Cognitive factors in early language development. In Schiefelbusch RL (Ed): *Bases of Language Intervention.* Baltimore: University Park Press, pp 67–96

Leonard L, Bolders J, Miller J (1976): An examination of the semantic relations reflected in the language usage of normal and language-disordered children. *J Speech Hear Res* 19:371–392

Leonard L, Miller JA, Brown H (1980): Consonant and syllable harmony in the speech of language disordered children. *J Speech Hear Disord* 45:336–345

Leonard L, Prutting C, Perozzi J, Berkley R (1978): Nonstandard approaches to the assessment of language behaviors. *ASHA* 20(5):371–379

Leopold WF (1939): *Speech Development of Bilingual Child,* vol 1. Evanston: Northwestern University Press

Leopold WF (1954): A child's learning of two languages. Georgetown University Round Table on Languages and Linguistics 7:19–30. Washington DC: Georgetown University Press

Levi-Strauss C (1962): *The Savage Mind.* Chicago: University Park Press

Levi-Strauss C (1963): *Structural Anthropology.* New York: Basic Books

Levy J (1974): Psychological implication of bilateral asymmetry. In Dimond SJ, Beaumont JF (Eds): *Hemisphere Function in the Human Brain.* New York: John Wiley & Sons, pp 121–183

Lewis MM (1959): *How Children Learn to Speak.* New York: Basic Books

Lewis M, Cherry L (1977): Social behavior and language acquisitions. In Lewis M, Rosenblum

L (Eds): *Interaction Conversation, and the Development of Language.* New York: John Wiley & Sons, pp 227–243

Lewis M, Freedle R (1973): Mother–infant dyad: The cradle of meaning. In Pliner P, Krames L, Alloway T (Eds): *Communication and Affect: Language and Thought.* New York: Academic Press

Lewis M, Lee-Painter S (1974): An interactional approach to the mother–infant dyad. In Lewis M, Rosenblum LA (Eds): *The Effect of the Infant on its Caregiver.* New York: John Wiley & Sons, pp 21–48

Liben LS (1978): Developmental perspectives on the experiential deficiencies of deaf children. In Liben LS (Ed): *Deaf Children: Developmental Perspectives.* New York: Academic Press, pp 195–216

Liberman AM, Cooper FS, Shankweiler DP, Studdert-Kennedy M (1967): Perception of the speech code. *Psychology Review* 74:431–461

Liberman IY, Shankweiler D (1979): Speech, the alphabet, and teaching to read. In Resnick L, Weaver P (Eds): *Theory and Practice of Early Reading.* Hillsdale, NJ: Lawrence Erlbaum Assoc, pp 109–132

Liberman IY, Shankweiler D, Fischer FW, Carter B (1974): Explicit syllable recognition and phoneme segmentation in the young child. *J Exper Child Psychol* 18:201–212

Liberman IY, Shankweiler D, Liberman AM, Fowler C, Fischer FW (1977): Phonetic segmentation and reading in the beginning reader. In Reber AS, Scarborough D (Eds): *Reading Theory and Practice.* Hillsdale, NJ: Lawrence Erlbaum Assoc, pp 207–225

Licklider JCR, Miller GA (1951): The perception of speech. In Stevens SS (Ed): *Handbook of Experimental Psychology.* New York: John Wiley & Sons

Lieberman P (1967): *Intonation, Perception, and Language.* Cambridge, Mass: MIT Press

Lillywhite HS, Bradley D (1969): *Communication Problems in Mental Retardation: Diagnosis and Management.* New York: Harper & Row

Limber J (1973): The genesis of complex sentences. In Moore TE (Ed): *Cognitive Development and the Acquisition of Language.* New York: Academic Press, pp 169–186

Ling D (1976): *Speech and the Hearing-Impaired Child: Theory and Practice.* Washington, DC: Alexander Graham Bell Assoc for the Deaf

Lloyd L, Dahle A (1976): Detection and diagnosis of a hearing impairment in the child. *Volta Review* 78:12–22

Loban WD (1963): *The Language of Elementary School Children* (Research Report No 1). Champaign, Ill: National Council of Teachers of English

Loban WD (1966): *Problems in Oral English* (Research Report No 5). Champaign, Ill: National Council of Teachers of English

Longhurst TM, Siegel GM (1973): Effects of communication failure on speaker and listener behavior. *J Speech Hear Disord* 16:128–140

Lotter V (1967): Epidemiology of autistic conditions in young children: II. Some characteristics of parents and children. *Soc Psychol* 1:163

Lovaas O (1977): *The Autistic Child.* New York: Irvington

Lovaas O, Schreikman L, Koege R (1973): A behavior modification approach to the treatment of autistic children. In Schopler E, Reichler R (Eds): *Psychopathology and Child Development.* New York: Plenum Press, pp 291–310

Lovell K, Hoyle H, Sidall M (1968): A study of some aspects of the play and language of young children. *J Child Psychol Psychiatry* 9:41–50

Lowe A, Campbell R (1965): Temporal discrimination in aphasoid and normal children. *J Speech Hear Disord* 8:313–314

Lubert N (1981): Auditory perceptual impairments in children with specific language disorders: A review of the literature. *J Speech Hear Disord* 46:3–9

Luria AR (1961): *The Role of Speech in the Regulation of Normal and Abnormal Behavior.* Oxford: Pergamon Press

Luria AR (1966): *Higher Cortical Function in Man.* New York: Basic Books

Lyle JG (1970): Certain antenatal, perinatal, and developmental variables and reading retardation in middle class boys. *Child Development* 41:481–491

Lynch J (1972): A longitudinal study of spontaneous language recovery in a seven-year-old following partial removal of the left temporal lobe. Paper presented at ASHA convention, San Francisco

Lynch J (1978): Evaluation of linguistic disorders in children. In Singh S, Lynch J (Eds): *Diagnostic Procedures in Hearing Speech and Language.* Baltimore: University Park Press, pp 327–378

Lynch J (1979): Use of prescreening checklist to supplement speech, language, and hearing screening. *Lang Speech Hear Serv Sch* 10:249–258

Lynch J, Hayden ME (in preparation): Psycholinguistic recovery of left-handed boy following left hemisphere injury: A seven year followup

Lyons J (1970): *Noam Chomsky.* New York: Viking Press

MacDonald J, Blott J (1974): Environmental language intervention. The rationale for a diagnostic and training strategy through rules, context, and generalization. *J Speech Hear Disord* 39:244–256

MacGinitie WH (1964): Ability of deaf children to use different word classes. *J Speech Hear Res* 7:141–150

MacNamara J (1967): The bilingual's linguistic performance—a psychological overview. *J Soc Issues* 23:58–77

MacNeilage PJ (1972): Speech physiology. In Gilbert JH (Ed): *Speech and Cortical Functioning.* New York: Academic Press, pp 1–72

Mahler M, Furer M (1972): Child psychosis: A theoretical statement and its implications. *J Aut Child Schizo* 2:213–218

Malkin SF, Freeman RD, Hastings JO (1976): *Aud Hear Educ* 2:21–29

Mann RA, Baer DM (1971): The effects of receptive language training on articulation. *J Appl Behav Anal* 4:291–298

Mark HJ, Hardy WG (1958): Orienting reflex disturbances in central auditory or language handicapped children. *J Speech Hear Disord* 23:237–242

Marler P (1967): Acoustical influences in bird song development. *The Rockefeller University Review,* Sept/Oct, pp 8–13

Mattingly IG (1972): Reading, the linguistic process, and linguistic awareness. In Kavanagh JF, Mattingly IG (Eds): *Language by Ear and by Eye.* Cambridge, Mass: MIT Press, pp 133–148

McCabe R (1978): *McCabe's Test Handbook.* Tigard, Oregon: C. C. Publications

McCarthy D (1954): Language development in children. In Carmichael L (Ed): *Manual of Child Psychology* (ed 2). New York: John Wiley & Sons

McDonald ET (1980): Early identification and treatment of children at risk for speech development. In Schiefelbusch RL (Ed): *Nonspeech Language and Communication.* Baltimore: University Park Press, pp 50–79

McDonald ET, Schultz AR (1973): Communication boards for cerebral palsied children. *J Speech Hear Disord* 38:73–88

McGinnis ME (1963): *Aphasic Children.* Washington, DC: Alexander Graham Bell Assoc for the Deaf

McGuigon FT (1966): Thinking: Studies of covert language processes. New York: Appleton-Century-Crofts

McLean J, Snyder LK (1978): *A Transactional Approach to Early Language Training.* Columbus, Ohio: Charles E. Merrill

McLean L, McLean J (1978): A language training program for nonverbal autistic children. In Lahey M (Ed): *Readings in Childhood Language Disorders.* New York: John Wiley & Sons

McNamara J, McNamara B (1977): *The Special Child Handbook.* New York: Hawthorn Books

McNeill D (1966): Developmental psycholinguistics. In Smith F, Miller GA (Eds): *The Genesis of Language.* Cambridge, Mass: MIT Press

McNeill D (1968): On theories of language acquisition. In Dixon TR, Horton DL (Eds): *Verbal Behavior and General Behavior Theory.* Englewood Cliffs: Prentice-Hall, pp 406–421

McNeill D (1970): *The Acquisition of Language.* New York: Harper & Row

Mead GH (1934): *Mind, Self and Society.* Chicago: University of Chicago Press

Mecham M, Jex J, Jones J (1967): *Utah Test of Language Development.* Salt Lake City: Communication Research Assoc

Menolascino FS, Egger ML (1978): *Medical Dimensions of Mental Retardation.* Lincoln, Nebraska: University of Nebraska Press

Menyuk P (1963): Syntactic structures in the language of children. *J Child Dev* 34:407–422

Menyuk P (1964a): Comparison of grammar of children with functionally deviant and normal speech. *J Speech Hear Res* 7:109–121

Menyuk P (1964b): Syntactic rules used by children from preschool or through first grade. *J Child Dev* 35:533–546

Menyuk P (1969): *Sentences Children Use.* Cambridge, Mass: MIT Press

Menyuk P (1971): *The Acquisition and Development of Language.* Englewood Cliffs: Prentice-Hall

Menyuk P (1977): *Language and Maturation.* Cambridge, Mass: MIT Press

Menyuk P (1978a): Language: What's wrong and why. In Rutter M, Schopler E (Eds): *Autism: A Reappraisal of Concepts and Treatment.* New York: Plenum Press, pp 105–116

Menyuk P (1978b): Linguistic problems in children with developmental dysphasia. In Wyke MA (Ed): *Developmental Dysphasia.* New York: Academic Press, pp 135–158

Menyuk P, Looney PL (1972): A problem of language disorder: Length versus structure. *J Speech Hear Res* 15:264–279

Mercer J (1972): IQ: The lethal label. *Psychology Today* 6:44–47, 95–97

Merleau-Ponty M (1962): *Phenomenology of Perception.* London: Routledge

Miller A, Miller E (1973): Cognitive-developmental training with elevated boards and sign language. *J Aut Child Schizo* 3:65–85

Miller GA (1956): The magical number seven, plus or minus two: Some limits on our capacity for processing information. *Psychological Review* 63:81–97

Miller GA (1962): Some psychological studies of grammar. *American Psychologist* 17:748–762

Miller GA (1963): *Language and Communication.* New York: McGraw-Hill

Miller GA (1965): Some preliminaries to psycholinguistics. *American Psychologist* 20:15–20

Miller GA (1967): Some psychological studies of grammar. In De Cecco JP (Ed): *The Psychology of Language, Thought, and Instruction.* New York: Holt, Rinehart & Winston, pp 38–56

Miller GA (1978): Semantic relations among words. In Halle M, Bresnan J, Miller GA (Eds): *Linguistic Theory and Psychological Reality.* Cambridge: MIT Press, pp 60–118

Miller GA, Ervin SM (1964): The development of grammar in child language. In Bellugi U, Brown R (Eds): The Acquisition of Language. *Monographs of the Society for Research in Child Development,* 29:9–33

Miller GA, Isard S (1963): Some perceptional consequences of linguistic rules. *J Verbal Learn Verbal Behav* 2:217–228

Miller JF (1978): Assessing children's language behavior: A developmental process approach. In Schiefelbusch RL (Ed): *Bases of Language Intervention.* Baltimore: University Park Press, pp 270–318

Miller JF (1981): *Assessing Language Production in Children: Experimental Procedures.* Baltimore: University Park Press

Miller JF, Chapman RS (1981): The relation between age and mean length of utterance in morphemes. *J Speech Hear Res* 24:154–161

Miller JF, Chapman RS, Branston MB, Reichle J (1980): Language comprehension in sensori-motor stages V and VI. *J Speech Hear Res* 23:284–311

Miller JF, Yoder DE (1972): *The Miller-Yoder Test of Grammatical Comprehension.* Madison, Wis: Communication Development Group

Miller JF, Yoder DE (1974): An ontogenetic language teaching strategy for retarded children. In Schiefelbusch RL, Lloyd LL (Eds): *Language Perspectives—Acquisition, Retardation and Intervention.* Baltimore: University Park Press, pp 505–528

Miller L (1978): Pragmatics and early childhood. Language disorders: Communicative interventions in a half-hour sample. *J Speech Hear Disord* 43:419–436

Moerk EL (1977): *Pragmatic and Semantic Aspects of Early Language Development.* Baltimore: University Park Press

Monsees EK (1968): Temporal sequencing and expressive language disorders. *J Exceptional Child* 35:141–147

Monsen RB (1976): Second formant transitions of selected consonant–vowel combinations in the speech of deaf and normal-hearing children. *J Speech Hear Res* 19:279–289

Monsen RB (1978): Toward measuring how well hearing-impaired children speak. *J Speech Hear Res* 21:197–219

Monsen RB (1979): Acoustic qualities of phonation in young hearing-impaired children. *J Speech Hear Res* 22:270–288

Moog JS, Geers AV (1975): *Scales of Early Communication Skills for Hearing Impaired Children.* St. Louis: Central Institute for the Deaf

Moore T (1973): *Cognitive Development and the Acquisition of Language.* New York: Academic Press

Moores DF (1978): Current research and theory with the deaf: Educational implications. In Liben LS (Ed): *Deaf children: Developmental perspectives.* New York: Academic Press, pp 173–194

Morain GG (1978): *Kinesics and Cross-Cultural Understanding.* Arlington, Va: Center for Applied Linguistics

Moran MJ, Gilbert HG (1978): Speaking fundamental frequency characteristics of institutionalized adults with Down's syndrome. *Am J Ment Defic* 83:248–252

Morehead DM, Ingram D (1973): The development of base syntax in normal and linguistically deviant children. *J Speech Hear Res* 16:330–352

Morehead DM, Morehead AE (1974): From signal to sign: A Piagetian view of thought and language during the first two years. In Schiefelbusch RL, Lloyd LL (Eds): *Language Perspectives—Acquisition, Retardation, and Intervention.* Baltimore: University Park Press, pp 153–190

Morehead DM, Morehead K (1979): Delayed language development. *Tejas* IV: 7–9

Morris CG (1979): Intelligence and creativity. In *Psychology: An Introduction.* Englewood Cliffs: Prentice-Hall, pp 251–287

Morris CW (1938): Foundation of the theory of signs. In Naurath O (Ed): *International Encyclopedia of Unified Science.* Chicago: University of Chicago Press, pp 1–59

Morris CW (1946): *Signs, Language and Behavior.* Englewood Cliffs: Prentice-Hall

Moscovitch M (1977): The development of lateralization of language function and its relation to cognitive and linguistic development: A review and some theoretical speculations. In Segolowitz S, Gruber F (Eds): *Language Development and Neurological Theory.* New York: Academic Press

Moulton RD, Beasley DS (1975): Verbal coding strategies used by hearing impaired individuals. *J Speech Hear Res* 18:559–570

Mowrer OH (1958): Hearing and speaking: An analysis of language learning. *J Speech Hear Disord* 23:143–152

Mowrer OH (1960): *Learning theory and the symbolic processes.* New York: John Wiley & Sons

Muma JR (1973a): Language Assessment: The co-occurring and restricted structure procedure. *Acta Symbolica* 4:12–29

Muma JR (1973b): Language assessment: Some underlying assumptions. *ASHA* 15:331–338

Muma JR (1975): The communication game: Dump and play. *J Speech Hear Res* 40:296–309

Muma JR (1978): *Language Handbook: Concepts, Assessment, Intervention.* New York: Prentice-Hall

Muma JR (1979): Language training in speech–language pathology and audiology: A survey. *ASHA* 21:467–473

Murray S (1972): Investigation of three teaching methods for language training. Unpublished doctoral dissertation. Lawrence, Kansas: University of Kansas

Myklebust H (1954): *Auditory Disorders in Children.* New York: Grune & Stratton

Myklebust H (1957): Babbling and echolalia in language theory. *J Speech Hear Disord* 22:35–60

Myklebust H (1971): Childhood aphasia: An evolving concept. In Travis LE (Ed): *Handbook of Speech Pathology and Audiology.* New York: Meredith

Mysak ED (1966): *Speech Pathology and Feedback Theory.* Springfield, Ill: Charles C Thomas

Naremore R, Dever R (1975): Language performance of educable mentally retarded and normal children at five age levels. *J Speech Hear Res* 18:82–95

Nation J, Aram D (1977): *Diagnosis of Speech and Language Disorders.* St Louis: CV Mosby

Neisser U (1967): *Cognitive Psychology.* New York: Appleton-Century-Crofts

Nelson K (1973a): Some evidence for the cognitive primacy of categorization and its functional basis. *Merrill Palmer Quarterly* 19:21–39

Nelson K (1973b): Structure and strategy in learning to talk. *Monographs of the Society for Research in Child Development* Serial No. 179, *38* (1–2)

Nelson K (1974): Concept, word and sentence: Interrelations in acquisition and development. *Psychological Review* 81:267–285

Nelson K (1975): The nominal shift in semantic–syntactic development. *Cognitive Psychology* 7:461–479

Nelson K (1978): Early speech in its communicative context. In Minifie FD, Lloyd LL (Eds): *Communicative and Cognitive Abilities: Early Behavioral Assessment.* Baltimore: University Park Press, pp 443–473

Nelson KE, Nelson K (1978): Cognitive pendulums and their linguistic realization. In Nelson K (Ed): *Children's Language,* vol 1. New York: Gardner Press, pp 223–285

Neville H (1976): The functional significance of cerebral specialization. In Rieber RN (Ed): *The Neuropsychology of Language.* New York: Plenum Press, pp 193–227

Newport EL (1976): Motherese: The speech of mothers to young children. In Castellan JJ, Pisoni DB, Potts GR (Eds): *Cognitive Theory,* vol II. Hillsdale, NJ: Lawrence Erlbaum Assoc

Norman DA (1972): The role of memory in the understanding of language. In Kavanagh JF, Mattingly IG (Eds): *Language by Eye and by Ear.* Cambridge, Mass: MIT Press, pp 277–288

Northern JL, Downs MP (1974): *Hearing in Children.* Baltimore: Williams & Wilkins

Northern JL, Downs MP (1978): *Hearing in Children* (ed 2). Baltimore: Williams & Wilkins

O'Connor N (1975): Cognitive processes and language ability in the severely retarded. In Lenneberg E, Lenneberg E (Eds): *Foundations of Language Development: A Multidisciplinary Approach,* vol 1. New York: Academic Press, pp 311–322

Ochs E (1979): Transcription as theory. In Ochs E, Schieffelin B (Eds): *Developmental Pragmatics.* New York: Academic Press, pp 43–72

Odom PB, Blanton RL, Nunnally JC (1967): Some "cloze" technique studies of language capability of the deaf. *J Speech Hear Res* 10:816–827

Ogden CK, Richards IA (1953): *The Meaning of Meaning.* Harcourt, Brace & World

Oller DK (1978): Discussion summary: Origins of syntax, semantics, and pragmatics. In Minifie FD, Lloyd LL (Eds): *Communicative and Cognitive Abilities—Early Behavioral Assessment.* Baltimore: University Park Press, pp 475–480

Olson GM (1973): Developmental changes in memory and the acquisition of language. In Moore TE (Ed): *Cognitive Development and the Aquisition of Language.* New York: Academic Press, pp 145–157

Ong BH (1968): The pediatrician's role in learning disabilities. In Myklebust H (Ed): *Progress in Learning Disability.* New York: Grune & Stratton

Ornitz EM (1978): Neurophysiologic studies. In Rutter M, Schopler E (Eds): *Autism: A Reappraisal of Concepts and Treatment.* New York: Plenum Press, pp 117–140

Osgood CE (1967): The nature of meaning. In De Cecco JP (Ed): *The Psychology of Language, Thought and Instruction.* New York: Holt, Rinehart & Winston, pp 156–164

Osgood CE (1968): Toward a wedding of insufficiencies. In Dixon TR, Horton DL (Eds): *Verbal Behavior and General Behavior Theory.* Englewood Cliffs: Prentice-Hall, pp 495–521

Osgood CE, Miron MS (1963): *Approaches to the Study of Aphasia.* Urbana, Ill: University of Illinois Press

Palermo DS (1971): On learning to talk: Are principles derived from the learning laboratory applicable? In Slobin DI (Ed): *The Ontogenesis of Grammar: A Theoretical Symposium.* New York: Academic Press, pp 41–63

Palermo DS, Molfese DL (1972): Language acquisition from age five onward. *Psychological Bulletin* 78: 409–428

Paris S, Carter A (1973): Semantic and constructive aspects of sentence memory in children. *Dev Psychol* 9:109–113

Parker TB, Freston CW, Drew CJ (1975): Comparison of verbal performance of normal and learning disabled children. *J Learning Disabilities* 8:53–60

Pascual-Leone J (1970): A mathematical model for the transition rule in Piaget's developmental stages. *Acta Psychol* 32:301–345

Patterson F (1979): Linguistic capabilities of a lowland gorilla. In Schiefelbusch RL, Hollis JH (Eds): *Language Intervention from Ape to Child.* Baltimore: University Park Press, pp 325–356

Peñalosa F (1975): Chicano multilingualism and multiglossia. In Hernandez-Chavez E, Cohen D, Beltramo AF (Eds): *El Lenguage de los Chicanos.* Arlington, Va: Center for Applied Linguistics, pp 164–170

Penfield W (1965): Conditioning the uncommited cortex for language learning. *Brain* 88:787–798

Penfield W, Roberts L (1959): *Speech and the Brain Mechanism.* Princeton: Princeton University Press

Piaget J (1954): *The Construction of Reality in the Child.* New York: Basic Books

Piaget J (1955): *Language and Thought of the Child.* Cleveland: World

Piaget J (1962): *Play, Dreams and Imitation in Childhood.* New York: Norton

---

Piaget J (1969): *The Mechanism of Perception.* New York: Basic Books

Piaget J (1970): Piaget's theory. In Carmichael L (Ed): *Manual of Child Psychology.* New York: John Wiley & Sons, pp 703–732

Pierce CS (1932): Collected papers of Charles Sanders Pierce. In Hartshorne C, Weiss P (Eds): *Elements of Logic*, vol II. Cambridge, Mass: Harvard University Press

Pollack D (1970): *Educational audiology for the limited hearing infant.* Springfield, Ill: Charles C Thomas

Potter MC, Valian VV, Faulconer BA (1977): Representation of a sentence and its pragmatic implications: Verbal, imagistic, or abstract? *J Verbal Learn Verbal Behav* 16:1–112

Power DJ, Quigley SP (1973): Deaf children's acquisition of the passive voice. *J Speech Hear Res* 16:5–11

Pressnell LM (1973): Hearing impaired children's comprehension and production of syntax in oral language. *J Speech Hear Res* 16:12–21

Pronovost W, Wakstein MP, Wakstein DJ (1966): A longitudinal study of speech behavior and language comprehension of fourteen children diagnosed atypical or autistic. *J Expect Child* 33:19–26

Prutting CA (1979): Process /'prà/ses/n: The action of moving forward progressively from one point to another on the way to completion. *J Speech Hear Disord* 44:3–30

Prutting CA, Bagshaw N, Goldstein H, Juskowitz S, Umen I (1978): Clinician–child discourses: Some preliminary questions. *J Speech Hear Disord* 43:123–139

Prutting CA, Connolly JE (1976): Imitation: A closer look. *J Speech Hear Disord* 41:412–422

Prutting CA, Gallagher T, Mulac A (1975): The expression portion of the NSST compared to a spontaneous language sample. *J Speech Hear Disord* 40:40–48

Pulaski MAS (1971): *Understanding Piaget, An Introduction to Children's Cognitive Development.* New York: Harper & Row

Quigley SP, Wilbur RB, Montanelli DS (1974): Question formation in the language of deaf subjects. *J Speech Hear Res* 17:699–713

Quigley SP, Wilbur RB, Montanelli DS (1976): Compliment structures in the language of deaf students. *J Speech Hear Res* 19:448–466

Raffin MJM, Davis JM, Gilman LA (1978): Comprehension of inflectional morphemes by deaf children exposed to a visual English sign system. *J Speech Hear Res* 21:387–400

Ramer A (1976): Syntactic styles in emerging language. *J Child Lang* 3:49,62

Ramey CT, Farran DC, Campbell FA, Finkelstein NW (1978): Observations of mother–infant interactions: Implications for development. In Minifie FD, Lloyd LL (Eds): *Communicative and Cognitive Abilities—Early Behavorial Assessment.* Baltimore: University Park Press, pp 349–386

Raven R (1978): Two Norwegian children's acquisition of English syntax. In Hatch EM (Ed): *Second Language Acquisition.* Rowley, Mass: Newbury House, pp 148–154

Rees NS (1973a): Noncommunicative functions of language in children. *J Speech Hear Disord* 38:98–110

Rees NS (1973b): Auditory processing factors in language disorders: The view from Procrustes' bed. *J Speech Hear Disord* 3:304–315

Rees NS (1978): Pragmatics of language: Application to normal and disordered language development. In Schiefelbusch RL (Ed): *Basis of Language Intervention.* Baltimore: University Park Press, pp 196–268

Rescorla LA (1980): Overextension in early language development. *J Child Lang* 7:321–335

Richards JC (1969): Error analysis and second language strategies. In Schumann JH, Stenson N (Eds): *New Frontiers in Second Language Learning.* Rowley, Mass: Newbury House, pp 32–54

Richer J (1978): The partial non-communication of culture to autistic children: An application of human ethology. In Rutter M, Schopler E (Eds): *Autism: A Reappraisal of Concepts and Treatment.* New York: Plenum Press, pp 47–62

Richman LC (1979): Language variables related to reading ability of children with verbal deficits. *J Psychol Schools* 16:299–305

Ricks DM (1975): Vocal communication in pre-verbal normal and autistic children. In O'Connor N (Ed): *Language, Cognitive Deficits and Retardation.* London: Butterworth

Ricks DM, Wing L (1975): Language, communication and the use of symbols in normal and autistic children. *J Aut Child Schizo* 5:191–220

Ricks DM, Wing L (1976): Language communication and the use of symbols in normal and autistic children. In Wing L (Ed): *Early Childhood Autism.* Oxford: Pergamon Press, pp 93–134

Rimland B (1964): *Infantile Autism.* New York: Appleton-Century-Crofts

Ritvo E, Freeman BJ, Ornitz EM, Tanguay PE (Eds) (1976): *Autism: Diagnosis, Current Research and Management.* New York: Spectrum

Robinson NM, Robinson HB (1976): *The Mentally Retarded Child: A Psychological Approach.* New York: McGraw-Hill

Rohr A, Burr DB (1978): Etiological differences in patterns of psycholinguistic development of children of IQ 30 to 60. *J Ment Defic* 82:549–553

Rosch EH (1973): On the internal structure of perceptual and semantic categories. In Moore T (Ed): *Cognitive Development and the Acquisition of Language.* New York: Academic Press, pp 111–144

Rosenberger P (1978): Neurological processes. In Schiefelbusch RL (Ed): *Bases of Language Intervention.* Baltimore: University Park Press

Ruddell RB (1976): Language acquisition and the reading process. In Singer H, Ruddell RB: *Theoretical Models and Processes of Reading.* Newark, Del: International Reading Association, pp 22–38

Ruder KF (1978): Planning and programming for language intervention. In Schiefelbusch RL (Ed): *Bases of Language Intervention.* Baltimore: University Park Press, pp 319–372

Ruder KF, Smith MD (1974): Issues in language training. In Schielfelbusch RL, Lloyd LL (Eds): *Language Perspectives—Acquisition, Retardation and Intervention.* Baltimore: University Park Press, pp 565–605

Rupp RR, Smith M, Briggs P, Litvin K, Banachowski S, Williams R (1977): A feasibility scale for language acquisition routing for young hearing-impaired children. *J Lang Speech Hear Serv Sch* 8:222–233

Russell R, Esper M (1961): *Traumatic Aphasia.* New York: Oxford University Press

Rutter M (1965): Speech disorders in a series of autistic children. In Franklin AW (Ed): *Children with Communication Problems.* London: Pitman

Rutter M (1968): Concepts of autism. *J Child Psychol Psychiatry* 9:1–25

Rutter M (1972): Childhood schizophrenia reconsidered. *J Aut Child Schizo* 2:315–337

Rutter M (1978a): Diagnosis and definition. In Rutter M, Schopler E (Eds): *Autism: A Reappraisal of Concepts and Treatments.* New York: Plenum Press, pp 1–25

Rutter M (1978b): Language disorder and infantile autism. In Rutter M, Schopler E (Eds): *Autism: A Reappraisal of Concepts and Treatment.* New York: Plenum Press, pp 85–104

Rutter M, Bartak L (1971): Causes of infantile autism—Some considerations from recent research. *J Aut Child Schizo* 1:20–32

Rutter M, Lockyer L (1967): A five to fifteen year follow-up study of infantile psychosis I. Description of sample. *Br J Psychiatry* 113:1169–1182

Ryan J (1977): The silence of stupidity. In Morton J, Marshall J (Eds): *Psycholinguistics: Developmental and Pathological.* Ithaca: Cornell University Press, pp 99–124

Sachs JS (1967): Recognition memory for syntactic and semantic aspects of connected discourse. *Perception Psychophysics* 2:437–442

Sachs J, Truswell L (1978): Comprehension of two-word instructions by children in the one-word stage. *J Child Lang* 5:17–24

Safer DJ, Allen RP (1976): *Hyperactive Children.* Baltimore: University Park Press

Sander LW (1977): The regulation of exchange in the infant–caretaker system and some aspects of the context–content relationship. In Lewis M, Rosenblum LS (Eds): *Interaction, Conversation, and the Development of Language.* New York: John Wiley & Sons, pp 133–157

Sapir ET (1921): *Language: An Introduction to the Study of Speech.* New York: Harcourt Brace & World

Sawyer JB (1975): Spanish-English bilingualism in San Antonio, Texas. In Hernandez-Chavez E, Cohen AD, Beltramo AF (Eds): *El Lenguaje de los Chicanos.* Arlington, Va: Center for Applied Linguistics, pp 77–99

Schaeffer B (1980): Spontaneous language through signed speech. In Schiefelbusch RL (Ed): *Nonspeech Language and Communication Analysis and Intervention.* Baltimore: University Park Press, pp 423–446

Schaffer D, Chadwich O, Rutter M (1975): Psychiatric outcome of localized head injury in children. In *Outcome of Severe Damage to the Central Nervous System.* Ciba Foundation Symposium. New York: Elsevier North-Holland, pp 191–213

Schiefelbusch RL (1972): Language disabilities of cognitively involved children. In Irwin J, Marge M (Eds): *Principles of Childhood Language Disabilities.* Englewood Cliffs: Prentice-Hall, pp 209–234

Schiefelbusch RL, Hollis JH (1980): A general system for nonspeech language. In Schiefelbusch RL (Ed): *Nonspeech Language and Communication Analysis and Interventions.* Baltimore: University Park Press, pp 5–24

Schlanger BS (1973): *Mental Retardation.* Indianapolis: Bobbs-Merrill

Schlesinger HS (1978): The acquisition of signal and spoken language. In Liben LS (Ed): *Deaf children: Developmental perspectives.* New York: Academic Press, pp 69–86

Schlesinger HS, Meadow RD (1972): *Sound and Sign: Childhood Deafness and Mental Health.* Berkeley: University of California

Schlesinger IM (1971): Production of utterances and language acquisition. In Slobin D (Ed): *The Ontogenesis of Grammar.* New York: Academic Press

Schlesinger IM (1974): Relational concepts underlying language. In Schiefelbusch RL, Lloyd LL (Eds): *Language Perspectives—Acquisition, Retardation, and Intervention.* Baltimore: University Park Press, pp 129–151

Schopler E, Reichler RJ (1979): *Individualized Assessment and Treatment for Autistic and Developmentally Disabled Children: I. Psychoeducational Profile.* Baltimore: University Park Press

Schuler AL (1979): Echolalia: Issues and clinical applications. *J Speech Hear Disord* 44:411–434

Schuler AL (1980a): Aspects of communication. In Fay WH, Schuler AL: *Emerging Language in Autistic Children.* Baltimore: University Park Press, pp 89–111

Schuler AL (1980b): Guidelines for intervention. In Fay WH, Schuler AL: *Emerging Language in Autistic Children.* Baltimore: University Park Press, pp 167–189

Schuler AL, Fletcher EC, Davis-Welsh JD (1977): Language development in childhood autism: A case study. Paper presented at the annual meeting of the American Speech and Hearing Association, Chicago, November 1977

Schumann JH (1969): Implications of pidginization and creolization for the study of adult second language acquisition. In Schumann JH, Stenson N (Eds): *New Frontiers in Second Language Learning.* Rowley, Mass: Newbury House, pp 137–153

Schumann JH (1976): Second language acquisition: The pidginization hypothesis. *J Lang Learn* 26:391–408

Schwartz E (1974): Characteristics of speech and language development in the child with myelomingocele and hydrocephalus. *J Speech Hear Disord* 39:465–468

Schwartz RG, Leonard LB, Folger MK, Wilcox MJ (1980): Early phonological behavior in normal-speaking and language disordered children for a synergistic view of linguistic disorders. *J Speech Hear Disord* 45:357–377

Scott CM, Taylor AE (1978): A comparison of home and clinic gathered language. *J Speech Hear Disord* 43:482–495

Scott KG (1980): Learning theory, intelligence and mental development. *J Ment Defic* 82:325–336

Searle JR (1969): *Speech Acts.* London: Cambridge University Press

Searle JR (1976): Indirect speech acts. In Cole P, Morgan J (Eds): *Syntax and Semantics III.* New York: Academic Press, pp 59–82

Semmel MI, Barrett LS, Bennett SW (1970): Performance of EMR and nonretarded children on a modified cloze task. *Am J Ment Defic* 74:681–688

Semmel MI, Dolley DG (1971): Comprehension and imitation of sentences by Down's syndrome children as a function of transformational complexity. *Am J Ment Defic* 75(6):739–745

Shafer D, Lynch J (1981): Emergent language of six prelingually deaf children. *J Br Assoc Teach Deaf* 5:94–106

Shankweiler D, Liberman IY (1972): Misreading: A search for causes. In Kavanagh JF, Mattingly IG (Eds): *Language by Ear and by Eye.* Cambridge, Mass: MIT Press, pp 293–318

Shapiro T (1978): Therapy with autistic children. In Rutter M, Schopler E (Eds): *Autism: A Reappraisal of Concepts and Treatment.* New York: Plenum Press, p 363

Shapiro T, Charandi S, Fish B (1974): Thirty severely disturbed children: Evaluation of their language development for classification and prognosis. *Arch Gen Psychiatry* 30:819–825

Sheer D (1976): Focused arousal and 40 Hz EEG. In Knights RM, Bakken DJ (Eds): *The Neuropsychology of Learning Disorders.* Baltimore: University Park Press, pp 71–88

Shipley EF, Smith CS, Gleitman LR (1969): A study in the acquisition of language: Free responses to commands. *Language* 45:322–342

Siegel GM (1975): The use of language tests. *Lang Speech Hear Serv Sch* 4:211–217

Siegel GM, Broen P (1976): Language assessment. In Lloyd LL (Ed): *Communication Assessment and Intervention Strategies.* Baltimore: University Park Press, pp 73–122

Siegel GM, Spradlin JE (1978): Programming for language and communication therapy. In Schiefelbusch RL (Ed): *Language Intervention Strategies.* Baltimore: University Park Press, pp 357–398

Sigel IE, Cocking RR (1977): Cognition and communication: A dialectic paradigm for development. In Lewis M, Rosenblum LA (Eds): *Interaction, Conversation, and the Development of Language.* New York: John Wiley & Sons, pp 207–227

Silverman SR (1971): The education of deaf children. In Travis LE (Ed): *Handbook of Speech Pathology and Audiology.* New York: Appleton-Century-Crofts, pp 399–430

Simmons AA (1962): A comparison of the type–token ratio of spoken and written language of deaf and hearing children. *Volta Review* 64:417–421

Simmons FB (1980): Diagnosis and rehabilitation of deaf newborns: Part II. *ASHA* 22:475–479

Sinclair H (1971): Sensorimotor action pattern as a condition for the acquisition of syntax. In Huxley R, Ingram E (Eds): *Language Acquisition: Models and Methods.* London: Academic Press, pp 121–130

Sinclair-deZwart H (1973): Language acquisition and cognitive development. In Moore TE (Ed): *Cognitive Development and the Acquisition of Language.* New York: Academic Press, pp 9–25

Singh S, Lynch J (1978): *Diagnostic Procedures in Hearing, Speech and Language.* Baltimore: University Park Press

Skinner BF (1957): *Verbal Behavior.* New York: Appleton-Century-Crofts

Skinner BF (1967): A functional analysis of verbal behavior. In DeCecco JP (Ed): *The Psychology of Language, Thought, and Instruction.* New York: Holt, Rinehart & Winston, pp 318–325

Slobin DI (1966): Grammatical transformations and sentence comprehension in childhood and adulthood. *J Verbal Learn Verbal Behav* 5:219–227

Slobin DI (1967) (Ed): *A Field Manual for Cross-Culture Study of the Acquisition of Communicative Competence.* Berkeley: University of California

Slobin DI (1968): Imitation and grammatical development in children. In Endler NS, Boulter LR, Osser H (Eds): *Contemporary Issues in Developmental Psychology.* New York: Holt, Rinehart & Winston, pp 437–443

Slobin DI (1970): Suggested universals in the ontogenesis of grammar. Berkeley: University of California, unpublished working paper No. 32, Language Behavior Research Laboratory, April, 1970

Slobin DI (1971): On the learning of morphological rules: A reply to Palermo and Eberhart. In Slobin DI (Ed): *The Ontogenesis of Grammar.* New York: Academic Press, pp 215–225

Slobin DI (1972): On the nature of talk to children. In Lenneberg E (Ed): *Foundations of Language Development: A Multidisciplinary Approach* (vol 1). New York: Academic Press

Slobin DI (1973): Cognitive prerequisite for the development of grammar. In Ferguson CA, Slobin DI (Eds): *Studies of Child Development.* New York: Holt, Rinehart & Winston, pp 175–208

Slobin DI, Welsh CA (1973): Elicited imitations as a research tool in developmental psycholinguistics. In Ferguson CA, Slobin DI (Eds): *Studies of Child Language Development.* New York: Holt, Rinehart & Winston, pp 485–496

Smith A (1974): Dominant and nondominant hemispherectomy. In Kinsbourne M, Smith WL (Eds): *Hemispheric Disconnection and Cerebral Function.* Springfield, Ill: Charles C Thomas, pp 5–33

Smith CS (1970): An experimental approach to children's linguistic competence. In Hayes JR (Ed): *Cognition and the Development of Language.* New York: John Wiley & Sons, pp 109–135

Smith ME (1926): An investigation of the development of the sentence and the extent of vocabulary in young children. University of Iowa, *Studies in Child Welfare,* vol 3, no 5

Smith ME (1941): Measurement of size of general English vocabulary. *Genet Psychol Monograph* 24:311–345

Snow CE (1972): Mother's speech to children learning language. *Child Dev* 43:549–565

Snow CE (1977): The development of conversation between mothers and babies. *J Child Lang* 4:1–22

Snow CE, Hoefnagel-Höhle M (1978): Age differences in second language acquisition. In Hatch EM (Ed): *Second Language Acquisition.* Rowley, Mass: Newbury House, pp 333–346

Snyder M (1980): The many me's of the self-monitor. *Psychology Today* 10:33–40

Soeffing M (1977): New assessment techniques for mentally retarded and culturally different children: A conversation with Jane Mercer. In Drew CJ, Hardman M, Bluhm H (Eds): *Mental Retardation: Social and Educational Perspectives,* pp 55–61

Speaks C, Jerger J (1965): Method for measurement of speech identification. *J Speech Hear Res* 8:186–194

Spence MA (1976): Genetic studies. In Ritvo ER, Freeman BJ, Ornitz EM, Tanguay PE (Eds): *Autism: Diagnosis, Current Research and Management.* New York: Spectrum, pp 169–174

Spitz RA (1957): *No and Yes: On the Genesis of Human Communication.* New York: International Universities Press

Spreen O (1965a): Language function in mental retardation. *Am J Ment Defic* 69:482–494

Spreen O (1965b): Language function in mental retardation. *Am J Ment Defic* 70:351–352

Spreen O (1976): Neuropsychology of learning disorders: Post conference review. In Knights RM, Bakker DJ (Eds): *The Neuropsychology of Learning Disorders: Theoretical Approaches.* Baltimore: University Park Press, pp 445–467

Spring C (1976): Encoding speed and memory span in dyslexic children. *J Spec Ed* 10:35–40

Staats AW (1971): Linguistic–mentalistic theory versus an explanatory S–R learning theory of language development. In Slobin DI (Ed): *The Ontogenesis of Grammar.* New York: Academic Press, pp 102–150

Stark J, Poppen R, May MZ (1967): Effects of alterations of prosodic features on the sequencing performance of aphasic children. *J Speech Hear Res* 10:849–855

Stark RE, Tallal P (1981): Selection of children with specific language deficits. *J Speech Hear Res* 46:114–122

Starkweather C (1977): Disorders of nonverbal communication. *J Speech Hear Disord* 42:535–546

Stevens KN, Nickerson RS, Boothroyd A, Rollins AM (1976): Assessment of nasalization in the speech of deaf children. *J Speech Hear Res* 19:393–416

Strauss AA, Kephart NC (1955): *Psychopathology and Education of the Brain-Injured Child,* vol II. New York: Grune & Stratton

Strauss AA, Lehtinen LE (1947): *Psychopathology and Education of the Brain-Injured Child,* vol I. New York: Grune & Stratton

Stremel K, Waryas C (1974): A behavioral-psycholinguistic approach to language training. In McReynolds L (Ed): *Developing Systematic Procedures for Training Children's Language.* ASHA Monograph 18, pp 96–130

Sullivan R (1976): Current trends in services for autistic persons in the United States: An overview. In Ritvo E, Freeman BJ, Ornitz EM (Eds): *Autism: Diagnosis, Current Research and Management.* New York: Spectrum, pp 291–298

Swisher LP (1976): The language performance of the oral deaf. In Whitaker H, Whitaker HA (Eds): *Studies in Neurolinguistics,* vol 2. New York: Academic Press, pp 53–93

Swisher LP, Pinsker EJ (1971): The language characteristics of hyperverbal hydrocephalic children. *Dev Med Child Neurol* 13:746–755

Tallal P (1975): Perceptual and linguistic factors in the language impairment of developmental dysphasics. An experimental investigation with the token test. *Cortex* 11:196–205

Tallal P, Piercy M (1973): Developmental aphasia: Impaired rate of nonverbal processing as a function of sensory modality. *Neuropsychologia* 11:389–398

Tallal P, Piercy M (1978): Defects of auditory perception in children with developmental dysphasia. In Wyke MA (Ed): *Developmental Dysphasia.* New York: Academic Press, pp 63–84

Tallal P, Stark RE (1976): Relation between speech perception and speech production impairment in children with developmental dysphasia. *Brain and Language* 3:305–317

Tanner DC (1980): Loss and grief: Implications for the speech-language pathologist and the audiologist. *ASHA* 22:917–928

Taylor J (Ed): *Selected Writings of John Hughlings Jackson, vol II.* New York: Basic Books, pp 129–145

Templin MC (1957): *Certain Language Skills in Children, Their Development and Interrelationship.* Minneapolis: University of Minnesota Press

Templin MC (1963): Vocabulary knowledge and usage among deaf and hearing children. In *Proceedings of the International Congress on Education of the Deaf,* Washington, DC: US Government Printing Office

Tomlinson-Keasey C, Kelly RR (1974): The development of thought processes in deaf children. *Am Ann Deaf* 119:693–700

Tulving E, Patkau J (1962): Concurrent effects of contextual constraint and word frequency on immediate recall and learning of verbal material. *Can J Psychol* 16:83–89

Tyack D, Gottsleben R (1974): *Language Sampling, Analysis and Training: A Handbook for Teachers and Clinicians.* Palo Alto: Consulting Psychologists Press

Tyack D, Ingram D (1977): Children's production and comprehension of questions. *J Child Lang* 4:221–224

Uzgiris I, Hunt J McV: *Assessment in Infancy: Ordinal Scales of Psychological Development.* Urbana, Ill: University of Illinois Press

Vaisse L (1866): Des lourds-muets et de certains cas d'aphasie congenitale. *Ball Soc d'Anthropol de Paris* 1:146–150

Van Kleeck A, Carpenter RL (1980): The effects of children's language comprehension level on adults' child-directed talk. *J Speech Hear Res* 23:546–569

Vellutino FR (1978): Toward an understanding of dyslexia: Psychological factors in specific reading disability. In Benton AL, Pearl D (Eds): *Dyslexia, An Appraisal of Current Knowledge.* New York: Oxford University Press, pp 61–112

Ventry IM (1980): Effects of conductive hearing loss: Fact or fiction. *J Speech Hear Disord* 45:143–156

Verhone T (1972): A review of Chomsky's *Language and Mind. J Psycholinguistic Res* 2:183–195

Vernon M, Koh SD (1970): Early manual communication and deaf children's achievement. *Am Ann Deaf* 115:527–539

Vogel SA (1975): *Syntactic Abilities of Normal and Dyslexic Children.* Baltimore: University Park Press

von Bonin G (1960): *Some Papers on the Cerebral Cortex.* Springfield, Ill: Charles C Thomas, pp 49–72

Vygotsky LS (1962): *Thought and Language.* Cambridge, Mass: MIT Press, p 19

Wagner-Gough J (1978): Excerpts from comparative studies in second language learning. In Hatch EM (Ed): *Second Language Acquisition.* Rowley, Mass: Newbury House, pp 155–175

Walker S (1974): We're too cavalier about hyperactivity. *Psychology Today* 8:43–48

Wardhaugh R (1976): Theories of language acquisition in relation to beginning reading instruction. In Singer H, Ruddell RB (Eds): *Theoretical Models and Processes of Reading.* Newark, Del: Intl Reading Assoc, pp 52–66

Warrington EG (1971): Neurological disorders of memory. *Br Med Bull* 27:243–247

Waryas CL (1973): Psycholinguistic research in language intervention programming: The pronoun system. *J Psycholinguistic Res* 2:221–237

Washington DS, Naremore RC (1978): Children's use of spatial prepositions in two and three-dimensional tasks. *J Speech Hear Disord* 21:151–165

Wechsler D (1974): *Wechsler Intelligence Scale for Children.* New York: Psychological Corp

Weinberg B, Zlatin M (1970): Speaking fundamental frequency characteristics of five and six year old children with mongolism. *J Speech Hear Res* 13:418–425

Weiner N (1948): *Cybernetics.* New York: John Wiley & Sons

Weiner P (1969): The perceptual level functioning of dysphasic children. *Cortex* 5:440–457

Weinreich U (1953): *Languages in Contact.* The Hague: Mouton

Weir CC (1980): Habilitation and rehabilitation of the hearing impaired. In Hixon TJ, Shriberg LD, Saxman JH (Eds): *Introduction to Communication Disorders.* Englewood Cliffs: Prentice-Hall, pp 531–572

Weir RH (1962): *Language in the Crib.* The Hague: Mouton

Wepman JM, Jones LV, Bock RD, van Pelt D (1960): Studies in aphasia: Background and theoretical formulations. *J Speech Hear Disord* 25:323–332

Werner H (1948): Comparative psychology of mental development. New York: Science Editions

Werner H (1965): Introduction. In Wapner S, Werner H (Eds): *The Body Percept.* New York: Random House

Wernicke C (1963): The Breslau School and the history of asphasia. *Brain Function* 3:1–16

Westby CE (1980): Assessment of cognitive and language abilities through play. *Lang Speech Hear Serv Sch* 11:154–168

Wetstone HS, Friedlander BZ (1973): The effect of word order on young children's responses to simple questions and commands. *Child Dev* 44:734–740

Whatmough J (1956): *Language: A Modern Synthesis.* New York: Mentor Books

Whitaker H (1976): A case of the isolation of the language function. In Whitaker H, Whitaker HA (Eds): *Studies in Neurolinguistics.* New York: Academic Press, pp 1–58

Whorf BL (1967): Science and linguistics. In De Cecco JP (Ed): *The Psychology of Language, Thought and Instruction.* New York: Holt, Rinehart & Winston, pp 68–74

Wiig EH, Semel EM (1976a): Development of comprehension of logico-grammatical sentences by grade school children. *Percept Motor Skills* 38:171–176

Wiig EH, Semel EM (1976b): *Language Disabilities of School Age Children and Adolescents.* Columbus, Ohio: Charles E Merrill

Wiig EH, Semel EM, Crouse MB (1973): The use of English morphology by high-risk and learning disabled children. *J Learn Disord* 6 (7): 457–465

Wilbur RB, Montanelli DS, Quigley SP (1976): Pronominalization in the language of deaf students. *J Speech Hear Res* 19:120–140

Wilbur RB, Quigley SP, Montanelli DS (1975): Conjoined structures in the language of deaf students. *J Speech Hear Res* 18:319–335

Wilde WR (1853): *Practical Observations on Aural Surgery and the Nature and Treatment of Diseases of the Ear.* Philadelphia: Blanchard and Lea

Wiley TL (1980): Hearing disorders and audiometry. In Hixon TJ, Shriberg LD, Saxman JH (Eds): *Introduction to Communication Disorders.* Englewood Cliffs: Prentice-Hall

Williams F (1970): *Language and Poverty: Perspectives on a Theme.* Chicago: Markham

Williams R, Wolfram W (1977): *Social Dialects: Differences vs. Disorders.* Washington, DC: American Speech and Hearing Association

Wing JK (1976): Kanner's Syndrome—A historical introduction. In Wing L (Ed): *Early Childhood Autism: Clinical, Educational and Social Aspects.* New York: Pergamon Press, pp 3–14

Wing L (1969): The handicaps of autistic children—A comparative study. *J Child Psychol Psychiatry* 10:1–40

Wing L (1971): Perceptual and language development in autistic children: A comparative study. In Rutter M (Ed): *Infantile Autism: Concepts, Characteristics and Treatment.* London: Churchill-Livingstone, pp 173–197

Wing L (1975): A study of language impairment in severely retarded children. In O'Connor N (Ed): *Language, Cognitive Deficits and Retardation.* London: Butterworths, pp 87–112

Wing L (1976a): Diagnosis, clinical description and prognosis. In Wing L (Ed): *Early Childhood Autism: Clinical, Educational, and Social Aspects.* New York: Pergamon Press, pp 15–48

Wing L (1976b): Epidemiology and theories of aetiology. In Wing L (Ed): *Early Childhood Autism: Clinical, Educational, and Social Aspects.* New York: Pergamon Press, pp 65–92

Wing L (1978): Social, behavioral and cognitive characteristics: An epidemiological approach.

In Rutter M, Schopler E (Eds): *Autism: A Reappraisal of Concepts and Treatment.* New York: Plenum Press, pp 27–45

Wing L, Gould J, Yeates JR, Brierly LM (1977): Symbolic play in severely mentally retarded and in autistic children. *J Child Psychol Psychiatry* 18:167–178

Winitz H (1978): A reconsideration of comprehension and production in language training. *Allied Health Behav Sci* 1:272–314

Winitz H, Reeds J (1972): The OHR method of language training. Kansas City Working Paper in Speech Science and Linguistics No 3, University of Missouri at Kansas City

Winitz H, Reeds J (1975): *Comprehension and Problem Solving as Strategies for Language Training.* The Hague: Mouton

Wode H (1977): Four early stages in the development of L_1 negation. *J Child Lang* 4:87–102

Wode H (1978): Developmental sequences in naturalistic L_2 acquisition. In Hatch EM (Ed): *Second Language Acquisition.* Rowley, Mass: Newbury House, pp 101–117

Wolf M, Risley R, Mees J (1964): Application of operant conditioning procedures to the behavior problems of an autistic child. *Behav Res Ther* 1:305–312

Wolf M, Risley T, Johnston M, Harris F, Allen E (1967): Application of operant conditioning procedures to the behavioral problems of an autistic child: A follow-up and extension. *Behav Res Ther* 5:103–111

Wolff S, Chess S (1965): An analysis of the language of fourteen schizophrenic children. *J Child Psychol Psychiatry* 6:29–41

Wulbert M, Inglis S, Kriegsmann E, Mills B (1975): Language delay and associated mother–child interactions. *Dev Psychol* 11:61–70

Yarrow MR (1975): Some perspectives on research on peer relations. In Lewis M, Rosenblum LA (Eds): *Friendship and Peer Relations, The Origins of Behavior,* vol 4. New York: John Wiley & Sons, pp 298–305

Yeni-Komshian GH (1977): A long-term study of dichotic speech perception and receptive language skills. In Segalowitz S, Gruber FA (Eds): *Language Development and Neurological Theory.* New York: Academic Press, pp 171–191

Yoder D, Miller J (1972): What we may know and what we can do: Input toward a system. In McLean J, Yoder D, Schiefelbusch R (Eds): *Language Intervention with the Retarded.* Baltimore: University Park Press, pp 89–107

Zangwill OL (1978): The Concept of Developmental Aphasia. In Wyke MA (Ed): *Developmental Dysphasia.* New York: Academic Press, pp 1–11

Zedler E (1972): Social management. In Irwin J, Marge M (Eds): *Principles of Childhood Language Disability.* Englewood Cliffs: Prentice-Hall, pp 355–391

Zellweger H, Ionasescu V (1978): Genetics of mental retardation. In Carter CH (Ed): *Mental Aspects of Mental Retardation.* Springfield, Ill: Charles C Thomas, pp 123–193

Zimbardo PG, Ruch FL (1977): *Psychology and Life.* Glenview, Ill: Scott, Foresman

Zimmerman I, Steiner V, Evatt R (1969): *Preschool Language Scale.* Columbus, Ohio: Charles E Merrill

author index*

*Individuals mentioned only once in the text have not been included in this index.

subject index

Tests (*continued*)
 standardized, 232–234
  use and misuse of, 236–238
Theories of language development
 activity, 139
 behavioristic, 111–112
 cerebral dominance and, 338–339
 critique and integration of, 112–113
 deficit, 97–98
 difference, 97
 explanatory, 286–298
 for extending words, 140–142
 innate, 112
 of linguistic delay versus deviance, 293–298
 mediation in, 118
Time, concepts of, 47
Transformational grammar (TG), 28
Transformations, 22–23
 development of, 167–169
Turn-taking in conversation, 190–192

Underextension, 141
Utterance, mean length of, 247–249, 447–448

Verb modulation, 162–163
Visual memory, 43. *See also* Memory
Vocabulary. *See also* Speech; First words; Words
 atypical development of, 409–410
Vocal code, 6

Women, speech of, 189
Word order, 172
 complexity and, 156–157
Words, 19. *See also* Language; Language
  development
 combining, 148–150
 first, 142–144
  attrition of, 146–147
  styles of learning, 145–146
 knowledge of, 134
 order of acquisition of, 123–126
 schedule of development of, 150–151
 strategies for learning, 138–142
 taboo, 188
 theories for extending, 140–142
Writing, 19